How 2 Get Fit 4 Later Life!

EXERCISE & NUTRITION
FOR PEOPLE AGED 60+

How 2 Get Fit 4 Later Life!

EXERCISE & NUTRITION
FOR PEOPLE AGED 60+

GAV O'BRIEN
THE FITNESS COACH

THIS BOOK IS DEDICATED TO THE MEMORIES OF MY GRANDPARENTS & GREAT GRANDPARENTS

3Fs PUBLISHING

First published in 2020 by 3Fs Publishing.

Foreword

Thank you for purchasing **How 2 Get Fit 4 Later Life**. This is a general guide for people aged 60 and above. I hope that you will find it a useful, practical tool for a healthier and more active lifestyle. How regularly you exercise and what you eat, are the two main ingredients for improving your general health and fitness. Inside you will find a step-by-step guide to a wide range of exercises many with accompanying illustrative photos. You will also find an enlightening section covering food and nutritional advice, with suggestions based on my go-to foods and drinks for boosting energy levels, aiding weight loss and boosting your immune system, three issues that can affect all of us as we grow older. If you have any questions about anything covered in this book and or topic suggestions for future books please email me **gav@3fspt.co.uk**.

I'm not that keen about using the terms Older Adults, Seniors or Older People. Our society always seems to want to stick a limiting label on us. As a personal trainer, I see age in factual terms of how our bodies grow and develop, plateau and then decline. From birth until around 25 your body develops, from here until 35 there's a fairly stable period, then from 35 unless you work at it, your body is on the decline. However, on Google it's hard to ignore how people search for information of the type you'll find in this book, and for that reason alone, I often use these terms. I'd simply rather leave it as Adults.

A Bit About Gav

I'm a personal trainer and founder of 3Fs Personal Training. I'm 53 and have lived in Hove, East Sussex for several years. My passion for a career in all things fitness and nutrition arrived relatively late in my life, although I've been exercising my whole adult life. I've established myself as one of the top personal trainers in Brighton and Hove with a diverse client base. My clients enjoy the convenience of being trained in their home or office, outdoors in one of the many beautiful parks and gardens in the city and even by the beach. I studied for my Level 3 Diploma in Gym Instructing and Personal Training at YMCAfit in London. In addition to this, I have a further qualification Exercise for Older Adults.

Contents

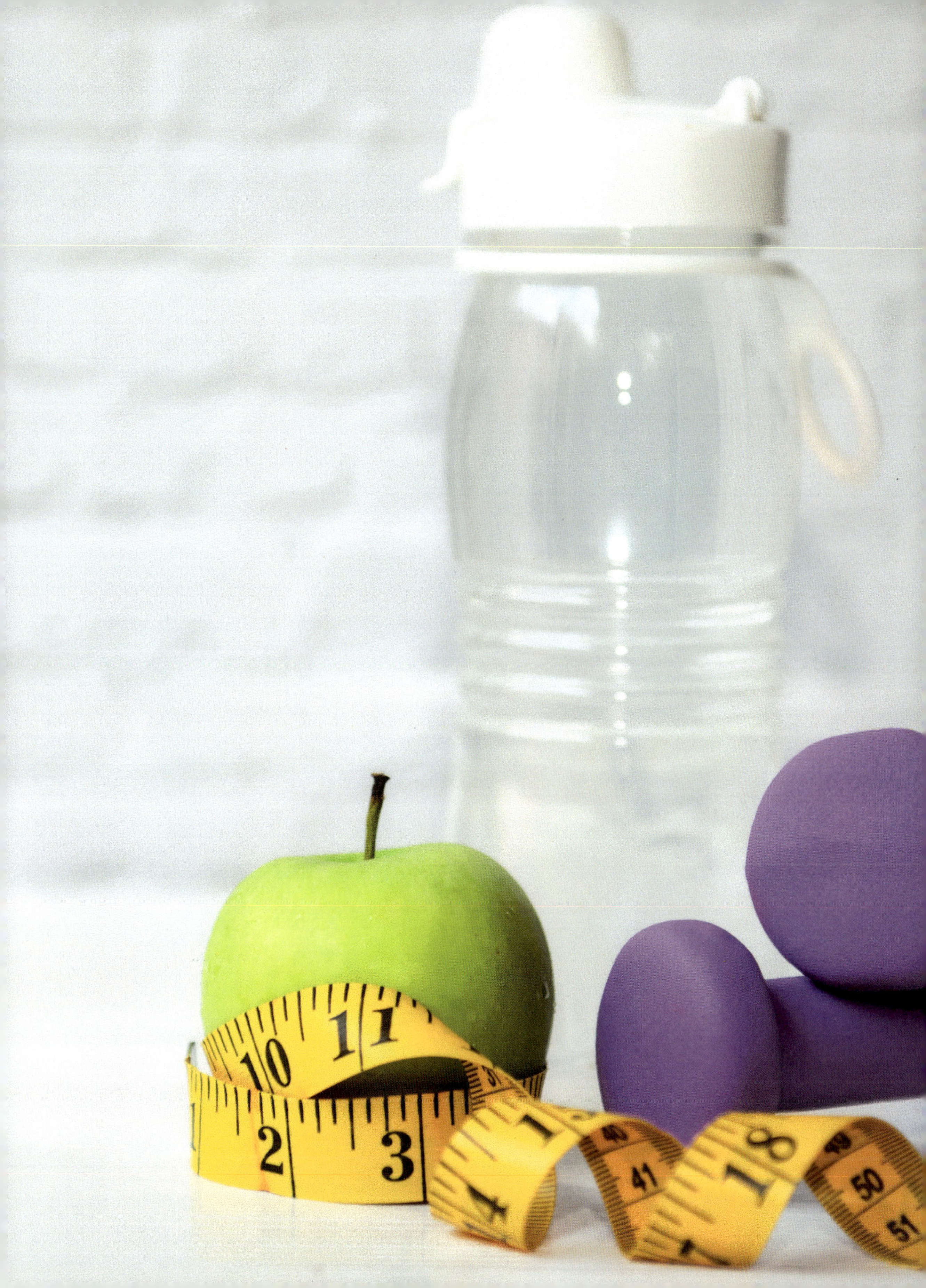

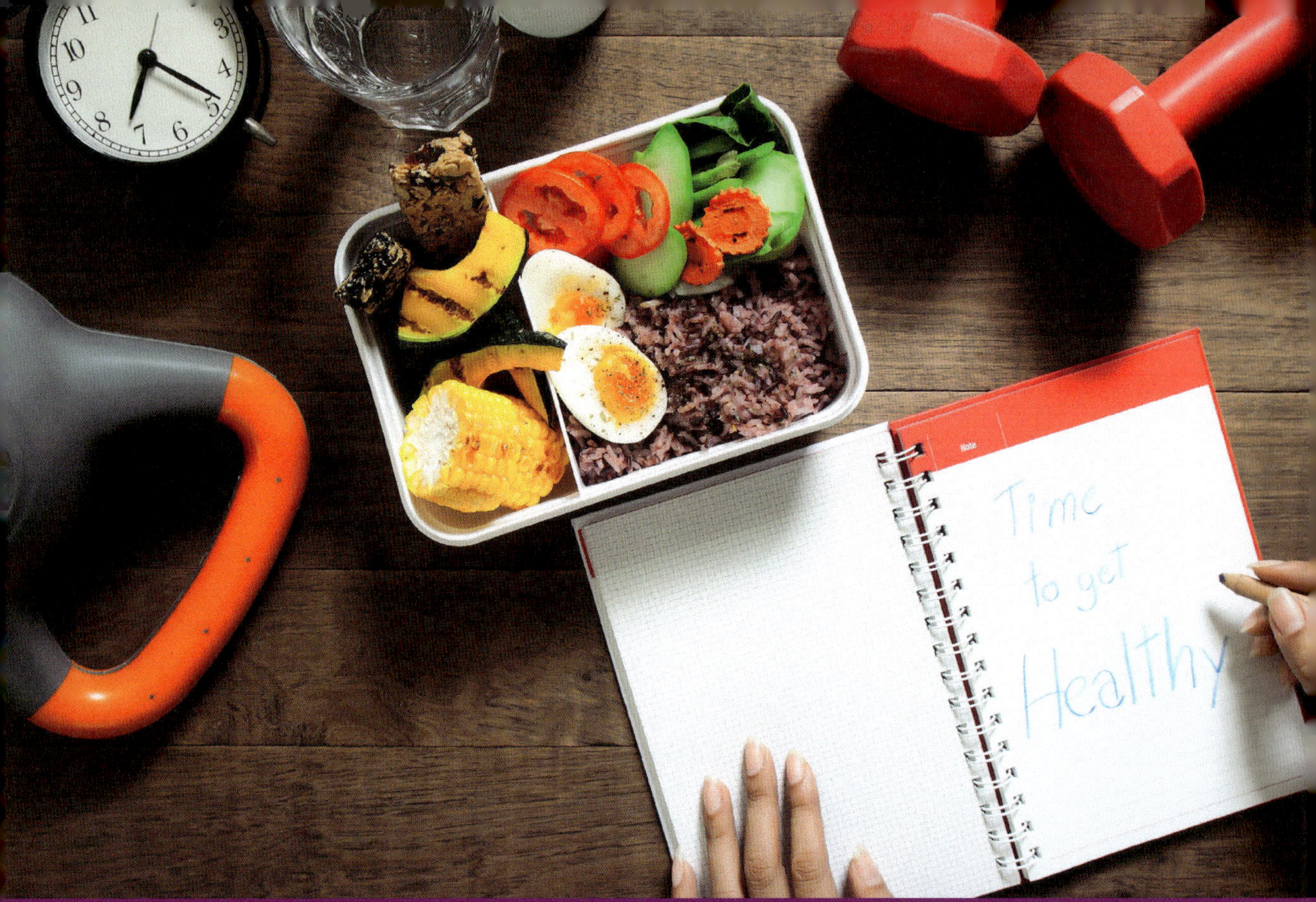

"Be good to your body, it's the only one you'll ever have!"

Introduction

Let's be honest, we all know that exercise is good for us. We may not all enjoy doing exercise but that's not the point. There are many reasons for starting or continuing to do exercise as we get older, including:

1. Live longer
2. Better bone density
3. Prevent trips and falls
4. Reduced risk of dementia
5. Reduced risk of heart attack or stroke
6. Prevent, delay, better manage health conditions
7. More confidence and maintain independent living

Long before I became a personal trainer based in Brighton and Hove, I spent a year working as a domiciliary care worker helping mainly older adults live as independently as possible in their own home. It struck me that for some, making different lifestyle choices earlier in their lives might have saved them from having to rely on the care that carers like me provided daily. When I decided my vocation was to be a personal trainer, it was a natural choice for me to want to work with older adults. Now exercise isn't the cure-all for every illness and known medical condition. More is the pity. However, it can delay, prevent or at least help you to better manage a wide range of illnesses and medical conditions. I've previously written blogs on this subject, and the following are just a few of the illnesses and medical conditions where regular exercise can be beneficial:

- Anxiety
- Arthritis
- Cancer
- Cold and Flu
- COPD
- Depression
- Fibromyalgia
- Heart Disease
- High Blood Pressure
- High Cholesterol
- Obesity
- Osteoporosis
- Type II Diabetes

Sadly, the Covid-19 pandemic has affected millions of people around the World, while the statistical data is far from being fully analysed, early indications show that obese individuals have been particularly badly affected. 2020 will be a year that we are unlikely to forget. Perhaps when the worst of this dreadful episode is behind us, people of all ages will reflect on their health and where necessary make changes for the better. For my part, the Covid-19 lockdown has given me the time to write this book, trying to make something positive that I can share.

Recommended Guidelines

In the UK, the Chief Medical Officer recommends target minimal levels of exercise for different groups. For adults and older adults, the recommendations are for physical activity of moderate intensity of at least 150-minutes each week or of higher intensity for 75-minutes each week. The guidelines go on to recommend building strength on at least two days a week to keep muscles, bones and joints strong. Further guidance for older people is to improve their balance on at least two days a week, and for everyone to reduce the amount of time and frequency of sitting around doing nothing. Put simply, if on five days of the week you do 30-minutes of exercise, and you focus on flexibility, balance and strength on at least two of those days, you'll achieve the recommended minimum guidelines.

Before You Start Exercise

If you are new to exercise, or it's been a while since you have exercised and or you have an underlying medical condition, please consult your doctor to see if it's safe for you to start. For the vast majority of older adults, it will be safe to take up walking as a starting point. However, please check with your doctor if you know you are at risk from trips and falls, or have a history of feeling dizzy or are currently taking any medication that has the potential side effect of making you feel dizzy and or drowsy. You should also check with your doctor if you have a chronic health condition, for example, COPD, osteoporosis, diabetes or a heart condition.

You may also want to use a fitness industry standard helpful questionnaire known as the Physical Activity Readiness Questionnaire or PAR-Q. This health questionnaire has been designed to enable people to decide whether or not they need to speak with their doctor before starting on or indeed increasing any exercise programme. If you would like a copy of the 3Fs Personal Training

PAR-Q please email your request to **gav@3fspt.co.uk**. This is just a series of questions to answer yes or no to. If you answer yes to one or more, go chat to your doctor about starting exercise.

You don't need a fancy gym membership, or expensive equipment to do exercise, in fact, you don't even have to step outside your front door. A space of around six square feet, a sturdy dining room chair, two tins of food of equal weight (these weigh around 0.5kg) and a large bottle of water or squash (these weigh around 1.0kg) is everything you need to get started. I give you some suggestions on how to upgrade these basics at relatively little expense in chapter 13 of this guide. This book is meant to be read in its entirety before you start any of the exercises. However, if you do get tempted to practice some of the exercises, please warm-up first, wear comfortable loose fitting clothing and non-slip footwear.

All The Equipment You Need To Get Started

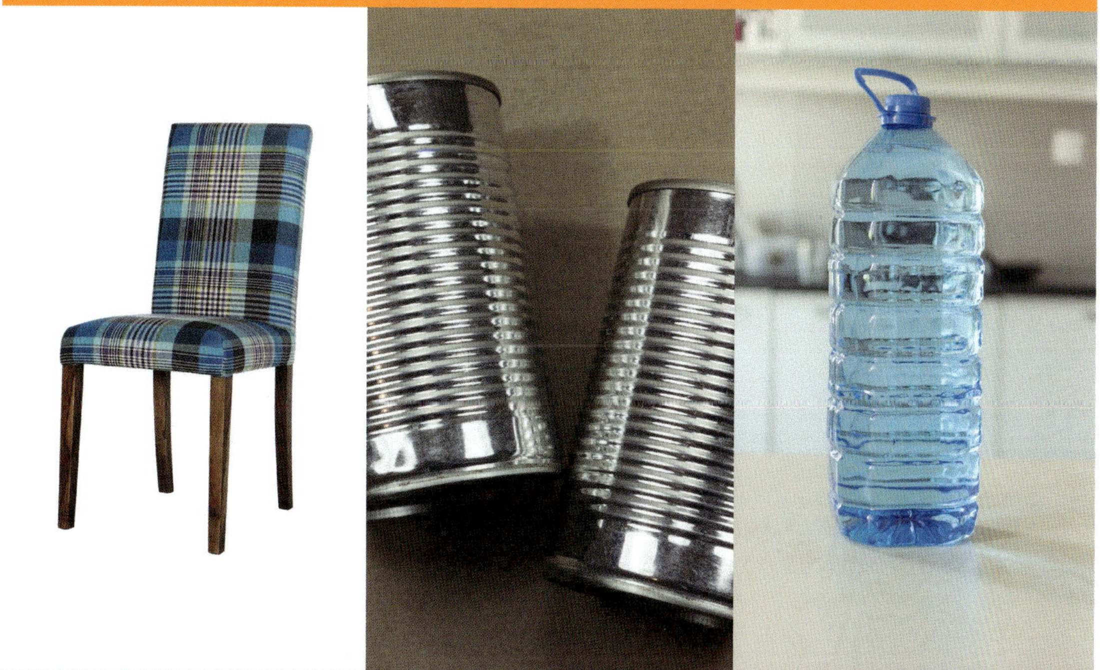

A STURDY DINING ROOM CHAIR | **TWO TINS OF FOOD OF EQUAL WEIGHT** | **LARGE BOTTLE OF WATER OR SQUASH**

How To Use This Book

As you read through this book, there are questions that you'll need to answer if you intend to do the **GET FITTER IN JUST 12-WEEKS CHALLENGE** to go from doing little or no exercise to achieving the recommended weekly target of 150 minutes. My wish for you is to take up my 12-week challenge and discover for yourself how great a healthier and fitter you feels. I know **YOU** can do it!

To help, you can download the **12-WEEKS EXERCISE PLANNER** (See chapter 10) or use the blank template in the **GET FIT TOOL KIT** to create your own using any combination of exercises in this book. Your 12-week challenge can be done with or without a calorie-controlled diet depending on whether you feel you need to lose weight. Calculate your Body Mass Index to guide you when making this decision as well as your Basal Metabolic Rate (See chapter 16) as this will help set your daily calorie limit for your diet. It is always advisable for you to chat through any change in exercise and or diet with your doctor first. To keep track of your answers as you read the book download the **GET FIT TOOL KIT** by visiting **www.3fspt.co.uk/toolkit**.

Inside the GET FIT TOOL KIT you will find:

- Your answers sheet
- Blank 3-day food diary
- Blank 12-week exercise planner
- Exercise planner as per the book
- A-z calorie counts for popular food list
- The individual step-by-step exercise sections:
  - >> Warm-up exercises
  - >> Aerobic exercises
  - >> Balance exercises
  - >> Chair-based exercises
  - >> Strength exercises
  - >> Core exercises
  - >> Stretching exercises

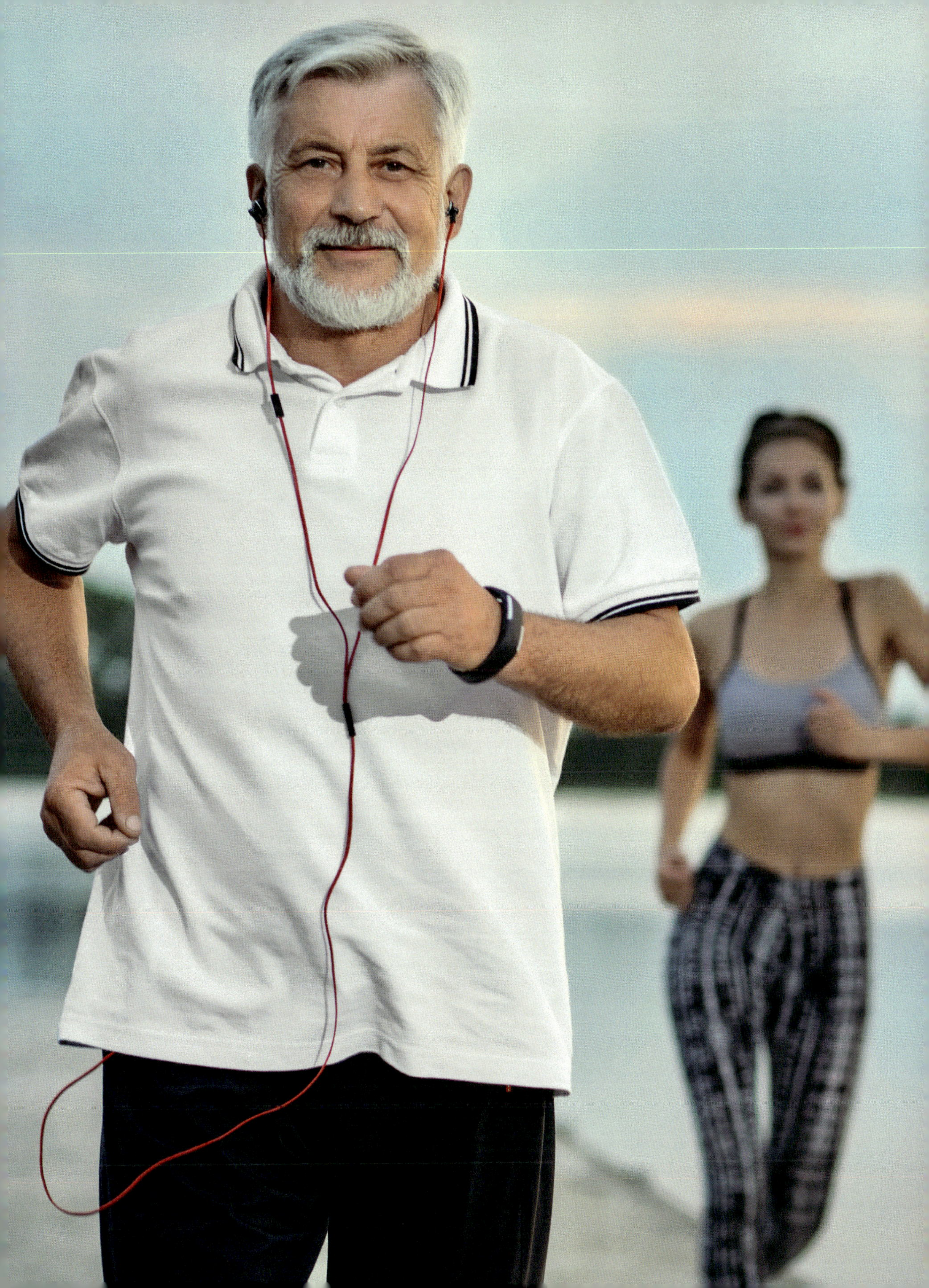

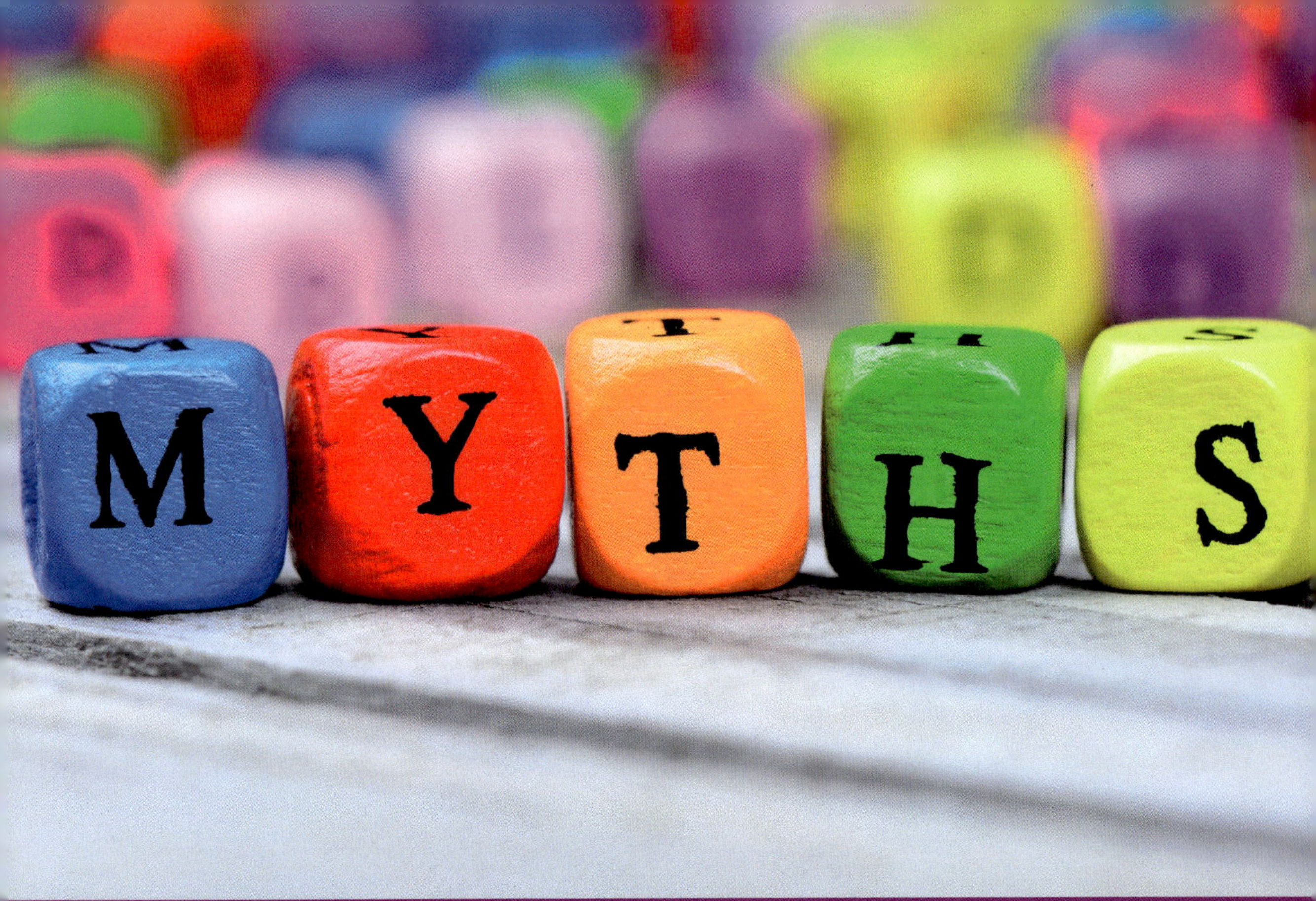

"Your body achieves what your mind believes."

CHAPTER 1

The Truth Behind The Myths Of Exercising & Ageing

Starting or maintaining a regular exercise routine can be a challenge at any age. You may feel that certain health problems, aches and pains, rule you out completely. Perhaps you're worried about trips and falls, or you have limited mobility through injury, illness or medical conditions. If you've never exercised before, you may not know where to begin, or perhaps you think you're too old or frail. Myths around starting exercise may resonate with your own beliefs. Here then is the truth behind the myths of exercising and ageing. Read on to take your first step on How 2 Get Fit 4 Later Life.

Exercise & Aging Myth no.1

>> There's no point to exercise as I'm too old anyway

TRUTH: You're never too old to gain a host of benefits from beginning regular exercise. Aerobic exercise and strength training exercise can help you look good and feel great as well as enabling you to stay active for longer, making activities for everyday living much easier. Regular exercise lowers your risk for many age-related medical conditions, including dementia, type 2 diabetes, high cholesterol, high blood pressure, heart disease, some cancers and obesity. So take inspiration from one of my clients. Early in 2020, he contacted me as he'd noticed that 'things were slowing down' for him. He decided that he needed a personal trainer, at the young age of 97.

Exercise & Aging Myth no.2

>> Older people shouldn't exercise at all and it's far better that they save their energy and rest

TRUTH: There's an enormous amount of scientific research that has shown a sedentary lifestyle is really unhealthy for older people. In-fact inactivity often causes seniors to lose the ability to do certain things on their own and can lead to frequent hospitalisations from falling over as well as the increased usage of medication to control illnesses and age-related medical conditions.

Exercise & Aging Myth no.3

>> Regular exercise can increase my risk of trips and of falling over

TRUTH: Regular exercise that includes strength and endurance exercises prevents loss of bone mass and improves flexibility and by adding balance exercises in the mix will actually reduce your risk of injury from trips and from falling over.

Exercise & Aging Myth no.4

>> I have an impairment to my mobility and or I use a wheelchair, I can't exercise sitting down

TRUTH: Chair bound adults do face certain challenges but you can lift light weights such as dumbbells as well as using resistance bands and do chair-based aerobics to increase your range of movement, improve your muscle tone, improve your flexibility and promote better cardiovascular health. In chapter 5 you'll find step-by-step guides to 12 chair-based exercises.

Exercise & Aging Myth no.5

>> I'm too unfit to go to an exercise class

TRUTH: Exercising in your home is good but exercising with others can actually be more motivating and fun. Right across the UK (when not in lockdown), there are scores of organisations of all types offering an astonishing range of exercise classes. Age UK for an example of a national charity that offers classes, and there is also Move It or Lose It a national company that offers keep fit classes for older people.

Exercise & Aging Myth no.6

>> I walk for half an hour each day, so it's okay for me to be a couch potato the rest of the day

TRUTH: Research has shown that even if you get the recommended amount of daily exercise your general health can still suffer if you sit down the rest of the time. Change your sedentary habits to incorporate much more movement, for example, by lifting light weights while you watch TV, walking around while talking on the phone, or meet a friend for a walk outdoors rather than sitting in a chair to chat over tea. Aim to be active on at least 5-days a week.

Tips for keeping motivated to exercise

Sometimes life has a habit of getting in the way and keeping motivated to do exercise after illness, injury and even the weather has interrupted your established exercise routines, you can find yourself right back to square one. Here are a few tips to help you get back your motivation to start exercising again:

Set short-term goals - By focussing on short-term goals, for example, increasing your energy levels, improving your mood rather than larger goals, for example, losing a lot of weight, which is likely to take a longer time, some quick wins can really help you commit for the longer term.

Rewards for making progress - When you've completed a challenge that you've set yourself, don't just ignore your success, reward yourself perhaps with your favourite non-alcoholic tipple, a nice long relaxing hot bath or a day out.

Enlist support - Encourage and motivate each other by working out with a partner, friend or member of your family. Share your achievements on social media so that your-extended circle of family and friends can offer you their encouragement and support too.

Keep a log - Writing down your activities in an exercise journal not only holds you accountable but is also a reminder of your accomplishments. Take photos as well, before and after shots can be a great way to help you keep motivation to maintain the new slimmer and fitter you. Again, share these on social media and you may even inspire others to follow your example. If you like technology and using gadgets then FitBit has some good options that will help track your activity, such as the number of steps you've walked. Visit **www.3fspt.co.uk/shop**.

Follow a plan - Go from ambling along to exercise hero in a few short weeks, see **Chapter 10 - GET FITTER IN JUST 12-WEEKS CHALLENGE**. Follow my plan and you can contact me for the motivation, support and advice by emailing **gav@3fspt.co.uk**.

Join my Facebook Group - Join the **HOW 2 GET FIT 4 LATER LIFE FACEBOOK GROUP**. I've set this up for everyone who takes up the 12-week challenge to provide peer support, motivation and to share progress. To join the Facebook Group use this link: **www.tiny.cc/H2GF4LL**

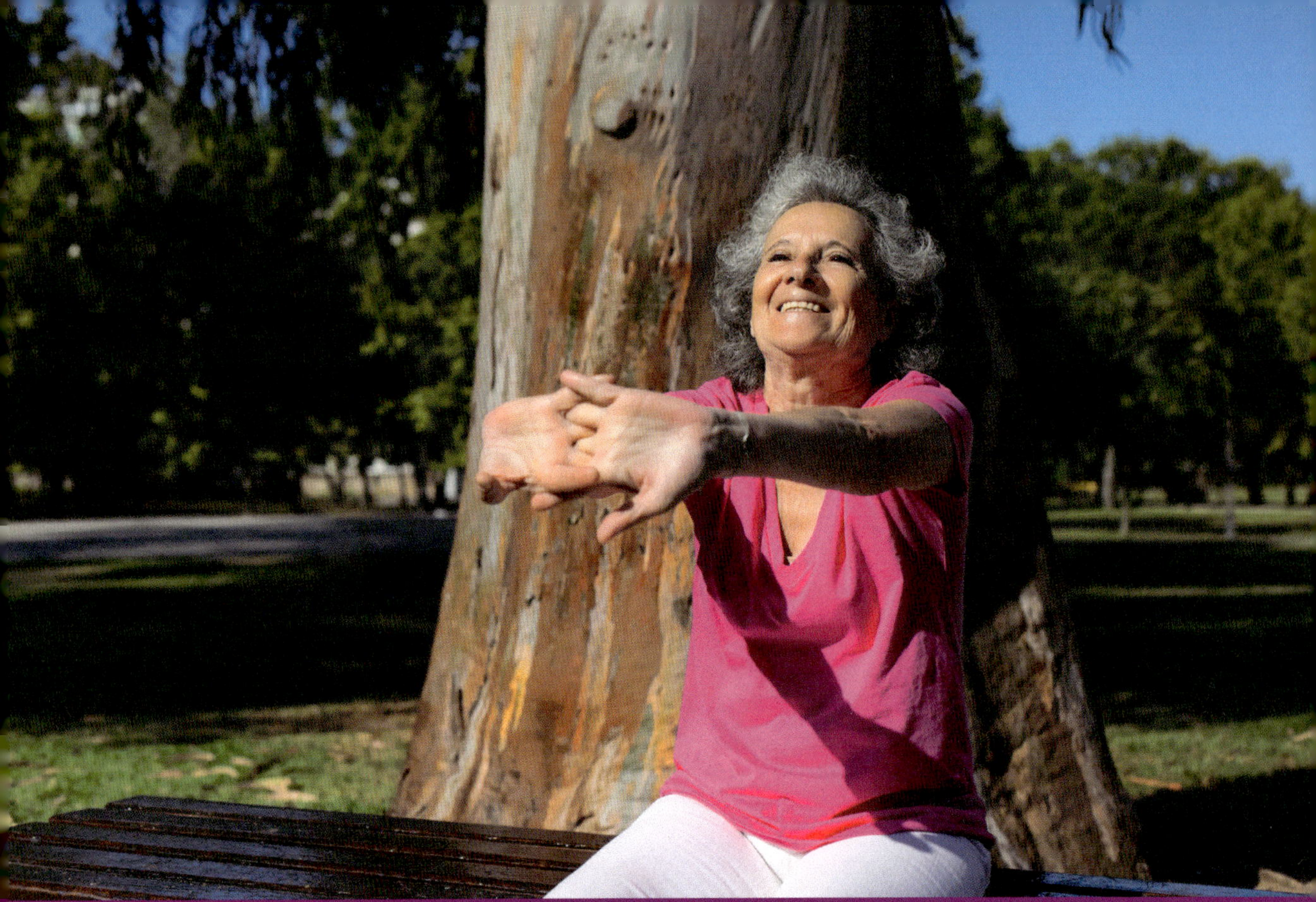

"You don't find
will power.
You create it."

CHAPTER 2

Step-By-Step Warm-Up Exercises

IMPORTANT: Each time you exercise please warm-up first. A good warm-up helps get your body ready to workout. Five to ten minutes should be enough to use most of your major muscles and all of your major joints from your neck right down to your toes. Wear comfortable loose-fitting clothes and non-slip footwear.

Warm-up Benefits

- Improved flexibility
- Better performance
- Improved blood flow
- Decreased muscle pain
- Decreased risk of injury
- Less muscle tension and pain
- Increased range of movement

Neck

- **EQUIPMENT:** N/A
- Head side to side, for this warm-up exercise, start by moving your left ear towards the top of your left shoulder, same on the right side, repeat several times
- Head left to right, to start, look over to your left and then to the right, repeat several times
- Head forwards and backwards, to start, look up towards the ceiling, then look down towards the floor, repeat several times
- Breathe normally

Shoulders

- **EQUIPMENT:** N/A
- Backward circles of both arms, for this warm-up exercise first make vertical circles with your arms going up right above your head and then down by your sides, and then horizontally to the same height as your shoulder starting with big circles and then getting smaller and smaller, repeat several times, and then do all over again but this time forwards
- Move your arms forwards across the chest as though giving yourself a big hug, alternate the crossing of hands, hands high, then hands lower clapping behind your back, clapping in front, repeat several times
- Shoulder rolls, hands down by your side, rolling shoulders forwards, upwards then down
- Breathe normally

Back

- **EQUIPMENT:** N/A
- For this warm-up exercise stand with feet about shoulders width apart. Rotating, swing your arms and wrap around waist tapping your bum, take your head around, repeat several times
- Side to side reach out as though you're trying to touch something, keep your hips still, repeat several times
- Forwards and backwards, back of hands facing forwards your arms are down by your side, as you-breathe in pull your shoulders back, opening up your chest. As you-breathe out fold your shoulders back to the starting position, repeat several times
- Breathe normally

Wrists

- **EQUIPMENT:** N/A
- For this warm-up exercise, start with your hands together, fingers interlaced, rotate hands in a circle, then forwards and backwards, repeat several times
- Single hand, circles, side-to-side, forwards and backwards, repeat several times
- Breathe normally

Hips - Upper

- **EQUIPMENT:** N/A
- For this warm-up exercise start with your hands on hips rotate round in a circle, go in both directions, repeat several times
- Hands-on hip move side to side, repeat several times
- Breathe normally

Hips – Lower

- **EQUIPMENT:** Chair (optional for support)
- For this exercise start by standing on one leg, hold on to the back of a chair for balance, make circles with the other leg, repeat several times
- Standing on one leg, hold on to the back of a chair for balance, move the other leg forwards and backwards, repeat several times
- Breathe normally

Knees

- **EQUIPMENT:** Chair (optional for support)
- For this warm-up exercise start standing on one leg, hold on to the back of a chair for balance, kick heel back behind the other, repeat several times
- Shallow squats, stand behind a chair in case you need help with balance, bend knees and squat down, straighten legs, repeat several times
- Breathe normally

Ankles

- **EQUIPMENT:** Chair
- Heel to toe taps, for this warm-up exercise, hold on to a chair and shift weight onto one foot. Bring the heel of your other foot off the ground so only your toes are touching. Then move the heel to touch the ground as you lift your toes up. Repeat several times, then change legs
- Breathe normally

Dynamic Stretching - Walking around arms open chest stretch

- **EQUIPMENT:** N/A
- For this warm-up exercise start walking a brisk pace
- Walking open arms taking one hand higher shoulder height, while the other lower, waist height, then alternate, repeat several times
- Breathe normally

Dynamic Stretching - Walking around 3 steps then 2 shallow squats

- **EQUIPMENT:** N/A
- For this warm-up exercise start walking a brisk pace walking 3 strides then squat twice, keep back flat, bottom out, repeat several times
- Breathe normally

Dynamic Stretching - Walking around 3 steps then oblique stretch

- **EQUIPMENT:** N/A
- For this warm-up exercise start walking a brisk pace walking 3 strides
- Stop and stand with feet shoulder-width apart reach up with the left arm, then change sides and reach up with the right arm, repeat several times
- Breathe normally

Heart Rate Pulse Raiser

- **EQUIPMENT:** Chair (optional)
- For this warm-up exercise start marching on the spot, can do this seated, march as briskly as you can for two minutes
- Knees into elbows, bring left knee up and right elbow down towards knee, change sides, bring right knee up and left elbow down, continue alternating at a brisk pace, can do this seated
- Breathe normally

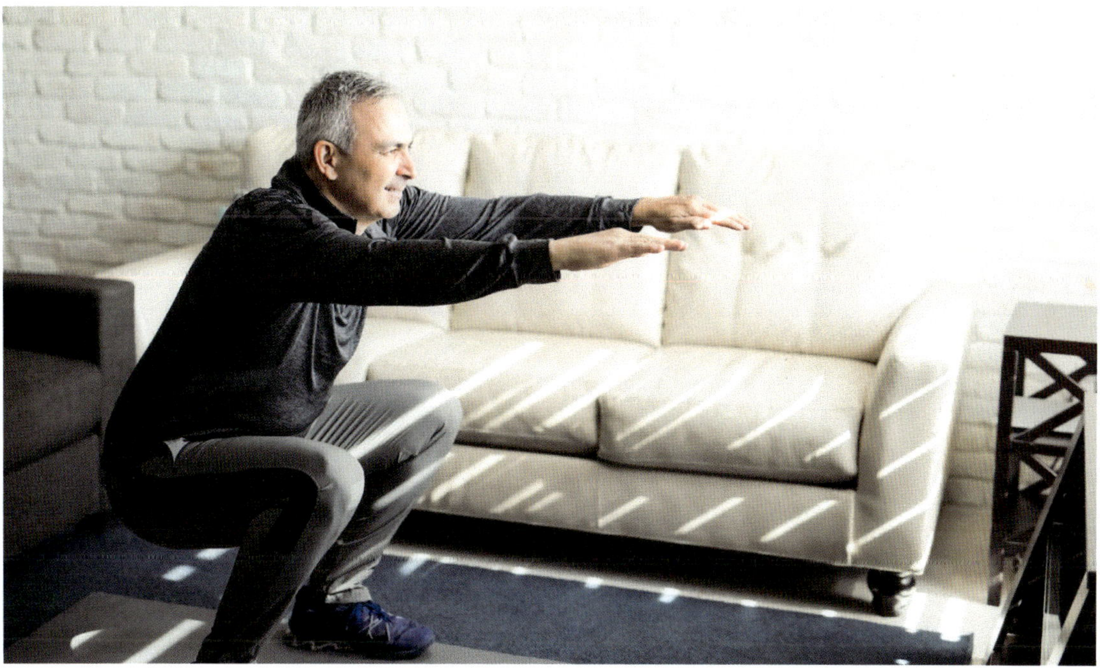

WARM-UP TIME GUIDELINES: You should spend at least 5 to 10 minutes warming up, longer if you feel you need to before you start your exercise routine.

Warm-up Tips

- Feel no pain. Stretch only to the point of mild tension, never to the point of pain. If a stretch hurts, stop immediately! Reset your position carefully after checking the step-by-step instructions, then try again.
- Pay attention to posture and good form. Posture counts whether you're sitting, standing or moving. Good form translates to better gains in flexibility and less likelihood of injury when stretching tight muscles.
- Focus on the muscle being stretched. You'll notice that one side of your body often is tighter than the other. Work on balancing this over time.
- Breathe comfortably while stretching or use yoga breathing.
- Practice often. You'll make the best gains if you stretch frequently even daily, or on as many days of the week as possible. At the very least, aim to do stretching two or three times a week.

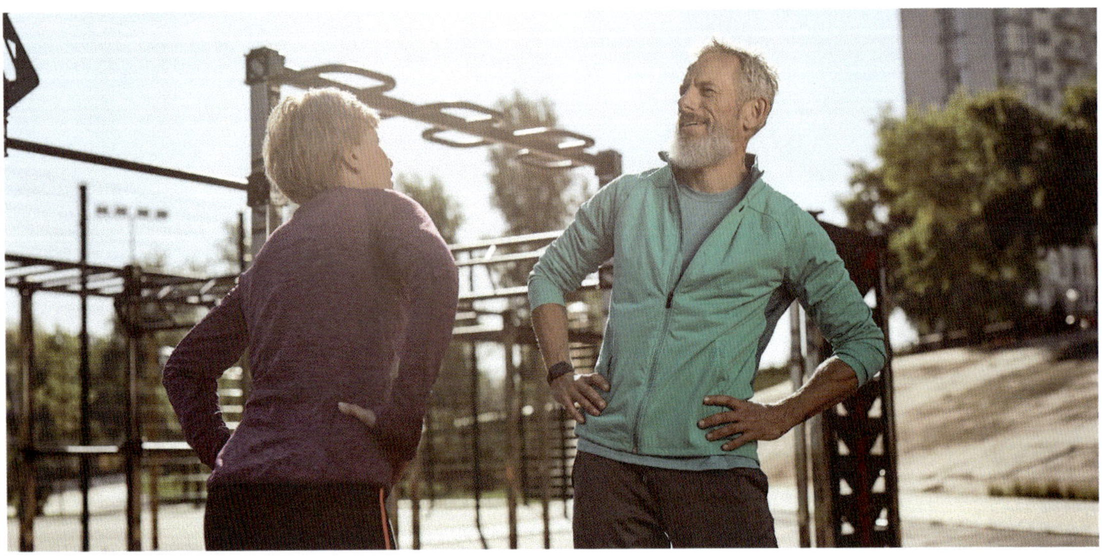

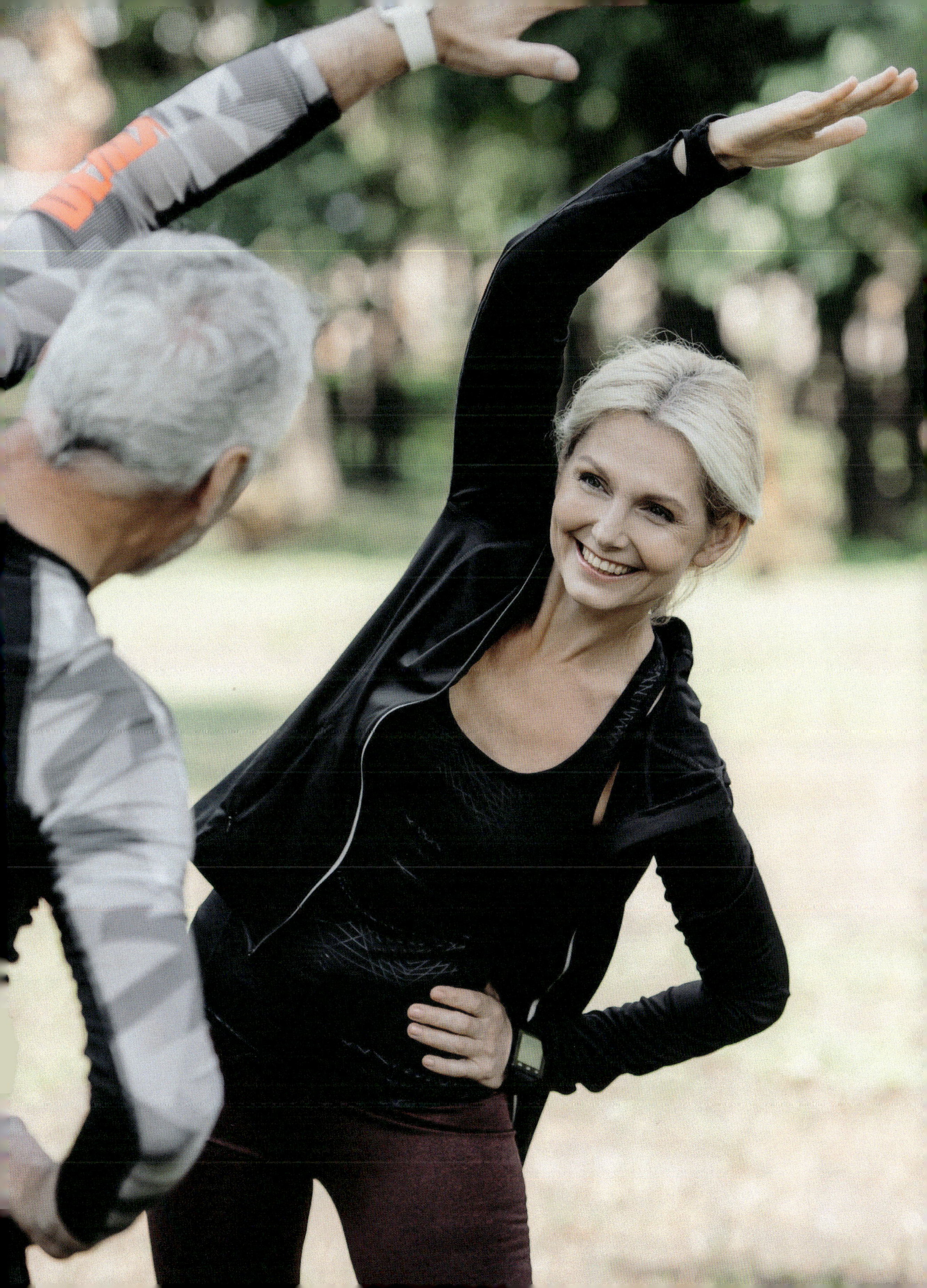

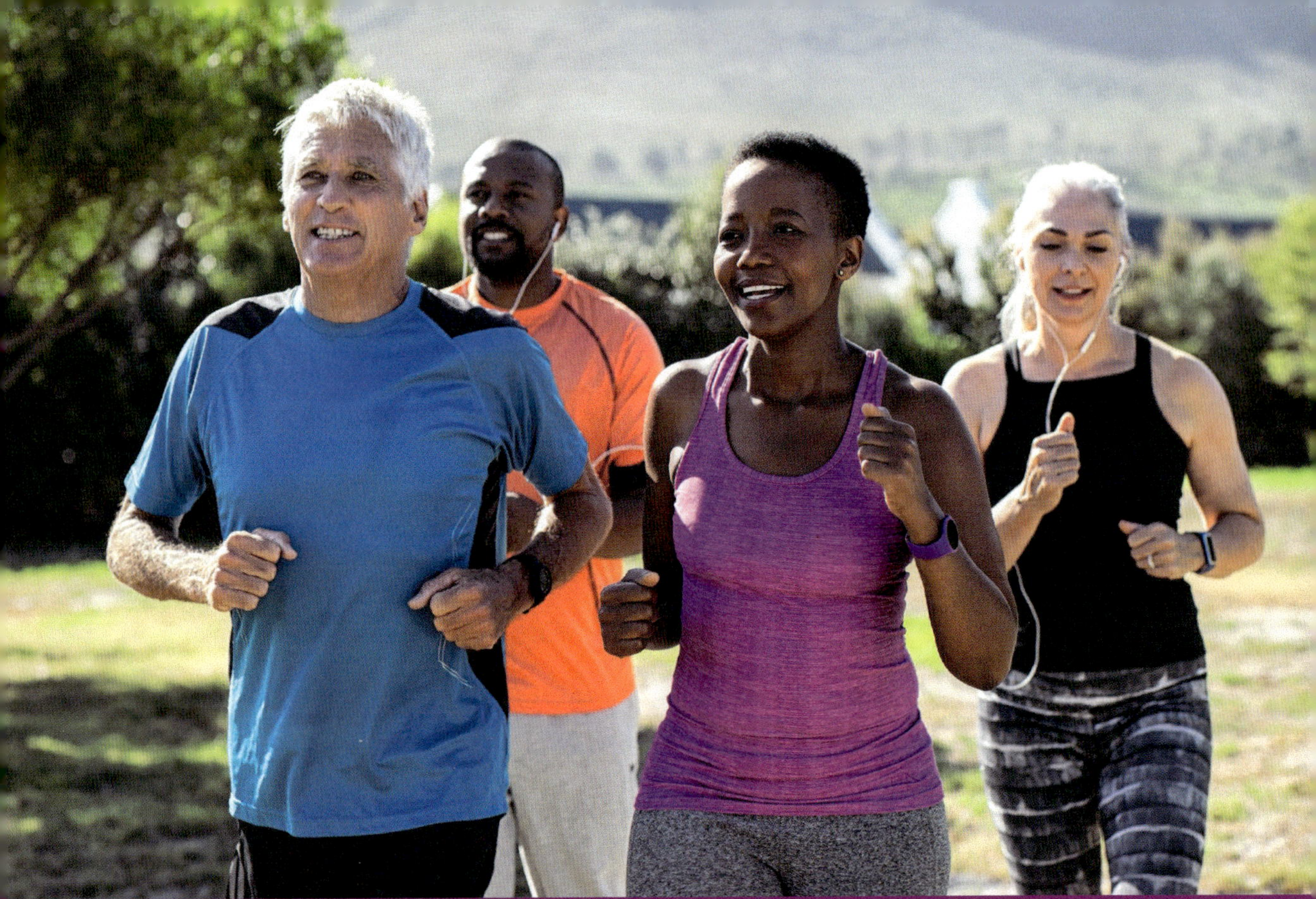

"Every workout counts even if it's just for 10 minutes."

CHAPTER 3

Step-By-Step Aerobic Exercises

Older adults probably have the most to gain by starting or continuing with an exercise programme that includes aerobic exercises. Not only will aerobic exercise strengthen your heart and lungs. It will also give you increased energy, help focus your mind, better manage your weight and even help to reduce symptoms of anxiety and depression.

The most convenient and affordable form of aerobic activity is walking. Studies have shown that brisk walking for at least half an hour, five times a week, has nearly the same health benefits as more vigorous exercise. People who take brisk walks have a lower risk for heart disease, diabetes, high blood pressure, high cholesterol, osteoporosis and perhaps other diseases. Even mental health problems are less frequent in regular walkers. Although it hasn't been studied, many regular walkers also believe that this simple exercise makes them feel more energetic.

Aerobic Training Benefits

- Live longer
- Boost your mood
- Keep arteries clear
- Reduce health risks
- Ward off viral illnesses
- Keep excess pounds at bay
- Manage chronic conditions
- Strengthen heart and lungs
- Stay active and independent
- Increased endurance, fitness and strength

Knees into Elbows

- **EQUIPMENT:** N/A
- For this aerobic exercise, start by bringing your left knee up and right elbow down towards your knee
- Change sides, bring right knee up and left elbow down
- Continue alternating at a brisk pace
- You can do a variation of this seated
- Breathe normally

High Knees Marching on the Spot

- **EQUIPMENT:** N/A
- For this aerobic exercise, stand with your back straight and your head up looking forward
- Begin with your feet together and hands straight down by the side of your body
- Lift one foot at a time bringing your knee up to the height of your waist
- Move alternate hands forwards and backwards as though you are jogging
- You can do a variation of this seated
- Breathe normally

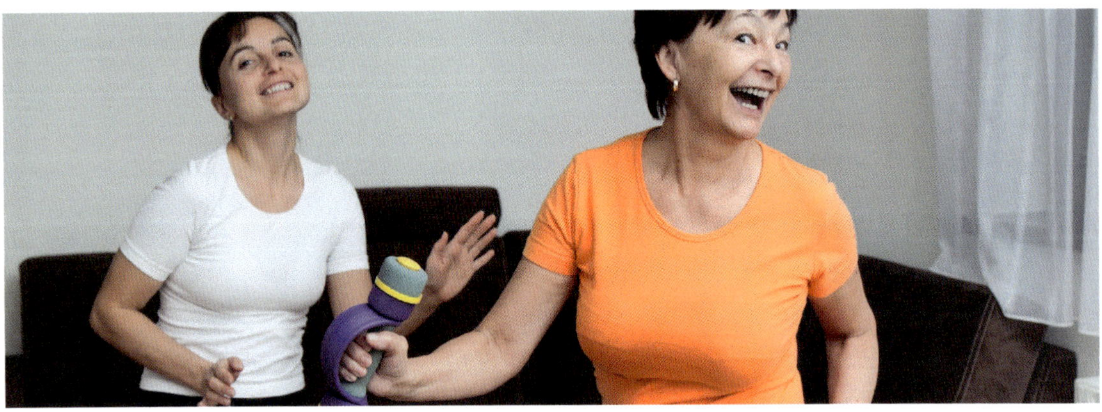

Step-Ups

- **EQUIPMENT:** Steps
- For this aerobic exercise, start on the bottom step of a set of steps or on your staircase. Step up onto the first step with your left foot, and then step up with your right foot, pause briefly
- Next, step back down with your right leg and then with your left leg
- Repeat on the other side
- You can make this a little more challenging by using weights; tins of food or dumbbells in each hand
- Breathe normally

Dancing

- A simple dance step of a brisk side to side, tap inside with your foot for a few minutes will do the job nicely
- You can of course, use any dance step; a Jive or Cha Cha etc as dancing is a great and indeed fun way to do aerobic exercise
- Put on your favourite music and let your feet loose and fancy-free for a nifty aerobic workout
- If dancing appeals, why not see if there's a local dance class to sharpen your moves as you get fit and have fun while doing it

Every Day Activities

- Any activity that leaves you slightly out of breath counts as aerobic exercise as you work towards your 150-minute weekly target
- Digging the vegetable garden, mowing and raking up the lawn, hand washing the car, brisk walk to the shops and carrying your shopping home, brisk walk with the dog, sports, for example, tennis and swimming

ACTIVITY TIME GUIDELINES: Older adults should aim to be active daily. Over a week, your activity should add up to at least 150-minutes of moderate-intensity activity in bouts of 10 minutes or more. One way to achieve this would be to do 30 minutes on at least 5 days of the week.

Aerobic Training Tips

- Before starting aerobic training talk to your doctor if you have any health conditions or concerns.
- Pick an activity that you enjoy and that's accessible, for example, walking, jogging, swimming and tennis.
- If it has been a while or if you've never exercised before, start with 5 to 10 minutes of cardio 2 to 3 times a week and gradually build-up to the above guidelines.
- Keep the intensity of your exercise to a moderate pace, so that you can always hold a conversation.
- Always warm-up before you start with 5 to 10-minutes of light warm-up exercises, or more if you feel you need to.
- Always stretch out after you've finished your workout to reduce muscle soreness.

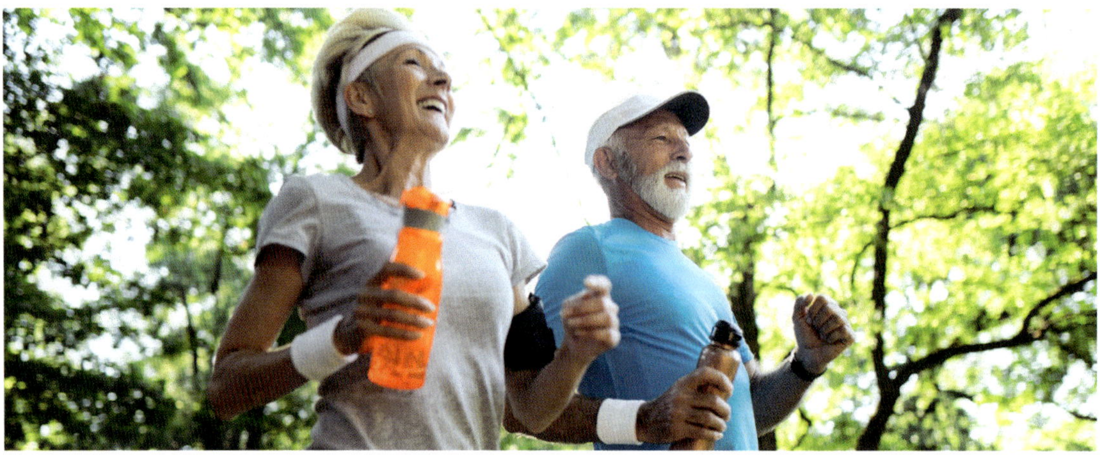

Question

Thinking about the last 7-days, how much moderate-intensity exercise of blocks of 10 minutes or more have you done?

NONE	30 mins or less	30 - 60 mins	60 - 90 mins	90 - 120 mins	120 - 160 mins	160 mins plus

Question

Thinking about the last 7-days, how many days of the week did you do moderate-intensity exercise of blocks of 10 minutes or more?

NONE	1	2	3	4	5	6 or 7

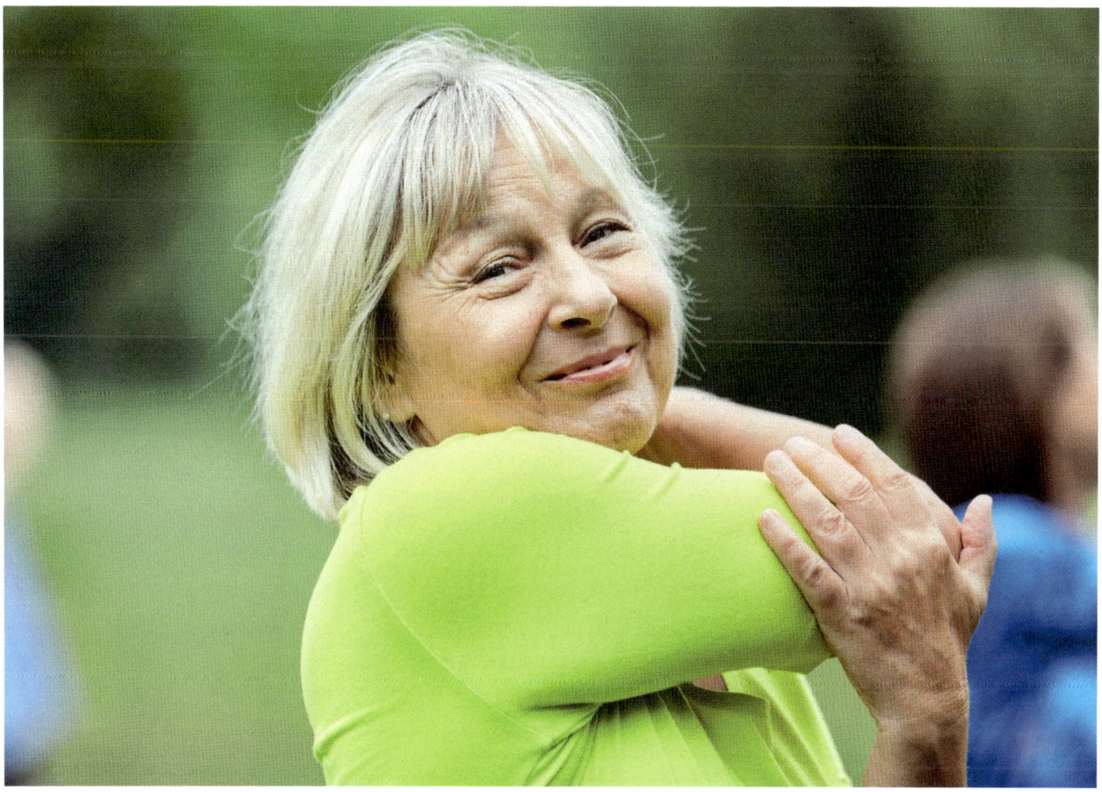

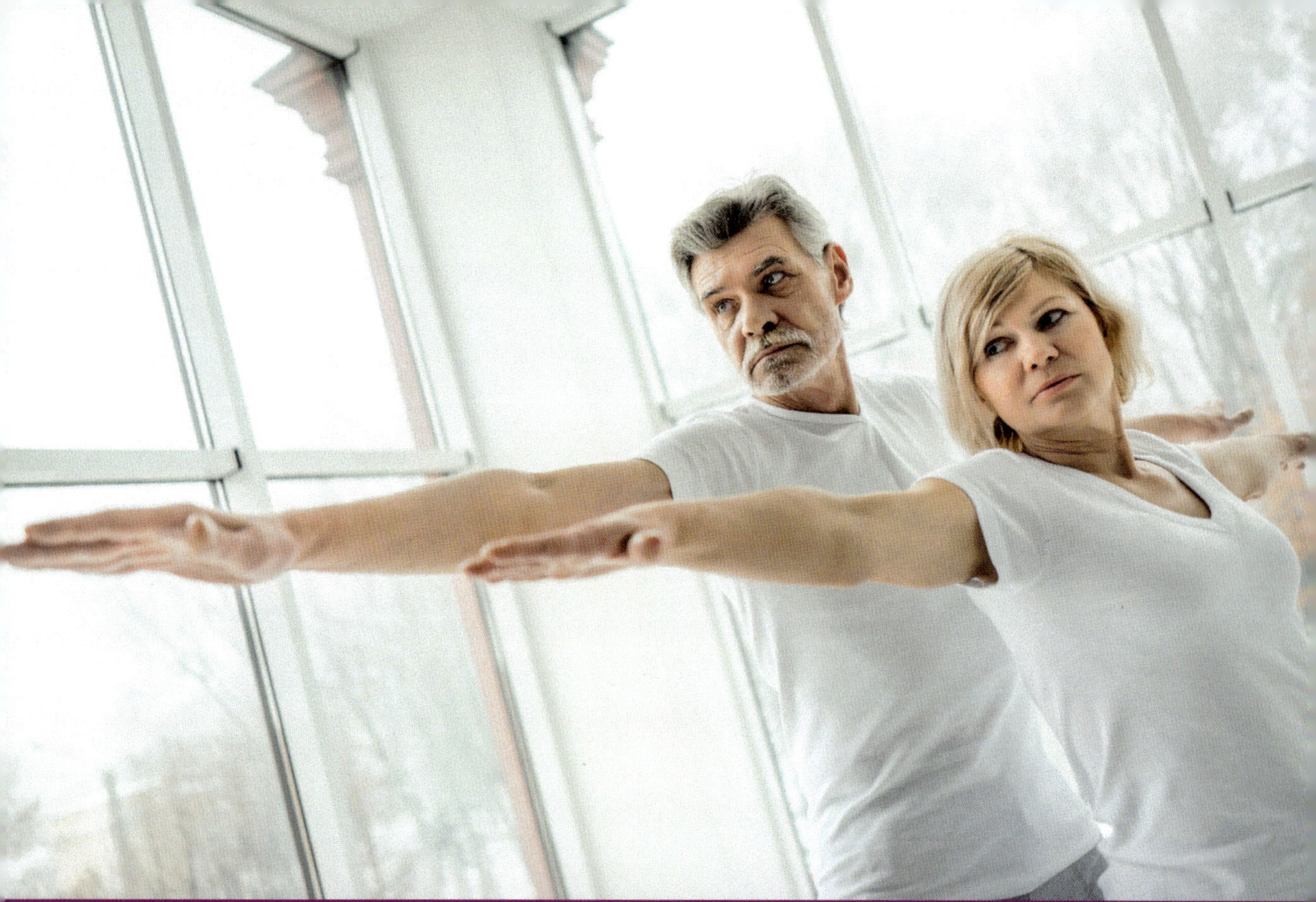

"Once you stop making excuses, success will follow."

CHAPTER 4

Step-By-Step Balance Exercises

As we grow older one of the body's systems that declines is our ability to balance, which in turn increases our risk of trips and falls. Trips and falls are perhaps one of the biggest threats to independent living. However, simply by doing some gentle balance exercises at least twice a week can significantly improve your ability to balance and therefore greatly reducing your risk of trips and falls.

Balance Training Benefits

- More muscle
- Stronger bones
- Faster reaction time
- Better brain function
- Improved coordination
- Reduced risk of trips and falls

Single Limb Stance

- **EQUIPMENT:** Chair
- For this balance exercise, start by standing behind a sturdy dining room chair and hold firmly on to the back initially using both hands, raise your right foot off of the floor and then balance on your left foot
- Hold the Single Limb Stance position for as long as you can, then change feet and repeat
- Your aim should be to stand in the Single Limb Stance position without holding onto the chair and hold it steady for up to one minute
- Breathe normally

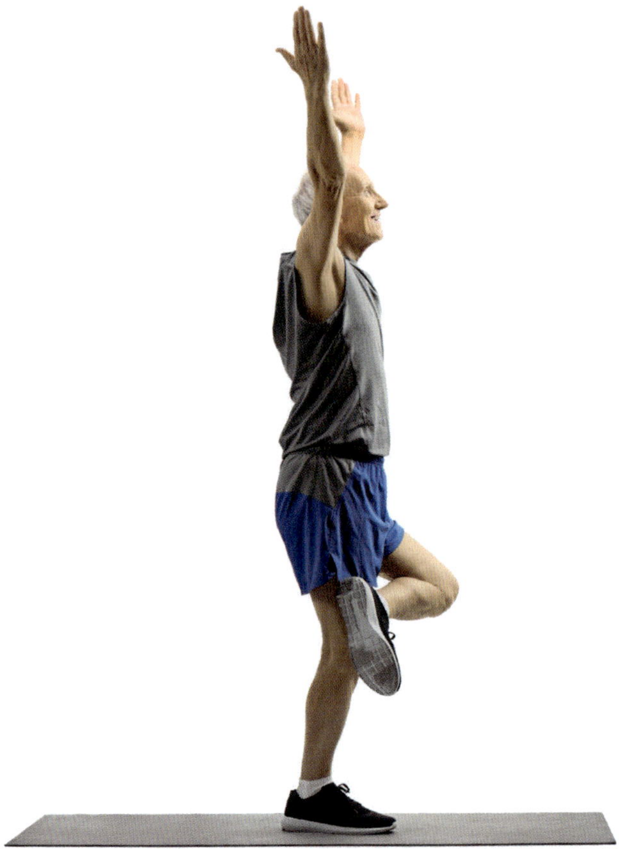

Rock the Boat

- **EQUIPMENT:** N/A
- For this balance exercise, start by standing with your feet about hip-width apart, with both feet pressed firmly on the floor
- Next stand up straight with your head level looking out forward, then transfer your weight onto your right foot and slowly lift your left leg off of the ground. Hold that position for as long as possible aiming for up to 30 seconds
- To finish the Rock the Boat exercise carefully place your foot back onto the floor, transferring your weight to this foot, then slowly lift your other leg
- Begin by doing the Rock the Boat exercise five times each side, then gradually work your way up to more repetitions
- Breathe normally

Walking Heel to Toe

- **EQUIPMENT:** N/A
- For this balance exercise, start by placing your right foot in front of left foot so that the heel of the right foot touches the top of the toes of the left foot
- Next, move your left foot in front of your right foot, putting your full weight on the heel, shift weight to your toes
- Repeat the step with the left foot, walk this way for 20 steps, turn around and walk back
- Tip; doing this balance exercise in a hallway with walls either side can make this feel safer, or have someone with you to watch you to keep you safe and support you as you Walk Heel to Toe
- Breathe normally

Back Leg Raises

- **EQUIPMENT:** Chair
- For this balance exercise, start by standing behind the dining chair
- Next start lifting your right leg straight backwards, avoid bending at the knees and remain in this balanced position for a couple of seconds before returning the leg back down
- Repeat for the other leg to complete your Back Leg Raises exercises, aim for 8 to 12 reps for each leg
- Breathe normally

Side Leg Raises

- **EQUIPMENT:** Chair
- For this balance exercise, start by standing behind a sturdy dining room chair or kitchen countertop with one or both hands resting on it for support
- Lift your right leg out to the side and then bring it back to the standing position, repeat 10 times for each leg to complete the exercise
- Breathe normally

Balancing Wand

- **EQUIPMENT:** Chair and Broom Handle (without the broom head)
- For this balance exercise, start seated holding the bottom of the broom handle so that it is flat on the palm of your hand, the aim of this exercise is to keep the broom handle upright for as long as possible
- Alternate between hands so that you practice your balance skills on both sides
- Breathe normally

Clock Reach

- **EQUIPMENT:** Chair
- For this balance exercise, pretend that you're standing in the middle of a large clock with 12 o'clock directly in front of you and with 6 o'clock directly behind you
- Start by holding onto the dining room chair with your left hand, lift up your right leg and extend your right arm so it points to 12 o'clock
- Next, point your arm towards 3 o'clock and then finally point your arm behind you towards 6 o'clock
- Bring your arm back to 3 o'clock and then back to 12 o'clock, looking straight out ahead throughout the exercise
- Repeat the Clock Reach exercise three times each side
- Breathe normally

Tip Toe Lifts

- **EQUIPMENT:** Chair or Counter (optional)
- For this balance exercise, start by standing up with your back straight extend your arms right out directly in front of you
- Lift yourself up on your toes as high as you can and then gently lower yourself down again
- Try not to lean too far forward
- Repeat lifting yourself up on your toes and lowering yourself down 20 times, repeat this for 2 to 3 sets
- Breathe normally

Marching on the Spot

- **EQUIPMENT:** Chair
- For this balance exercise, start by standing straight, lift your right knee as high as you can. Lower it then lift the left leg, lift and lower your legs 20 times
- Breathe normally

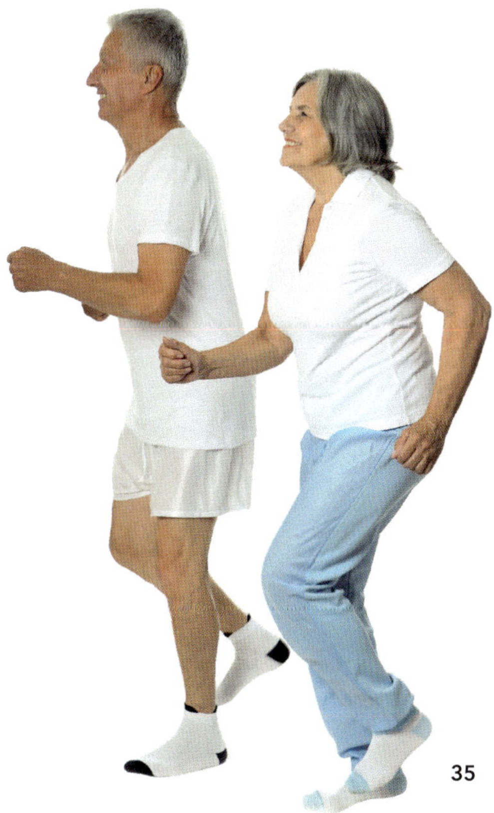

3-Way Hip Kick

- **EQUIPMENT:** Chair or Counter
- For this balance exercise, stand with your feet shoulder-width apart, firmly hold onto a chair or counter and extend your leg forward and return to your starting position
- Next repeat this movement to the side this time returning to the starting position
- Finally end the 3-way hip kick by extending your leg back before returning it to the starting position
- Perform the 3-way hip kick 8 to 12 times on each leg. Repeat for 2 to 3 sets
- Breathe normally

Mini Lunges

- **EQUIPMENT:** Chair or Counter
- For this balance exercise, stand with your feet shoulder-width apart. Firmly hold onto a chair or counter and step forward with your front knee slightly bent. Return your leg back to the starting position. Repeat with your other leg
- Please note that these lunges do not need to be that deep. If you feel any knee or hip pain use the chair or counter for more support and or take smaller lunge steps.
- Aim for 8 to 12 mini lunges on each leg. Repeat for 2 to 3 times sets
- Breathe normally

Grapevine

- **EQUIPMENT:** N/A
- For this balance exercise, begin by standing with your arms by your sides with your feet together
- Next step across in front of your right foot with your left leg, continue sideways across the floor uncrossing and crossing your leg
- To finish reverse directions only this time crossing your left leg behind your right leg back to your starting position
- Aim to do the Grapevine 3 times in each direction
- Breathe normally

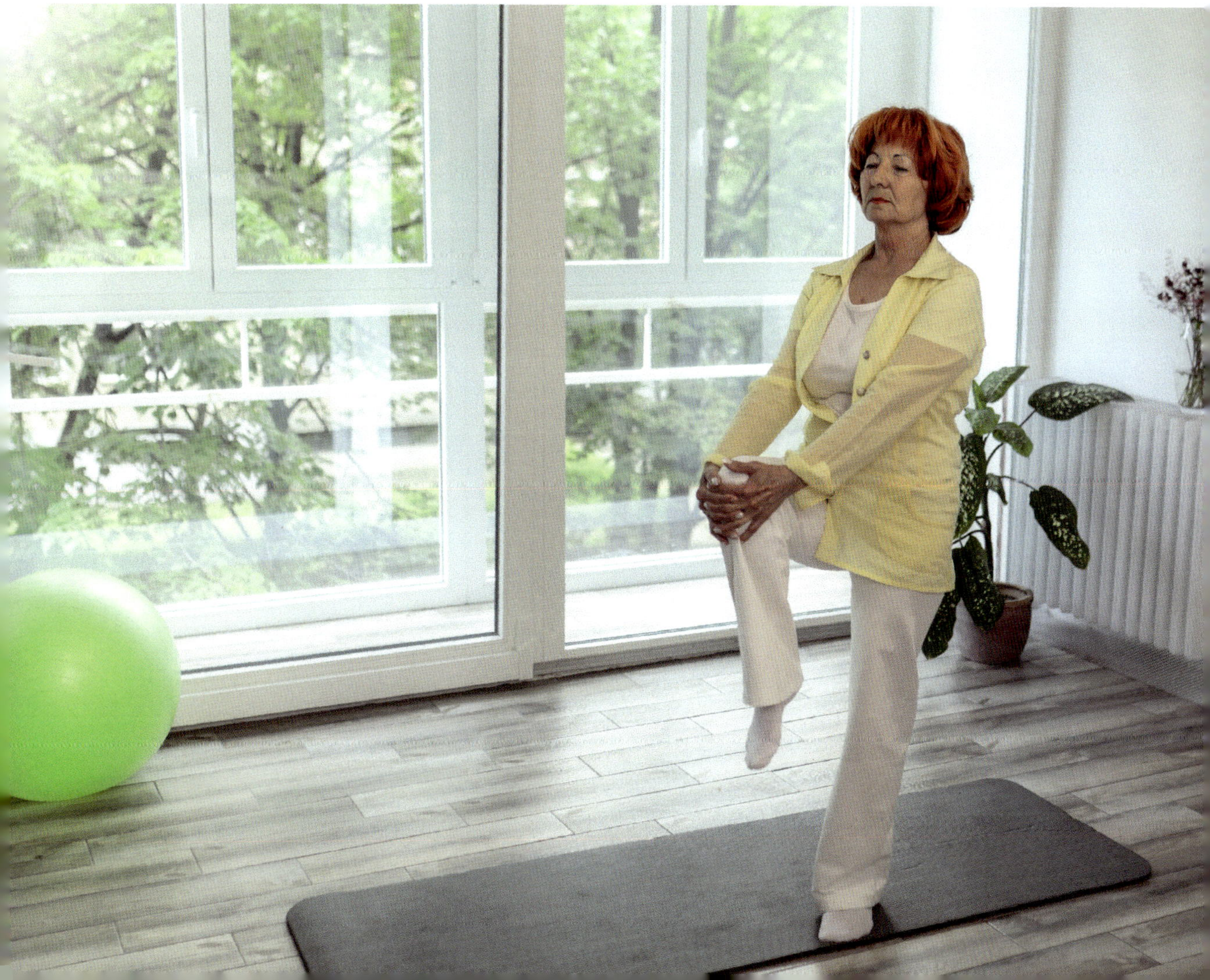

ACTIVITY TIME GUIDELINES: Older people should aim to do balance exercises at least twice a week, there is no set amount of time given but a sensible target would be at least 15 minutes each time.

Balance Training Tips

- As you move into retirement or semi-retirement keep up an active lifestyle with your increased free time, for example, join a local group; dancing, walking or rambling and tennis.
- Watch your weight as your diet can affect balance, consult a dietician, chat to your doctor or use established and well-respected sources, for example, the NHS Eatwell Guide: **www.nhs.uk/live-well/eat-well/the-eatwell-guide/**.
- Make sure you do some strength training (see Chapters 5 and 6) as some of these exercises can help you maintain or regain your balance.
- Make use of your walking aid, if your balance isn't what it used to be your doctor may have already recommended a walking aid, for example, a walking stick, use your walking aid as you undertake balance exercises.

Question

Thinking about the last 7-days, how much balance exercise, for example Tai Chi and Yoga, of blocks of 15 minutes or more have you done?

NONE	15 mins or less	15 - 30 mins	30 - 45 mins	45 - 60 mins	60 mins plus

Question

Thinking about the last 7-days, how many days of the week did you do balance exercise of blocks of 15 minutes or more?

NONE	1	2	3	4	5	6 or 7

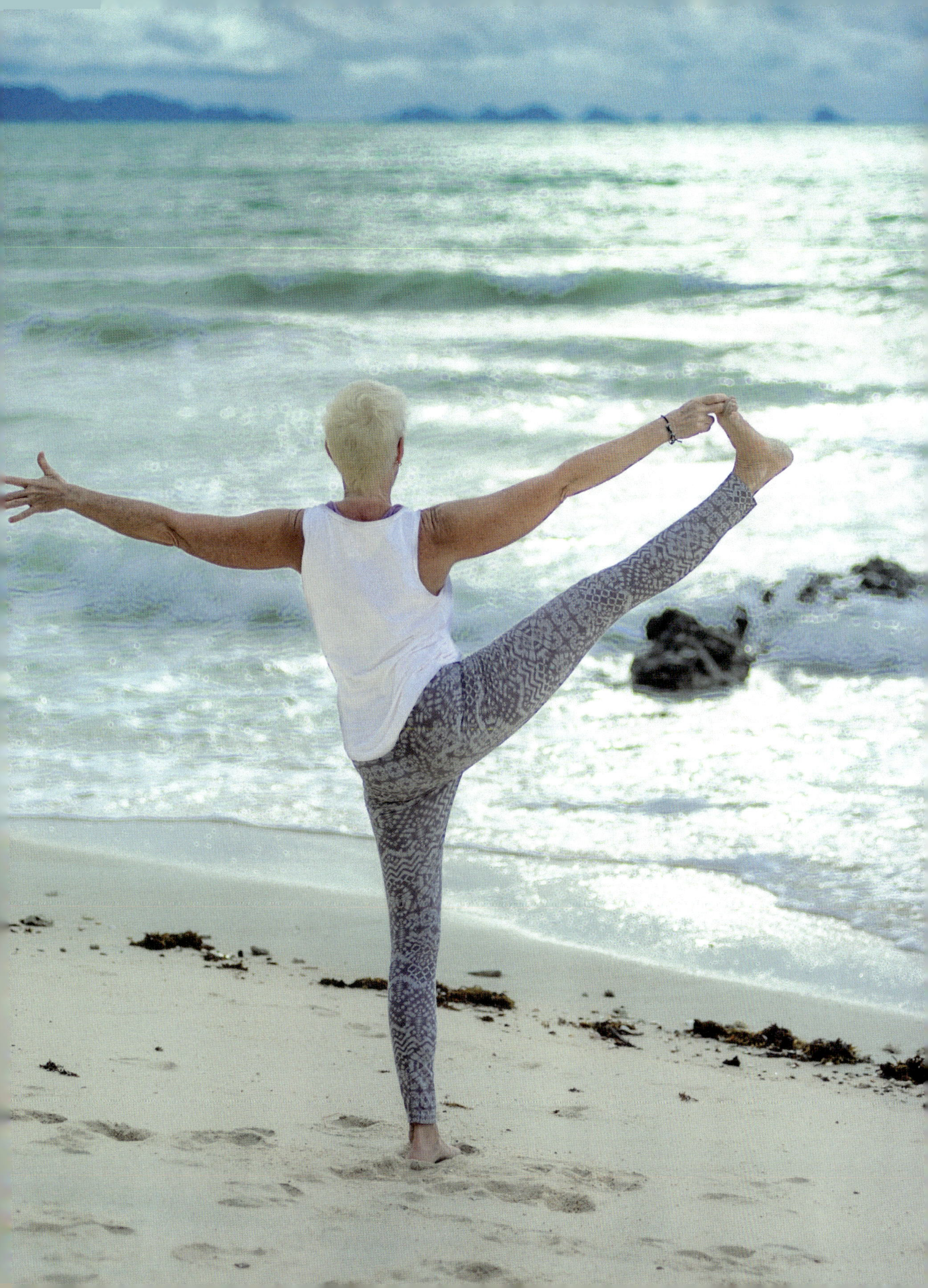

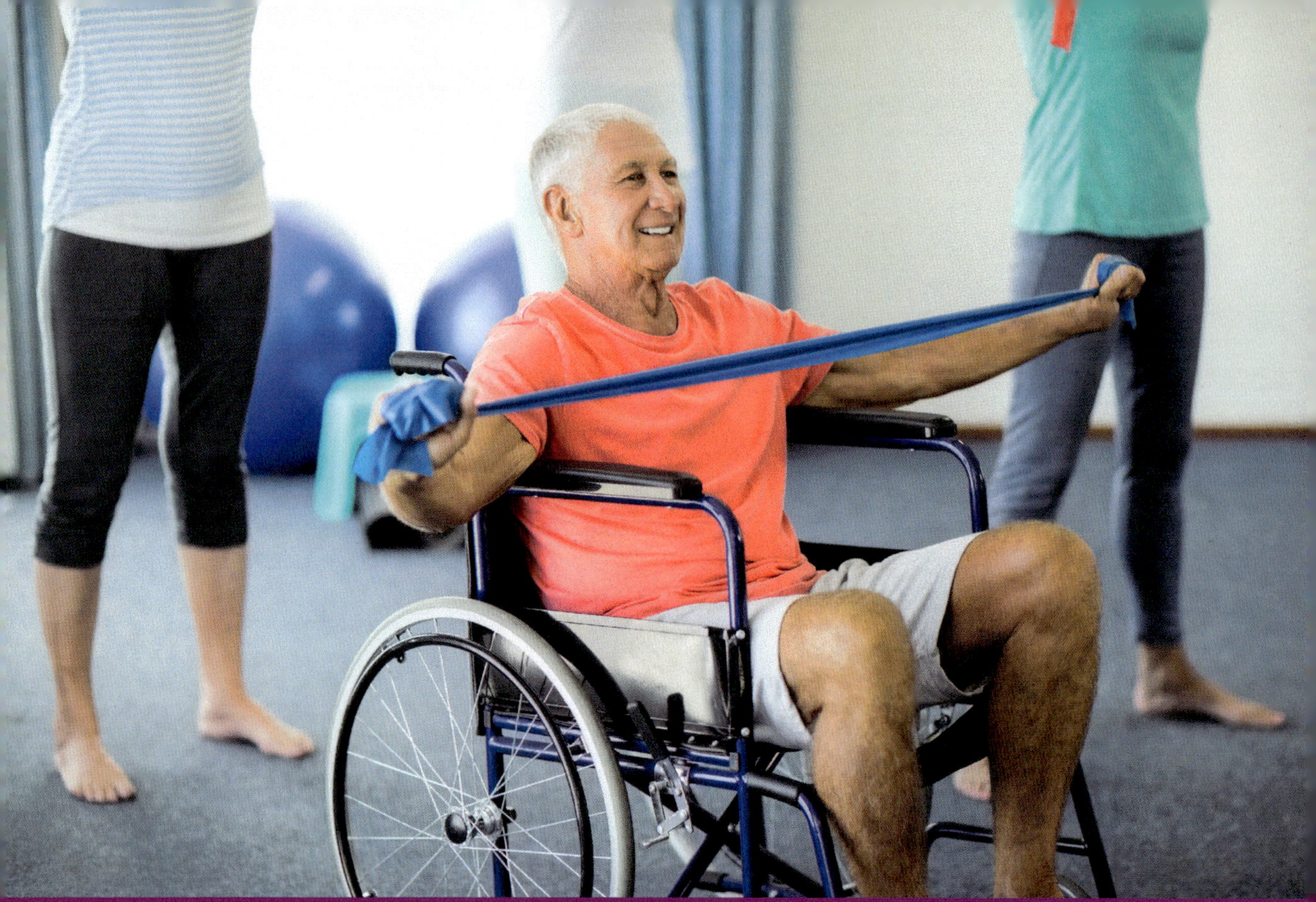

"Never give up,
amazing things
take time!"

CHAPTER 5

Step-By-Step Chair Based Exercises

Chair-based exercises can be just as challenging as regular standing up exercises, particularly for the upper body and abdominal muscles. Another advantage is that exercising while sitting requires less effort than standing and places a lot less pressure on lower body joints such as the knees and ankles, allowing adults who are less mobile to exercise.

Chair Based Training Benefits

- Sleep better
- Stronger bones
- Improved glucose control
- Keep excess pounds at bay
- Promote more independence
- Increased strength and muscle mass while raising metabolism
- Reduced symptoms of osteoarthritis, diabetes, osteoporosis, back pain and depression

Knees into Elbows

- **EQUIPMENT:** Chair
- For this aerobic exercise, start seated by bringing your left knee up and right elbow down towards the knee
- Change sides, bring right knee up and left elbow down
- Continue alternating at a brisk pace
- Breathe normally
- **TARGET**: As warm-up - 5 to 10 minutes, as aerobic exercise, 10 minutes and above

High Knees Marching on the Spot

- **EQUIPMENT:** Chair
- For this aerobic exercise, start seated sitting upright with your head up looking forward
- Begin with your feet together and hands straight down by the sides of the chair
- Lift one foot at a time bringing your knee up as high as you can
- Move alternate hands forwards and backwards as though you are jogging
- Breathe normally
- **TARGET:** As warm-up - 5 to 10 minutes, as aerobic exercise, 10 minutes and above

Bicep Curls

- **EQUIPMENT:** Chair, 2 Tins or 2 Dumbbells or Resistance Band
- For this strength exercise, sit towards the front of dining chair
- Holding a weight in each hand curl slowly upwards to your chest, keep your elbows fixed by your sides
- Lower the tins slowly, this is one complete rep
- Breathe in while lowering weights, breathe out while curling arms up
- **TARGET:** 2 to 3 sets of 8 to 12 repetitions

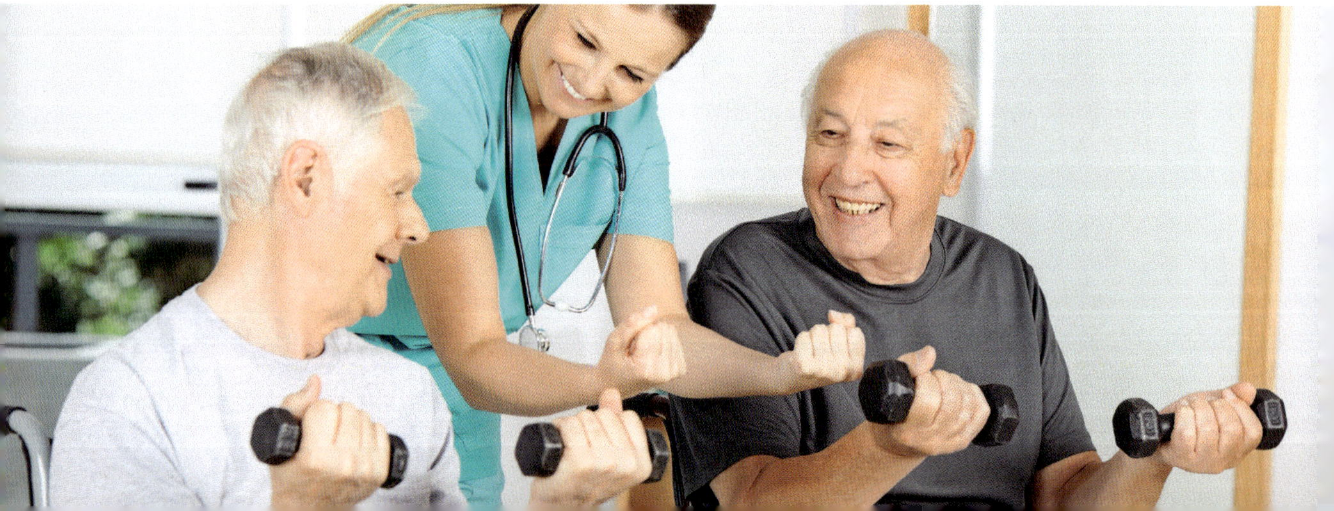

Triceps Extensions

- **EQUIPMENT:** Chair, Bottle of Water, Squash or a Dumbbell
- For this strength exercise, sit on a chair and hold the bottle in both hands extending it up overhead
- Keep your biceps close to your ears with your elbows pointing forward as you then lower the bottle behind your head until your elbows are at an angle of about 90-degrees
- Next straighten out your arms to the starting position, this is one rep
- Keep your abs engaged throughout the exercise, avoid arching your back
- Breathe in while lowering weight, breathe out while pushing arms up
- **TARGET:** 2 to 3 sets of 8 to 12 repetitions

Shoulder Rolls

- **EQUIPMENT:** Chair
- For this flexibility exercise, start seated and rotate your shoulders gently up towards the ceiling and then backwards and finally downwards
- Next, do the same movement but this time roll your shoulders upwards, forwards and then downwards
- Breathe normally
- **TARGET:** 2 to 3 sets of 8 to 12 repetitions

Upright Rows

- **EQUIPMENT:** Chair, 2 Tins or 2 Dumbbells or Resistance Band
- For this strength exercise, sit with a weight in each hand with your palms facing in towards your body
- Lift the weights by raising your elbows out to the sides until they line up with the height of your shoulders. Your hands should finish up just beneath your chin
- Next, slowly slide the weights down to your lap, this is one complete rep
- Breathe in while lowering weights, breathe out while moving arms up
- **TARGET:** 2 to 3 sets of 8 to 12 repetitions

Lateral Raises

- **EQUIPMENT:** Chair, 2 Tins or 2 Dumbbells or Resistance Band
- For this strength exercise, sit with a weight in each hand keep your arms down by your sides with your palms facing in
- Ensure that your shoulders are relaxed with your stomach muscles engaged
- Retaining this position, lift the weights out to the sides up to the height of your shoulders
- Pause and then slowly lower the weights back to your starting position, this is one complete rep
- Breathe in while lowering weights, breathe out while moving arms up
- **TARGET:** 2 to 3 sets of 8 to 12 repetitions

Front Raises

- **EQUIPMENT:** Chair, 2 Tins or 2 Dumbbells or Resistance Band
- For this strength exercise, sit with a weight in each hand with your arms down by your sides, palms facing your body
- Without bending your elbows, raise alternate arms straight up in front of the body until at shoulder-level height
- Lower the weights back down to starting position and then repeat with the other arm, this is one complete rep
- Breathe in while lowering weight, breathe out while moving arms up
- **TARGET:** 2 to 3 sets of 8 to 12 repetitions

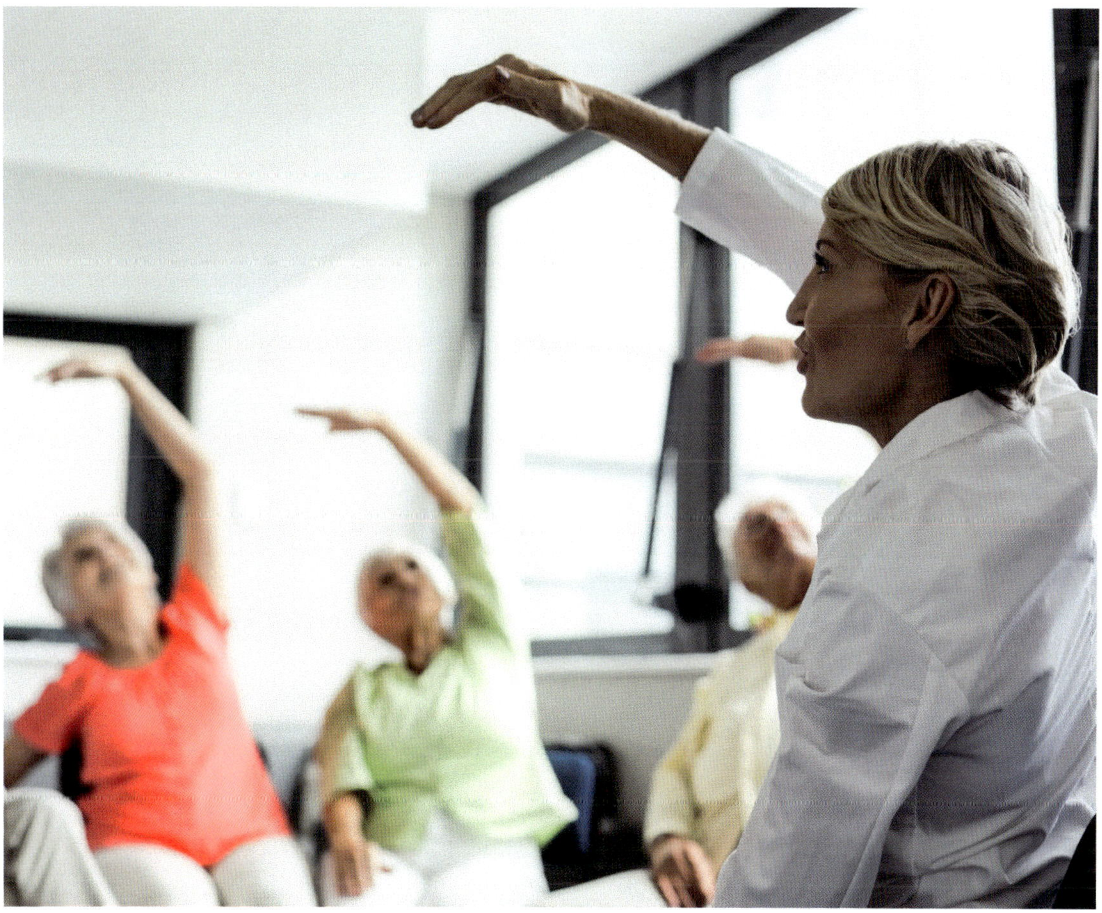

Stomach Twists

- **EQUIPMENT:** Chair
- For this strength exercise, start seated, holding the top and bottom of the bottle of water or squash in both hands close to your stomach and elbows bent slightly
- Slowly rotate your body to the right as far as you can comfortably go while keeping the rest of your body stable and the move back across your body to finish on your left side, return to the centre, this is one complete rep
- Breathe normally
- **TARGET:** 2 to 3 sets of 8 to 12 repetitions each side

Leg Extensions

- **EQUIPMENT:** Chair
- For this strength exercise, sit towards the front of the chair while keeping your left foot on the floor and with your upper body quite still
- Next, extend your right leg until its parallel with the floor and hold it up for the count of two
- Bend knee to lower your right leg back to the starting position, repeat with left leg, this is a complete rep
- Breathe in while lowering legs, breathe out while moving legs up
- **TARGET:** 2 to 3 sets of 8 to 12 repetitions each leg

Shin Extensions

- **EQUIPMENT:** Chair
- For this strength exercise, start by sitting on the edge of a dining chair with both your legs extended and your heels firmly planted on the floor, keep your knees slightly bent
- Next point your toes downwards and then flex them back upwards
- Breathe normally
- **TARGET:** 2 to 3 sets of 12 to 15 repetitions

Seated Calf Raises

- **EQUIPMENT:** Chair
- For this strength exercise, start seated with your hips back as far back as possible
- Place both your hands down by the sides of the dining chair holding the seat to keep yourself stable
- Keep both legs at an angle of about 90-degrees with the chair, with both feet flat on the floor
- Slowly, raise the heels of your feet upwards while pushing your toes on the ground and lifting your heels in the air
- Place both feet back to the starting position, this is one complete rep
- Breathe in while lowering down, breathe out while moving up
- **TARGET:** 2 to 3 sets of 15 to 20 repetitions

ACTIVITY TIME GUIDELINES: Older adults should aim to be active daily. Over a week, your activity should add up to at least 150 minutes of moderate-intensity activity in bouts of 10 minutes or more. One way to achieve this would be to do 30 minutes on at least 5 days of the week. Ideally, you should aim to build up a routine of 8 to 12 exercises that strength train the major muscle groups 2 to 3 times a week on non-consecutive days to allow for recovery.

Training Tips

- Before starting strength training speak with your doctor if you have any health conditions or concerns.
- Do not hold your weights too tightly and ensure that all movements are done in a controlled manner.
- You may get some muscular aches during exercise however stop immediately if you feel any sharp pain in your joints. You may get some muscular aches 24 to 48 hours after exercising. This is quite normal and will fade away.
- Keep the intensity of your exercise to a moderate pace, so that you can always hold a conversation.
- Always warm-up before you start with 5 to 10- minutes of light warm-up exercises, or more if you feel you need to.
- Always stretch out after you've finished your workout to reduce delayed onset muscle soreness.
- If you have limited mobility in your legs but are more able with your arms and hands, then you might want to consider buying a portable pedal exerciser. You can use this sitting at a table, using your arms and hands on the pedals, and this will provide you with a good aerobic workout in place of taking regular walks. Prices vary, but you can get a decent one from between £20 to £35. Drive DeVilbiss Healthcare has one at £24.99. This piece of equipment will enable you to do the **GET FIT IN JUST 12-WEEKS CHALLENGE**.

Question

Thinking about the last 7-days, how much chair-based exercise of blocks of 10 minutes or more have you done?

NONE	30 mins or less	30 - 60 mins	60 - 90 mins	90 - 120 mins	120 - 160 mins	160 mins plus

Question

Thinking about the last 7-days, how many days of the week did you do chair-based exercise of blocks of 10 minutes or more?

NONE	1	2	3	4	5	6 or 7

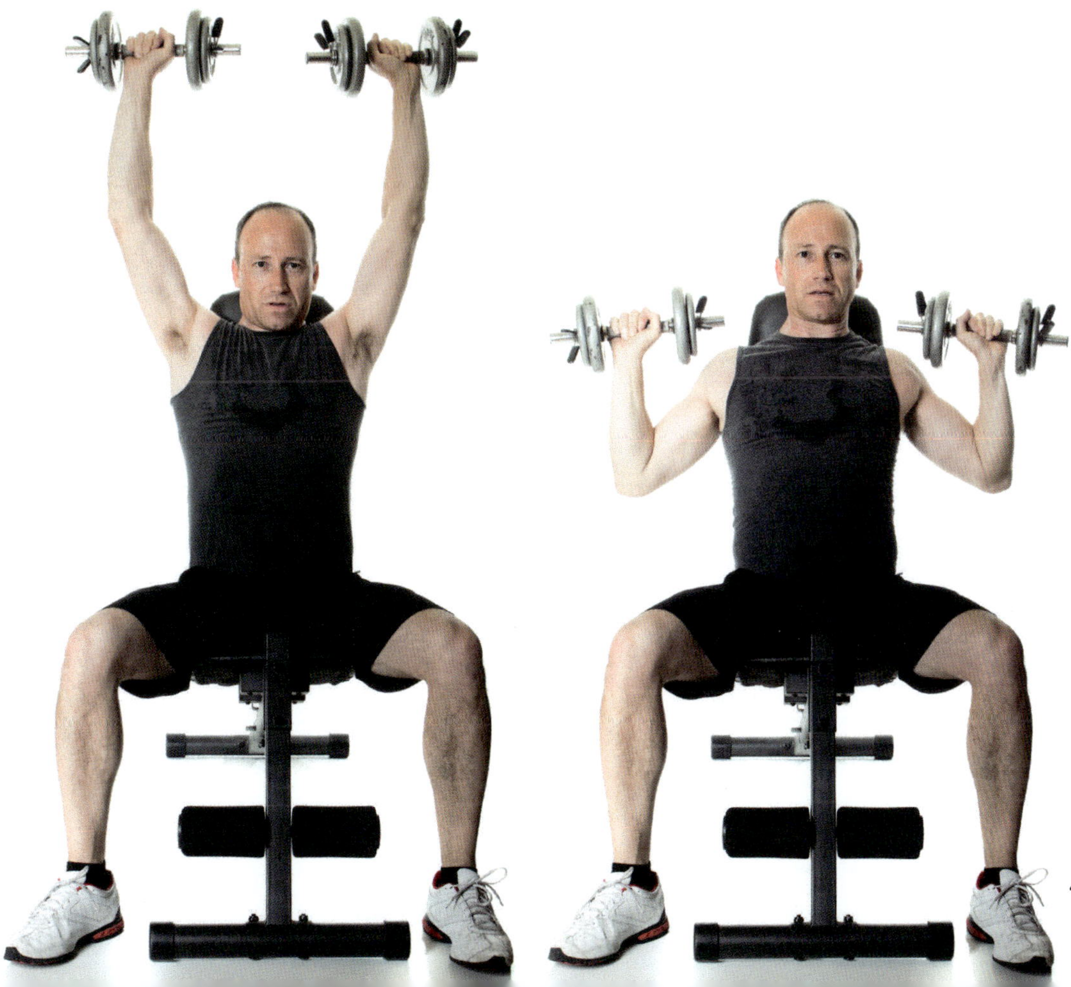

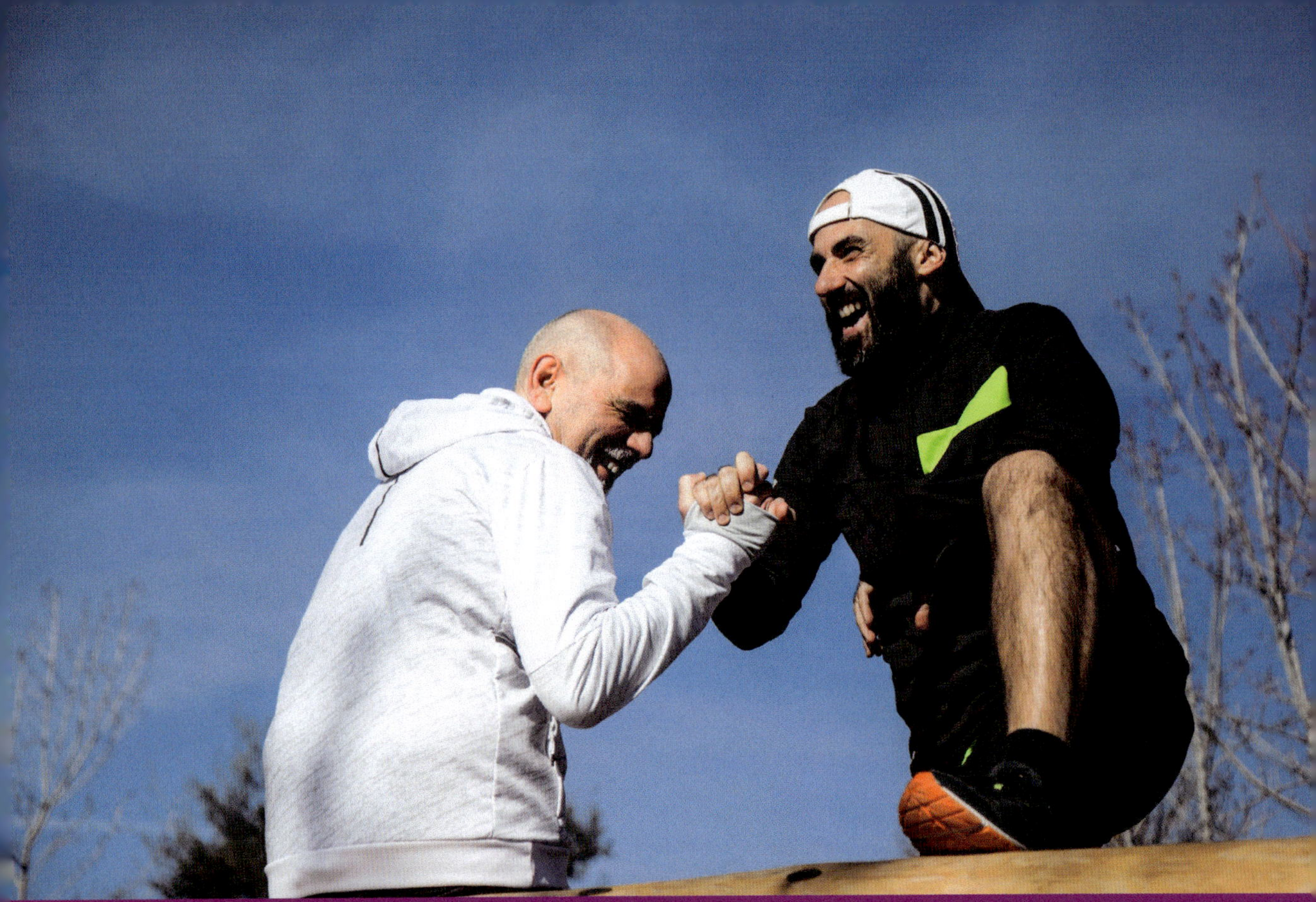

"If it doesn't challenge you,
it won't change you."

CHAPTER 6

Step-By-Step Strength Exercises

Strength training provides older people with some important benefits. Research has shown that it combats weakness and frailty if done regularly. Strength exercises build muscle strength and help to preserve bone density, important to fighting off osteoporosis.

Strength Training Benefits

- Sleep better
- Stronger bones
- Improved glucose control
- Keep excess pounds at bay
- Promote greater independence
- Increased strength and muscle mass while raising metabolism
- Reduced symptoms of osteoarthritis, diabetes, osteoporosis, back pain and depression

Wall Push-ups

- **EQUIPMENT:** N/A
- For this strength exercise, stand about an arm's length in front of the wall (for your safety make sure the wall does not have any paintings, decorations, windows or doors)
- Lean forward slightly and put your palms flat on the wall at the same height and slightly wider than your shoulders, keep your feet firmly on the floor as you slowly move your body towards the wall
- Gently push yourself back so that your arms are straight to your starting position, this is one rep
- Take a deep breath while lowering yourself to the wall, breathe out as you push back
- **TARGET**: 2 to 3 sets of 8 to 12 repetitions

Bicep Curls

- **EQUIPMENT:** 2 Tins or 2 Dumbbells or Resistance Band
- For this strength exercise, stand upright with your feet hip-width apart
- Holding a weight in each hand curl slowly upwards to your chest, keep your elbows fixed by your sides
- Lower the tins slowly, this is one complete rep
- Breathe in while lowering weight, breathe out while curling arms up
- **TARGET:** 2 to 3 sets of 8 to 12 repetitions

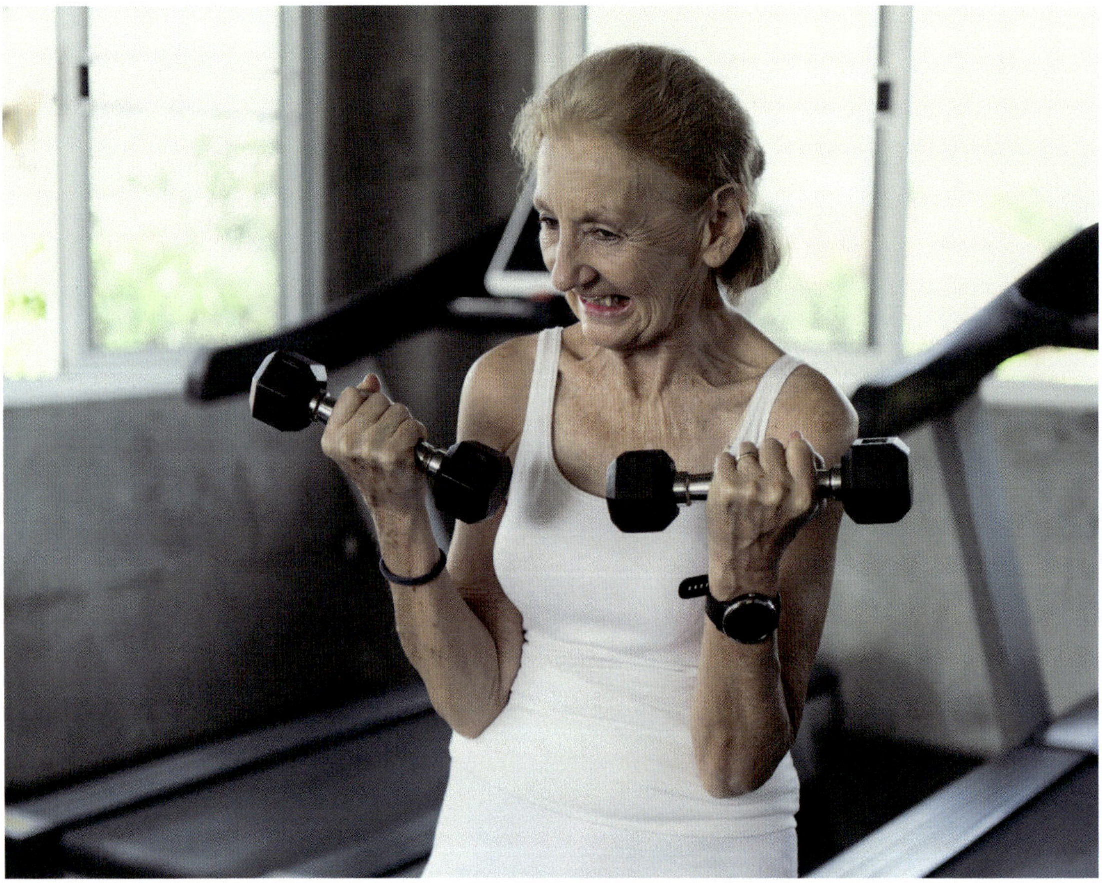

Triceps Extensions

- **EQUIPMENT:** Bottle of Water, Squash or a Dumbbell
- For this strength exercise, stand upright with your feet hip-width apart
- Keep your biceps close to your ears with your elbows pointing forward as you then lower the bottle behind your head until your elbows are at an angle of about 90-degrees
- Next straighten out your arms to the starting position, this is one rep
- Keep your abs engaged throughout the exercise, avoid arching your back
- Breathe in while lowering weight, breathe out while pushing arms up
- **TARGET:** 2 to 3 sets of 8 to 12 repetitions

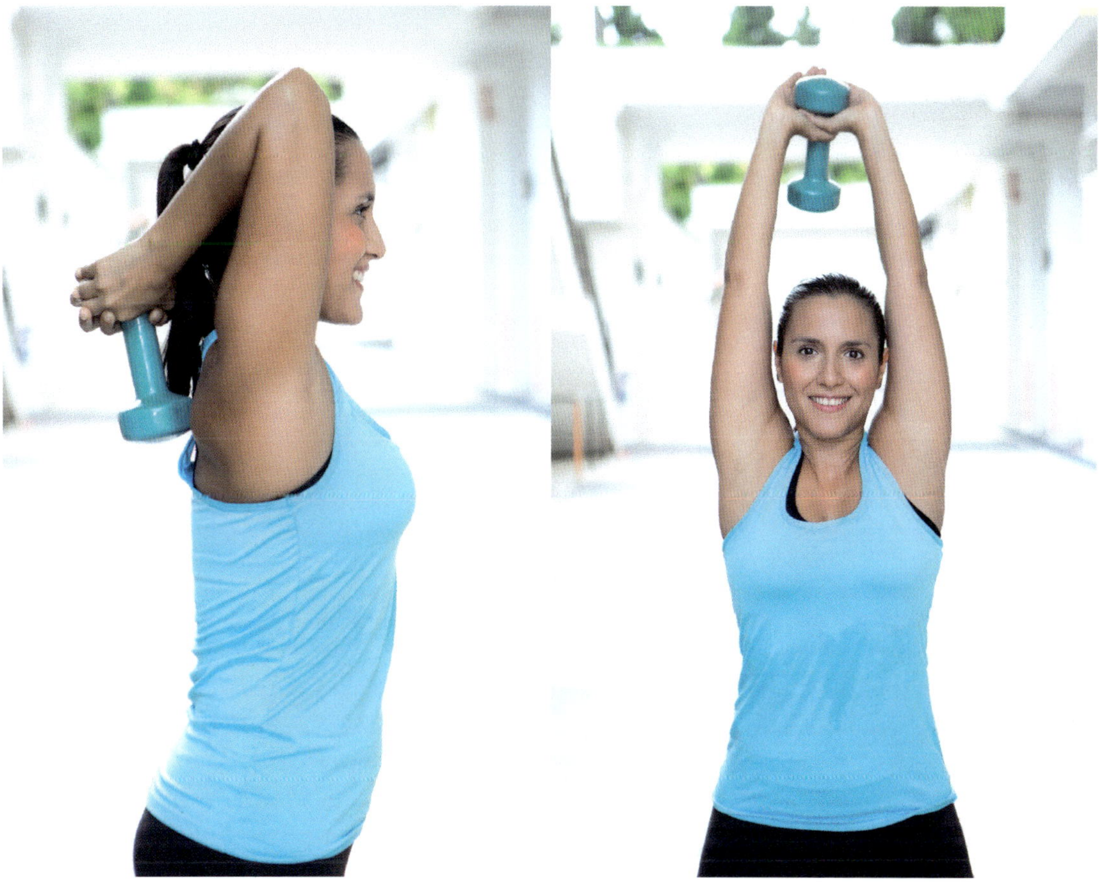

Upright Rows

- **EQUIPMENT:** 2 Tins or 2 Dumbbells or Resistance Band
- For this strength exercise, stand upright with your feet hip-width apart
- Lift the weights by raising your elbows out to the sides until they line up with the height of your shoulders. Your hands should finish up just beneath your chin
- Next, slowly slide the weights down to the starting position, this is one complete rep
- Breathe in while lowering weight, breathe out while moving arms up
- **TARGET:** 2 to 3 sets of 8 to 12 repetitions

Lateral Raises

- **EQUIPMENT:** 2 Tins or 2 Dumbbells or Resistance Band
- For this strength exercise, stand upright with your feet hip-width apart
- Ensure that your shoulders are relaxed with your stomach muscles engaged
- Retaining this position, lift the weights out to the sides up to the height of your shoulders
- Pause and then slowly lower the weights back to your starting position, this is one complete rep
- Breathe in while lowering weight, breathe out while moving arms up
- **TARGET:** 2 to 3 sets of 8 to 12 repetitions

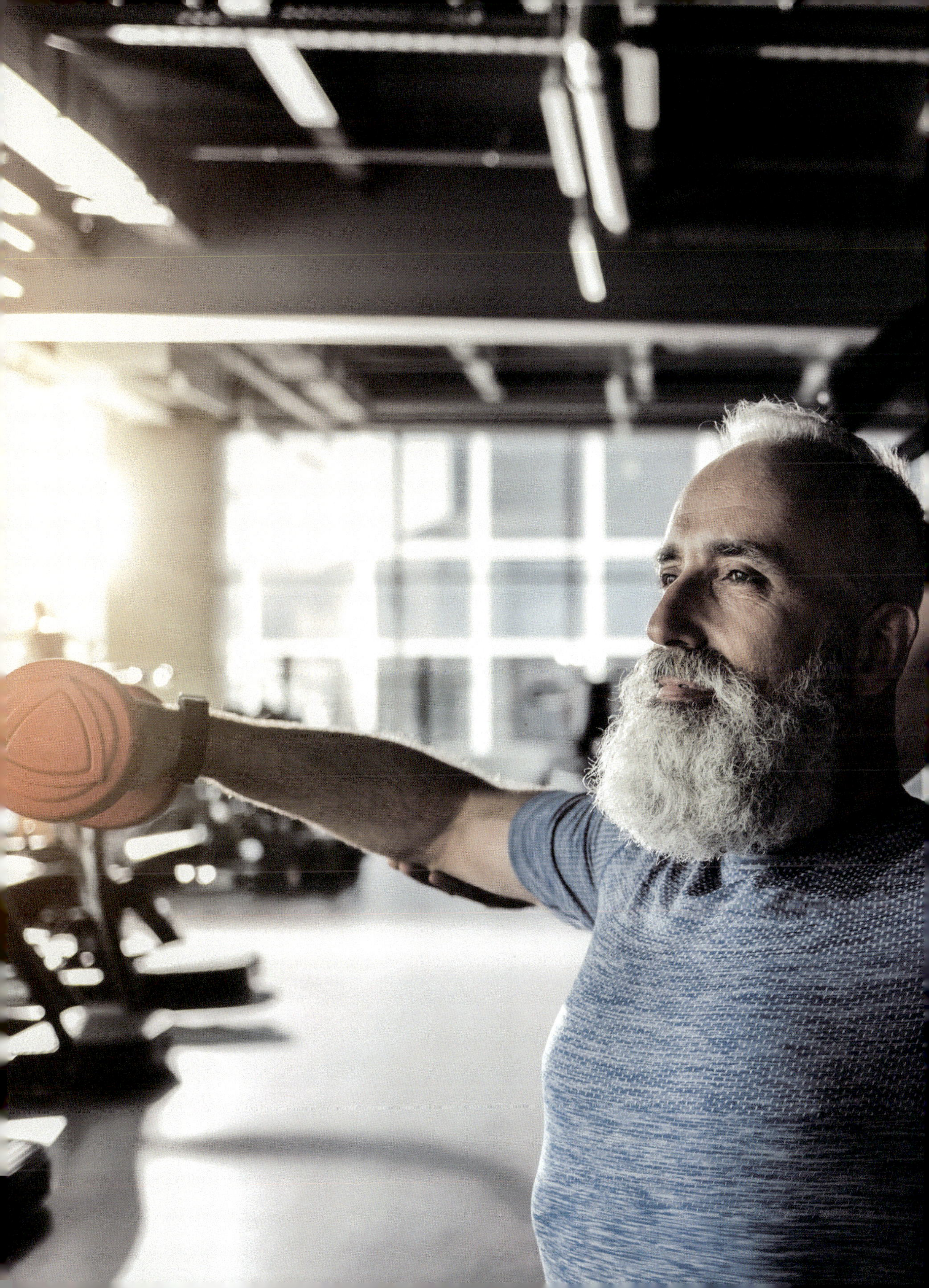

Front Raises

- **EQUIPMENT:** 2 Tins or 2 Dumbbells or Resistance Band
- For this strength exercise, stand upright with your feet hip-width apart
- Start with a tin in each hand with arms by sides and palms facing your body
- Raise alternate arms without bending at your elbows straight up in front of your body up to the height of your shoulders
- Lower the weights back down to the starting position and then repeat with your other arm, this is one complete rep
- Breathe in while lowering the weights and back out while moving your arms up
- **TARGET:** 2 to 3 sets of 8 to 12 repetitions

Shoulder Press

- **EQUIPMENT:** 2 Tins or 2 Dumbbells or Resistance Band
- For this strength exercise, start your Shoulder Press exercise with your feet shoulder-width apart, weights (either tins or dumbbells) in hand at chest level, palms forward.
- Extend your arms straight up over your head, then lower back down to the starting position, this is one rep
- Breathe in while lowering the weights and back out while moving your arms up
- **TARGET:** 2 to 3 sets of 8 to 12 repetitions

Sit Down Stand-Ups

- **EQUIPMENT:** N/A
- For this strength exercise, sit towards the front of the chair with your knees bent and both your feet flat on the floor about shoulder-width apart
- Next, lean back slightly with both your hands crossed over your chest, keep your back and your shoulders straight
- Breathe in slowly
- Bring your upper body forward until sitting upright as you breathe out, extend your arms so they are parallel to the floor and slowly stand up pushing up through your heel
- Breathe in as you sit back down slowly under control, this is one rep
- **TARGET:** 2 to 3 sets of 8 to 12 repetitions

Goblet Squats

- **EQUIPMENT:** Bottle of Water, Squash or a Dumbbell
- For this strength exercise, start by standing with your feet about shoulder-width apart
- Hold the weight with both hands in front of your chest
- Remember to keep your chest up with your heels down throughout
- Perform a standard squat and when on the upward move raise the weight up above your head, then lower back down to finish in front of your chest, this is one rep
- Breathe in as you slowly squat down under control, breathe out as you stand back up
- **TARGET:** 2 to 3 sets of 8 to 12 repetitions

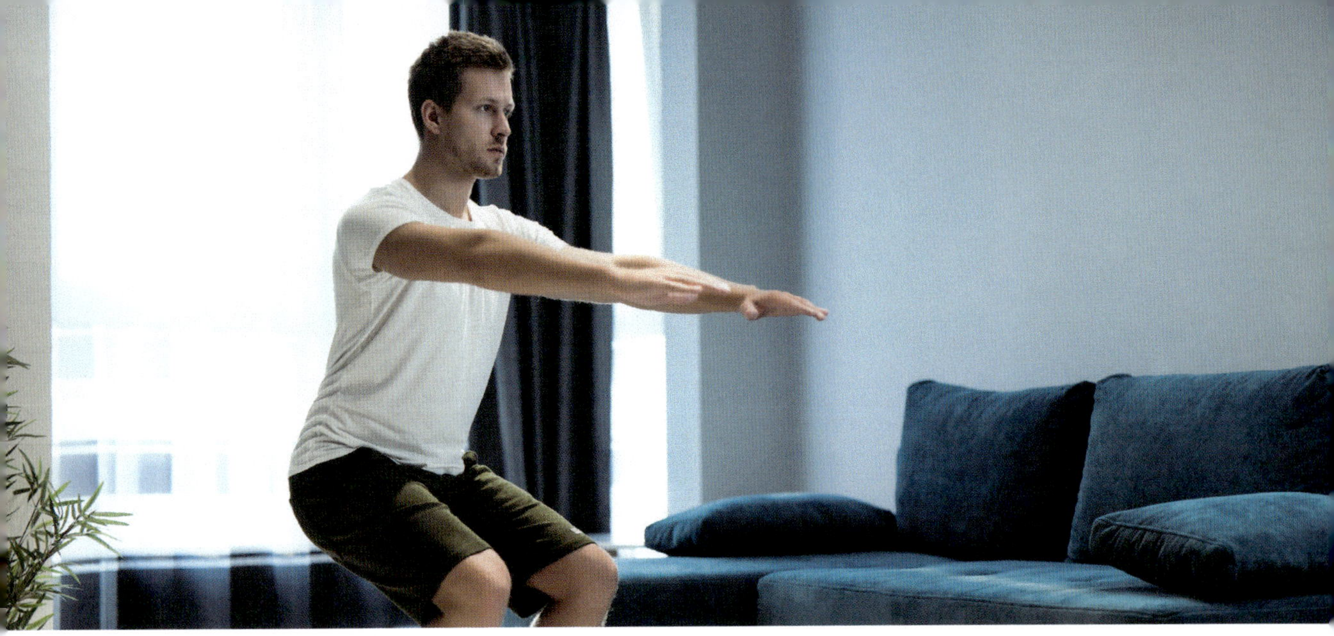

Squats

- **EQUIPMENT:** Chair for support (optional)
- For this strength exercise, start by standing up and using the dining chair as support
- Next, bend your knees as much as you can without your knees passing over your toes, then return to the starting position
- Breathe in as you slowly squat down, breathe out as you stand up
- **TARGET:** 2 to 3 sets of 8 to 12 repetitions

Standing Calf-Raises

- **EQUIPMENT:** Bottle of Water or Squash or a Dumbbell
- For this strength exercise, start by standing with your feet quite close together
- Hold the weight in front of you with both hands
- Push upwards through the balls of your feet and raise your heels until you are standing on your toes
- Next, lower slowly back to the start under control, this is one rep
- **TARGET:** 2 to 3 sets of 15 to 20 repetitions

Wrist Curls

- **EQUIPMENT:** Tin or Dumbbell, Chair with Arms
- For this strength exercise, start by placing your forearm on a chair's armrest with your hand hanging over the edge.
- Hold a tin with your palm facing upwards
- Slowly bend your wrist up and down and then repeat
- Change sides and perform with your other hand
- Breathe normally
- **TARGET:** 2 to 3 sets of 8 to 12 repetitions

Glute Bridges

- **EQUIPMENT:** Mat
- For this strength exercise, start by lying down on bed or floor with both your knees bent, your hips are in a neutral position
- Next, lift your bottom as high as you comfortably can off of the floor, pause briefly and then return the body to the starting position and repeat
- Breathe out completely and engage core before upward movement, breathe in during the downward movement
- **TARGET:** 2 to 3 sets of 8 to 12 repetitions

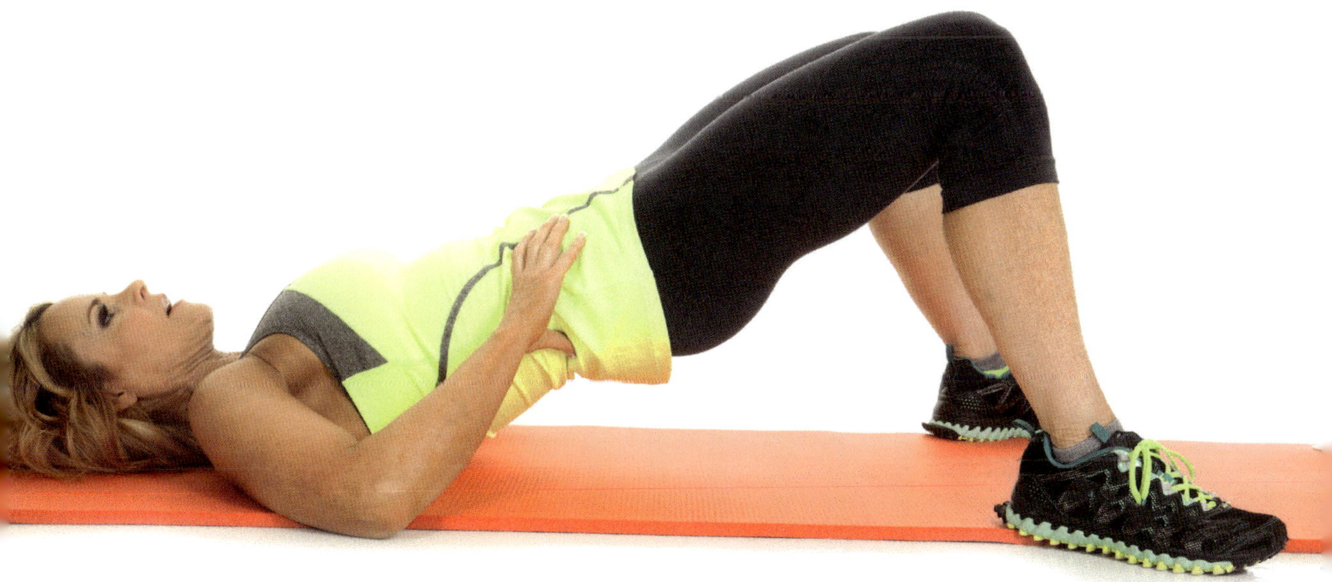

ACTIVITY TIME GUIDELINES: Older adults should aim to be active daily. Over a week, your activity should add up to at least 150 minutes of moderate-intensity activity in bouts of 10 minutes or more. One way to achieve this would be to do 30 minutes on at least 5 days of the week. Ideally, you should aim to build up a routine of 8 to 12 exercises that strength train the major muscle groups 2 to 3 times a week on non-consecutive days to allow for recovery.

Strength Training Tips

- Before starting strength training speak with your doctor if you have any health conditions or concerns.
- Do not hold your weights too tightly and ensure that all movements are done in a controlled manner.
- You may get some muscular aches during exercise. Stop immediately if you feel any sharp pain in your joints. You may get some muscular aches 24 to 48 hours after exercising; this is quite normal and will fade away.
- Keep the intensity of your exercise to a moderate pace, so that you can always hold a conversation.
- Always warm-up before you start with 5 to 10 minutes of light warm-up exercises, or more if you feel you need to.
- Always stretch out after you've finished your workout to reduce muscle soreness.

Question

Thinking about the last 7-days, how much strength training exercise of blocks of 10 minutes or more have you done?

NONE	30 mins or less	30 - 60 mins	60 - 90 mins	90 - 120 mins	120 - 160 mins	160 mins plus

Question

Thinking about the last 7-days, how many days of the week did you do strength exercise of blocks of 10 minutes or more?

NONE	1	2	3	4	5	6 or 7

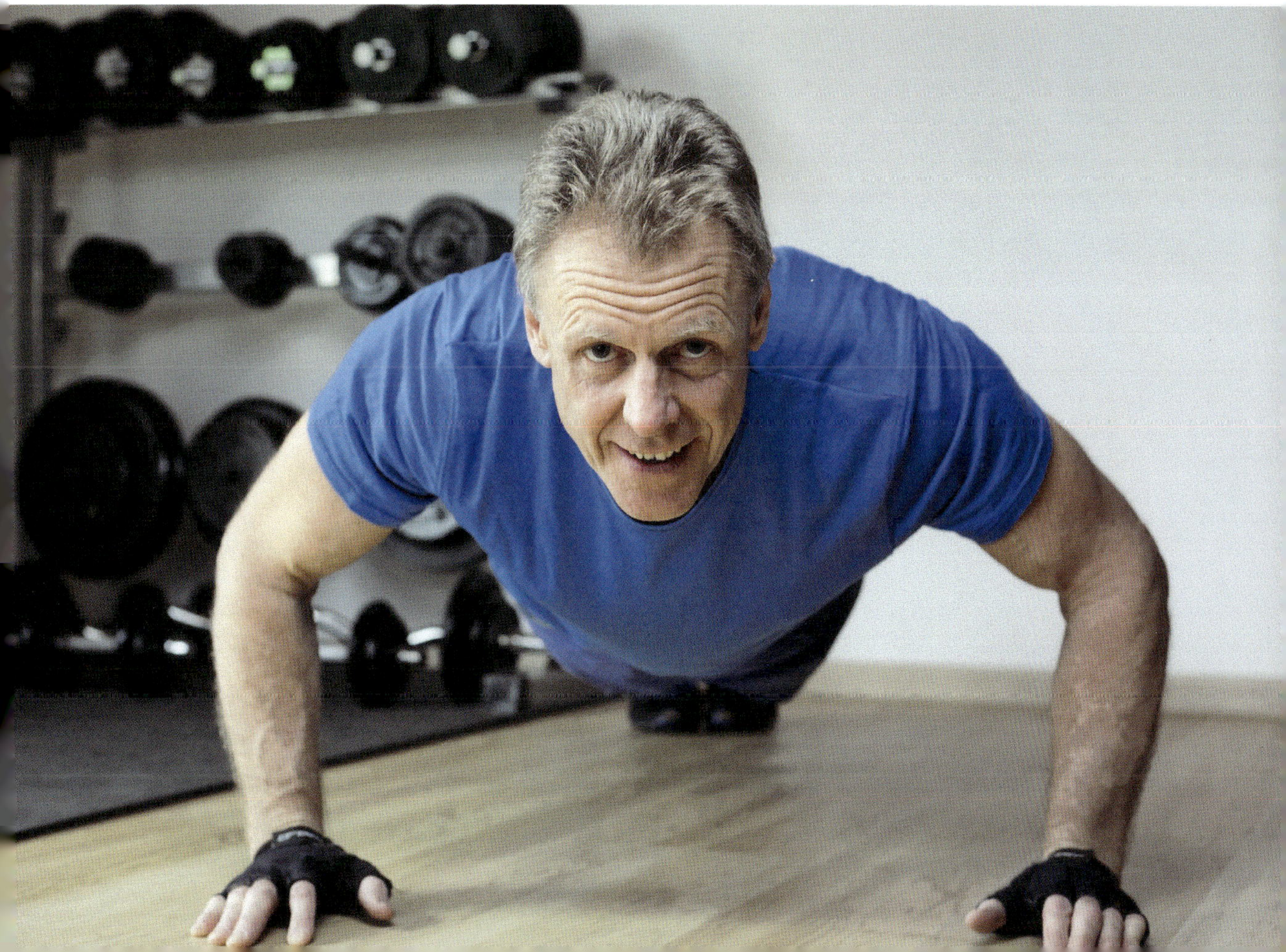

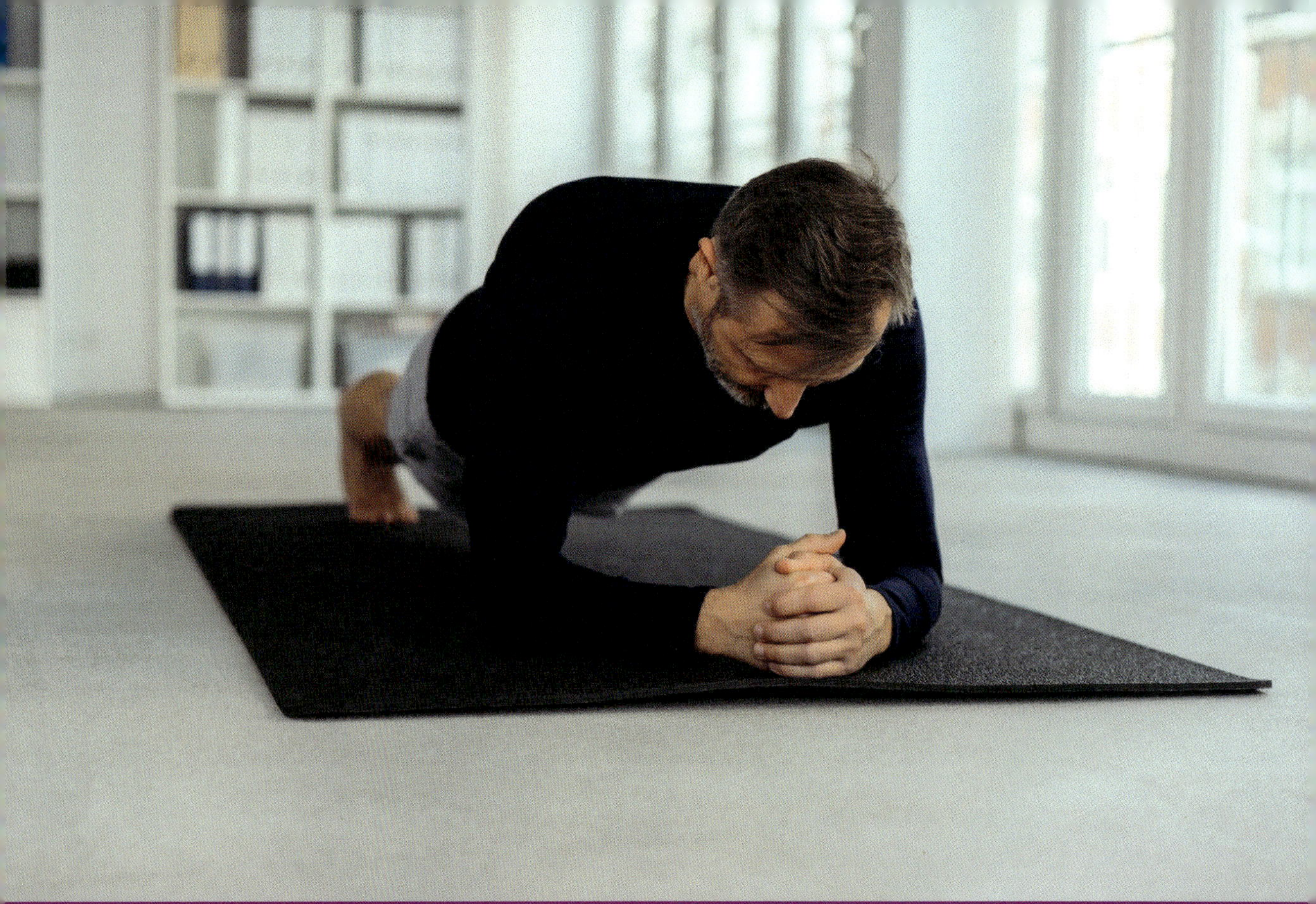

"Push yourself because no one else is going to."

CHAPTER 7

Step-By-Step Core Exercises

Many older adults suffer from lower back pain and core exercises can help stretch and strengthen these muscles, reducing pain, keeping you balanced and stable. Your core also helps support your spine which in turn aids balance and stability, reducing your risk of trips and falls.

Core Training Benefits

- Injury prevention
- Improved strength
- Makes daily tasks easier
- Managed and reduced pain
- Improved balance and stability
- Reduced injury risk from trips and falls

Lateral Side Bends

- **EQUIPMENT:** Chair, Tin or Dumbbell
- For this core exercise, start by holding a weight in your right hand
- Sit on the chair keeping your back straight and head held up, bend only at your waist
- Breathe in and bend down to your right side. Hold this position briefly and come back up to the starting position, keeping the rest of the body still, this is one rep
- Repeat the movement but bending towards your left side
- Breathe in while reaching down, breathe out while straightening up
- **TARGET:** 2 to 3 sets of 8 to 12 repetitions each side

Figure of Eights

- **EQUIPMENT:** Bottle of Water, Squash or Dumbbell
- For this core exercise, start seated on the chair with your feet about shoulder-width apart, bracing your stomach muscles, sitting up, holding the weight in both your hands, arms fully extended out
- With your arms fully extended draw big figures of eights, this is one complete rep
- Breathe normally
- **TARGET:** 2 to 3 sets of 8 to 12 repetitions

Leg Lifts

- **EQUIPMENT:** Mat
- For this core exercise, lie on your back with legs flat against the ground and feet relaxed
- Contract your abdominal muscles while raising one leg about 10 to 15 cm off the floor and hold for a few seconds
- Lower and repeat on your other leg
- Breathe in on the downward movement, breathe out while raising your leg back up
- **TARGET:** 2 to 3 sets of 8 to 12 repetitions

Seated Knee Lifts

- **EQUIPMENT:** Mat
- For this core exercise, begin seated on the floor
- Start by bringing both of your knees up towards your chest slowly under control, and continue by slowly extending your legs back out to the starting position, this is one complete rep
- Breathe in on the downward movement, breathe out while raising your leg back up
- **TARGET:** 2 to 3 sets of 8 to 12 repetitions

Air Bike

- **EQUIPMENT:** Mat
- For this core exercise, lie on your back with your hands behind your head
- Bend at your knees and lift both of your feet so that your calves are held parallel to the floor
- Next bring one knee towards your chest while reaching to it with the elbow from the opposite side, you should look as though you are pedalling a bike
- Breathe normally
- **TARGET:** 2 to 3 sets of 30-second bursts resting for one minute between sets

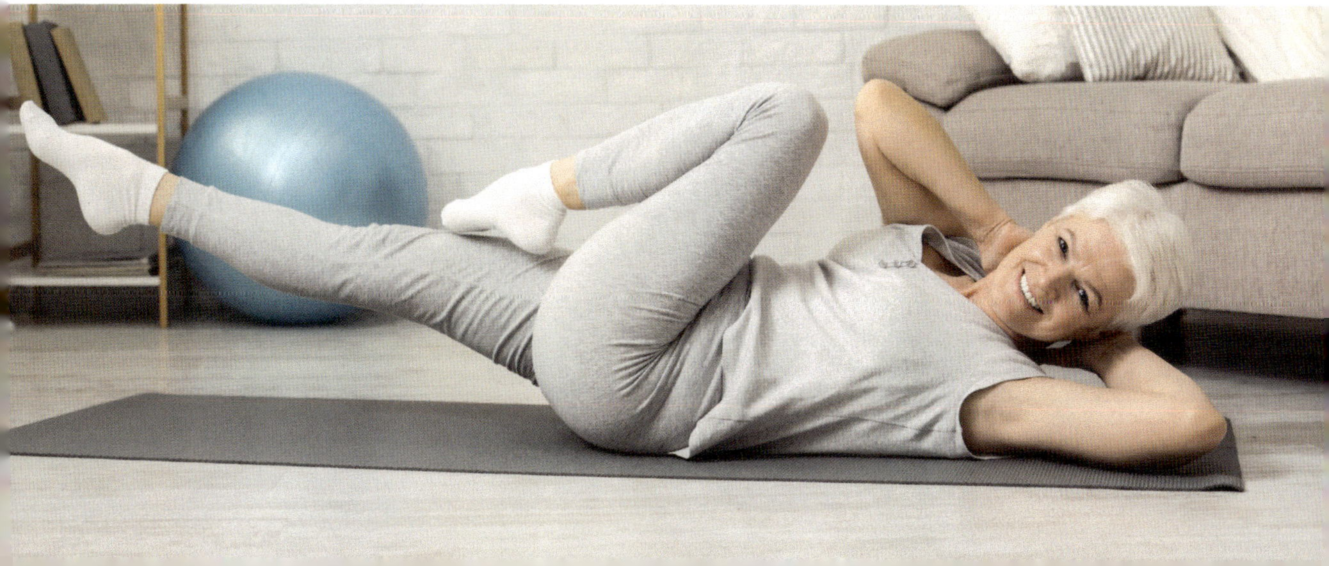

Seated Twists

- **EQUIPMENT:** Mat, note this exercise is for a more advanced person
- For this core exercise, start by sitting on a mat
- Bend your body to an angle of about 45-degrees from the floor, with your arms across your chest, leaning back, then move forward and slowly twist your body to the left then lean back slowly twisting back to the starting position
- Breathe normally
- **TARGET:** 2 to 3 sets of 12 to 15 repetitions

Semi-sits

- **EQUIPMENT:** Chair
- For this core exercise, start your Semi-sits exercise by standing in front of a chair, gently pulling in your stomach muscles
- Next slowly lower your bum, and bend your knees as though you are about to sit back down on a chair making only light contact with the chair seat and then return back up to the starting standing position, this is one complete rep
- Breathe in as you slowly sit down, breathe out as you slowly stand back up
- **TARGET:** 2 to 3 sets of 8 to 12 repetitions

Lumbar Rotation

- **EQUIPMENT:** Mat
- For this core exercise, start by lying on the floor with your legs bent and with both knees together on the floor over on your left side
- Next, extend both your arms out, but keep your shoulders firmly on the ground, pull your stomach muscles in
- Keeping your body still slowly roll your knees from the left, over to the right until they touch the floor or get close to touching the floor, hold this position just for a few seconds and then roll back, repeat
- Breathe normally,
- **TARGET:** 2 to 3 sets of 5 to 8 repetitions each side

Kneeling Rear Leg Raise

- **EQUIPMENT:** Mat
- For this core exercise, start by getting down on your hands and knees and engage your core muscles
- Next, extend your right leg back holding it slightly off the floor, toes pointing
- Lift your leg straight up as high as you can and then lower your leg back to the starting position, be careful not to arch your back
- Repeat this exercise with your other leg
- **TARGET:** 2 to 3 sets of 8 to 12 repetitions each leg

Wood Chops

- **EQUIPMENT:** N/A
- For this core exercise, start the Wood Chop exercise with your feet wider than shoulder-width apart clasping together both hands in front
- Next, pull your arms up to be level with one side of your head
- Squat down while doing a chopping movement with your arms diagonally downwards to the opposite side of your body
- Repeat by performing the chopping action back up towards the top, this is one rep
- Breath normally
- **TARGET:** 2 to 3 sets of 8 to 12 repetitions each side

Crunches

- **EQUIPMENT:** Mat
- For this core exercise, start by lying down with your back flat on the floor
- Place both of your feet on the floor about hip-width apart
- Next, bend both your knees, place both your hands behind your head, elbows pointing forwards while breathing in
- Breathe out and lift your torso slightly keeping your head and neck neutral
- To finish breathe out and return your body to the starting position
- **TARGET:** 2 to 3 sets of 12 to 15 repetitions

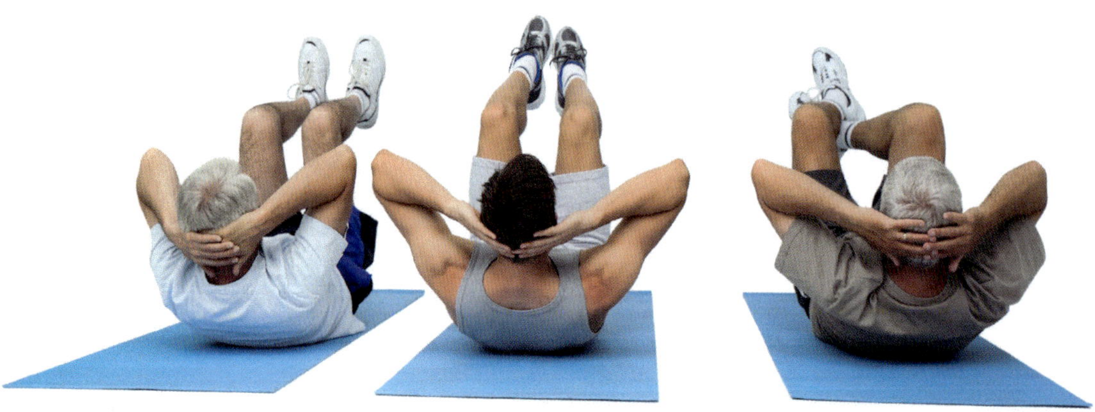

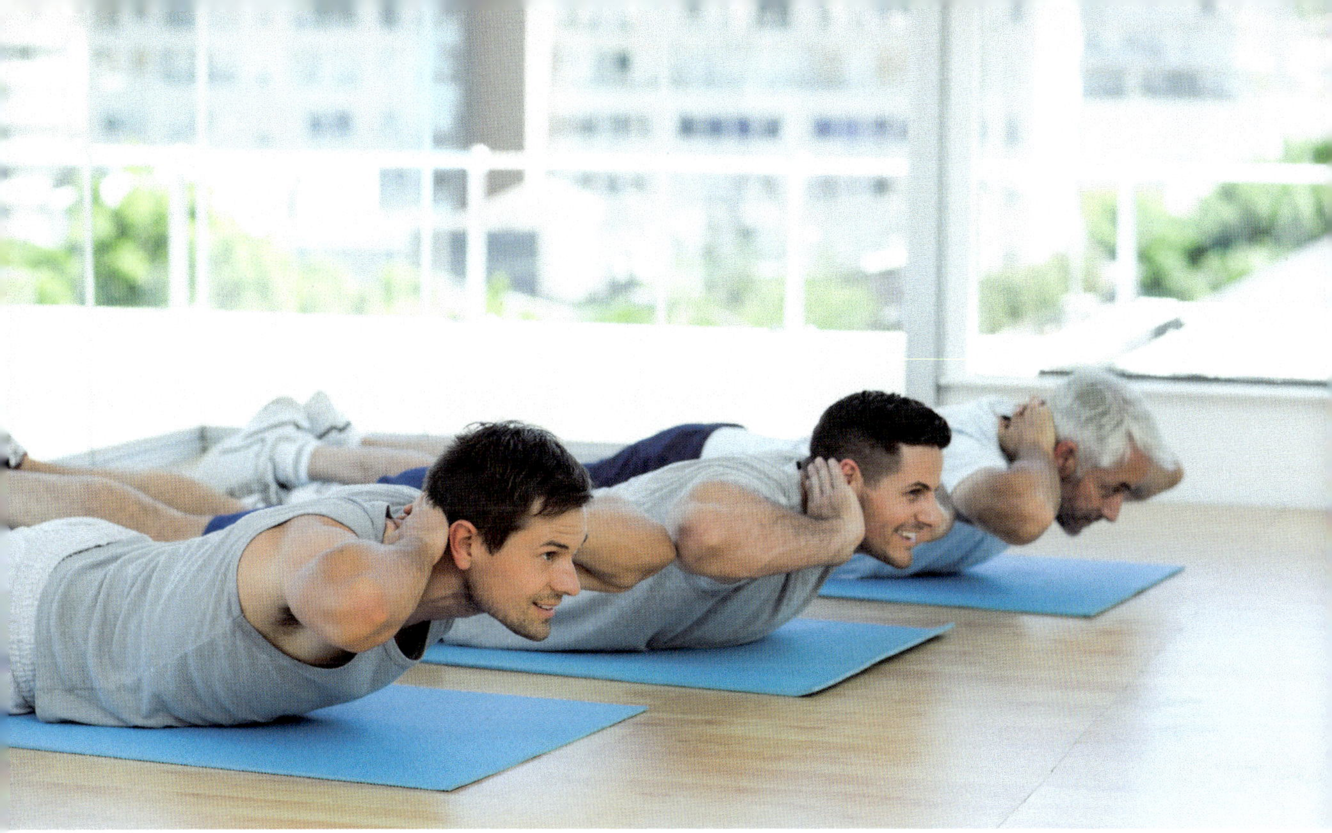

Superman

- **EQUIPMENT:** Mat
- For this core exercise, start the Superman exercise by lying on your stomach with your arms stretched out fully
- Next, raise your head, neck, and your right arm, as well as your left leg 5 cm off of the floor, lower and repeat on your other side
- During the exercise pull your stomach muscles in
- Breathe normally
- **TARGET:** 2 to 3 sets of 8 to 12 repetitions each side

ACTIVITY TIME GUIDELINES: Older adults should aim to be active daily. Over a week, your activity should add up to at least 150 minutes of moderate-intensity activity in bouts of 10 minutes or more. One way to achieve this would be to do 30 minutes on at least 5 days of the week. Ideally, you should aim to build up a routine of 8 to 12 exercises that strength train the major muscle groups 2 to 3 times a week on non-consecutive days to allow for recovery.

Core Training Tips

- Before starting core training speak with your doctor if you have any health conditions or concerns.
- You may get some muscular aches during exercise. Stop immediately if you feel any sharp pain in your joints and or back. You may get some muscular aches 24 to 48 hours after exercising; this is quite normal and will fade away.
- Keep the intensity of your exercise to a moderate pace, so that you can always hold a conversation.
- Always warm-up before you start with 5 to 10 minutes of light warm-up exercises, or more if you feel you need to.
- Always stretch out after you've finished your workout to reduce delayed onset muscle soreness.
- See Chapter 9 for a safe way of getting down to and back up from the floor to perform core exercises.

Question

Thinking about the last 7-days, how much core exercise of blocks of 10 minutes or more have you done?

NONE	30 mins or less	30 - 60 mins	60 - 90 mins	90 - 120 mins	120 - 160 mins	160 mins plus

Question

Thinking about the last 7-days, how many days of the week did you do core exercise of blocks of 10 minutes or more?

NONE	1	2	3	4	5	6 or 7

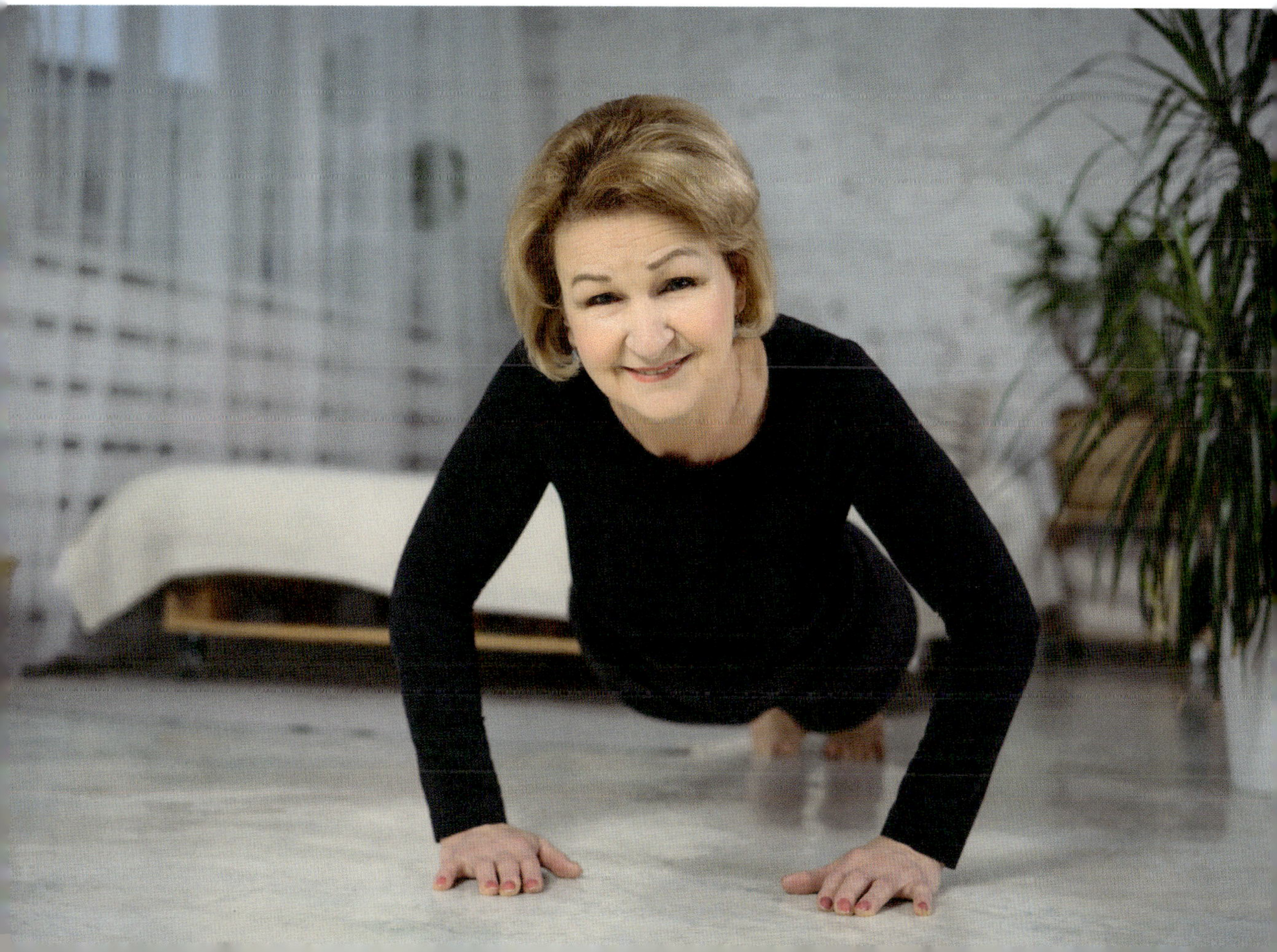

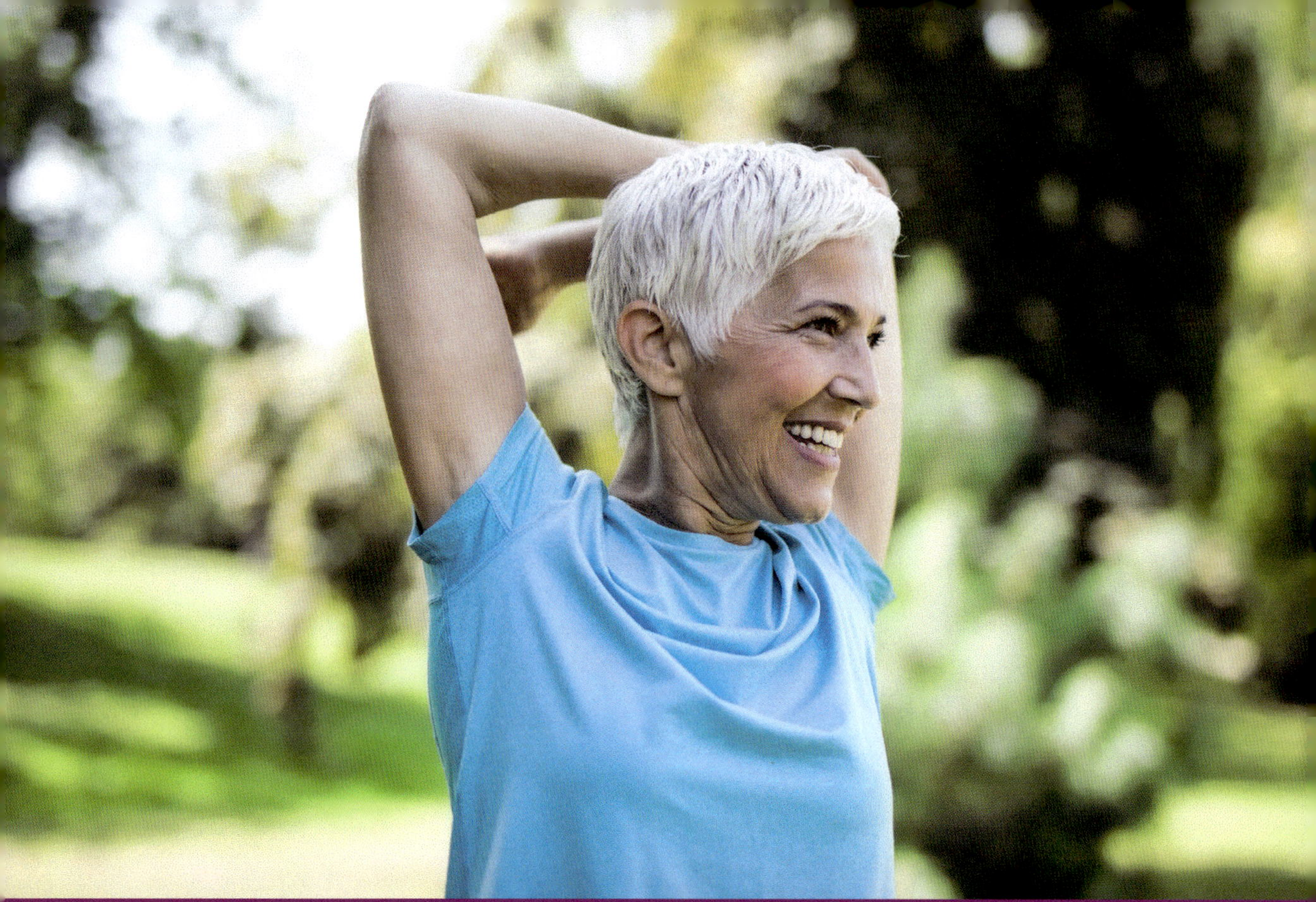

"A bad workout is the one that didn't happen."

CHAPTER 8

Step-By-Step Stretching Exercises

Stretching can help older adults stay flexible, mobile and most importantly of all, independent. Tight muscles, stiff joints and aches and pains; the ageing process can exact a heavy toll on the body. Regularly performing stretching exercises can help to reduce aches and pains while making daily tasks such as dressing or getting in and out of the bath easier to do.

Benefits of Stretching

- Reduced risk of injury
- Improved balance and coordination
- Helps to release muscle tension and soreness
- Helps increase circulation and muscle control
- Greater movement in joints and improves posture

Hamstring Seated Stretch

- **EQUIPMENT:** Chair
- For this stretching exercise, sit on the chair
- Straighten out one leg and place both hands on this bent leg
- Lean gently forwards
- Hold the position for about 10 to 15 seconds and ease further forwards, after about another 10 to 15 seconds ease forward once again
- Repeat with the other leg
- Breathe normally

Hamstring Bent Knee Seated Stretch

- **EQUIPMENT:** Chair
- For this stretching exercise, sit on the chair
- Straighten one leg out but keep it slightly bent, place both your hands on the bent leg and lean gently forwards
- Hold the position for about 10 to 15 seconds and ease further forwards, after about another 10 to 15 seconds ease forward once again
- Repeat with the other leg
- Breathe normally

Back & Shoulder Stretch

- **EQUIPMENT:** Chair
- For this stretching exercise, begin seated clasp both hands together in front with your arms extended out, next drop your head and shoulders forward and then push hands away from your body as far as you can
- Hold for about 10 to 15 seconds
- Breathe normally

Obliques Reaching Up Standing Stretch

- **EQUIPMENT:** N/A
- For this stretching exercise, stand with your feet about hip-distance apart keeping your spine neutral
- Place one hand just below your hip and reach with your other arm up right up above your head
- Next, lean over to one side
- Hold for about 10 to 15 seconds
- Repeat on your other side
- Breathe normally

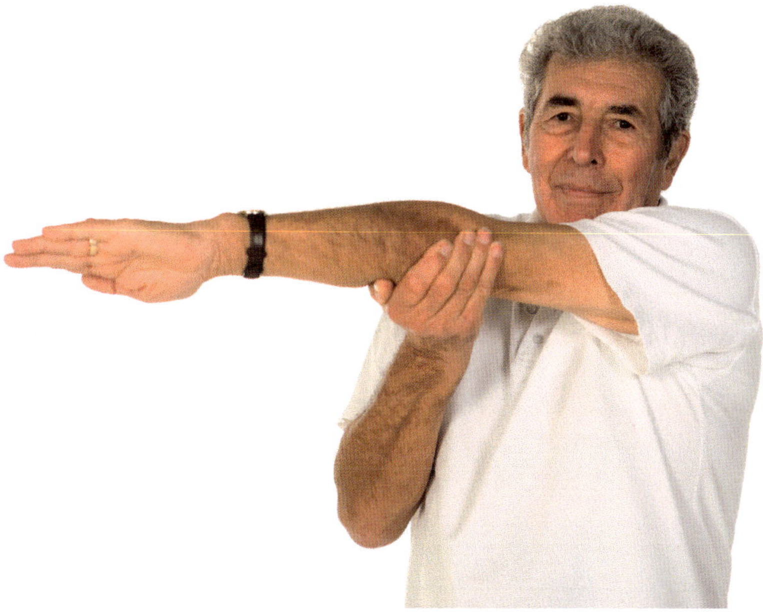

Arms Across Body Seated Stretch

- **EQUIPMENT:** Chair
- For this stretching exercise, sit on the chair, take one arm and fold it across the front of your body
- Place the palm of the other hand on the back of the upper arm and pull in and hold this position for about 10 to 15 seconds, release and then repeat on the other arm
- Breathe normally

Seated Chest Stretch

- **EQUIPMENT:** Chair
- For this stretching exercise, sit on the chair and place hands on small of your back
- Squeeze your shoulder blades so that they feel as though pinching together
- After about 10 to 15 seconds ease a little further into the stretch
- Breathe normally

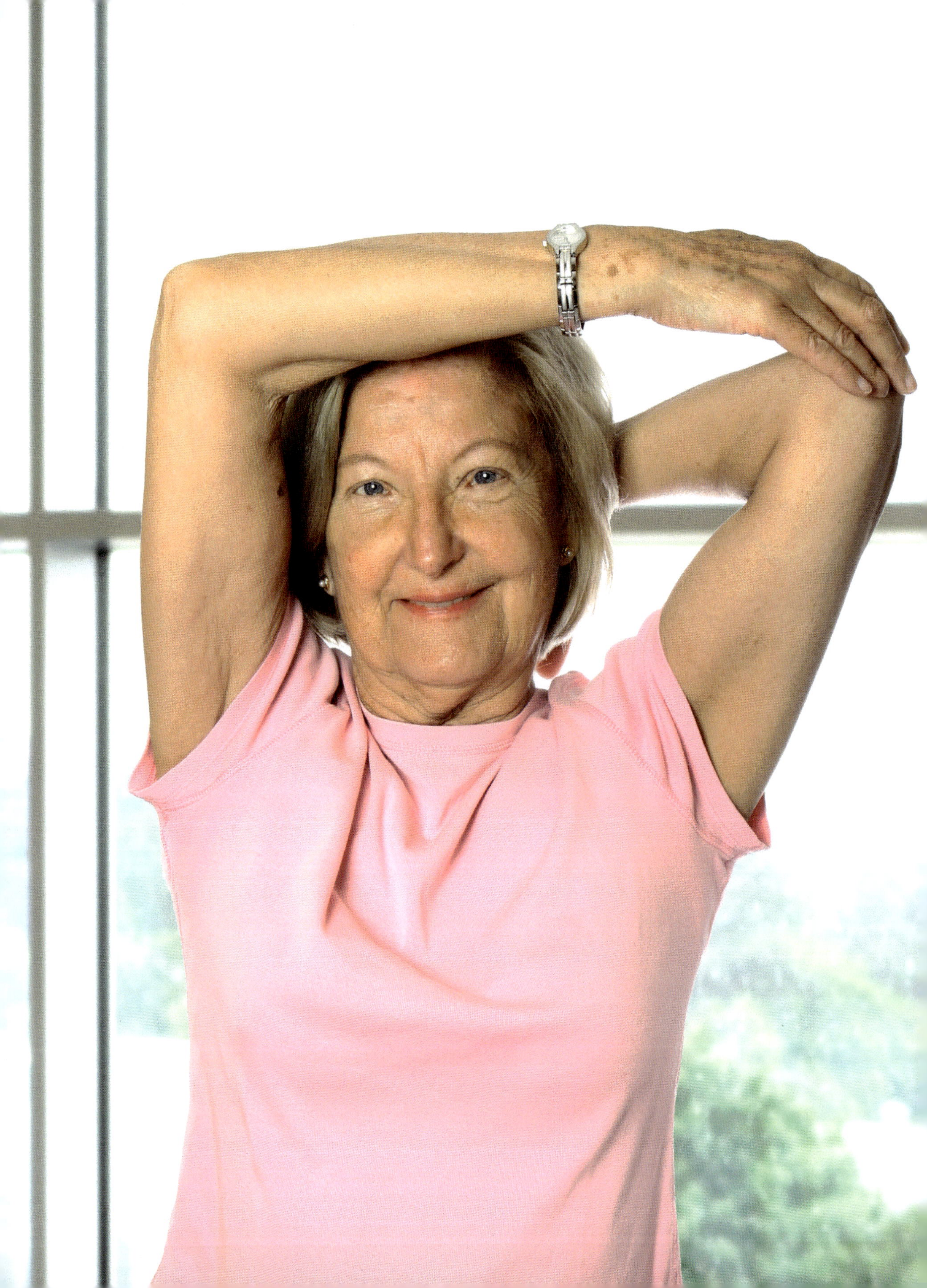

Triceps Stretch

- **EQUIPMENT:** Chair
- For this stretching exercise, sit on the chair and place one hand above the head and bend at the elbow, hand touching the back of your shoulder, with your other hand on the back of upper arm apply pressure
- Hold for about 10 to 15 seconds
- Breathe normally

Quads Leg Stretch

- **EQUIPMENT:** Chair (optional)
- For this stretching exercise, stand with feet hip-distance apart, neutral spine
- Hold on to chair or counter if needed, stand on one leg
- Raise one heel towards your bum and hold in your hand, or hold your trouser hem if easier
- After 10 to 15 seconds pull in a little further and hold for another 10 seconds
- Breathe normally

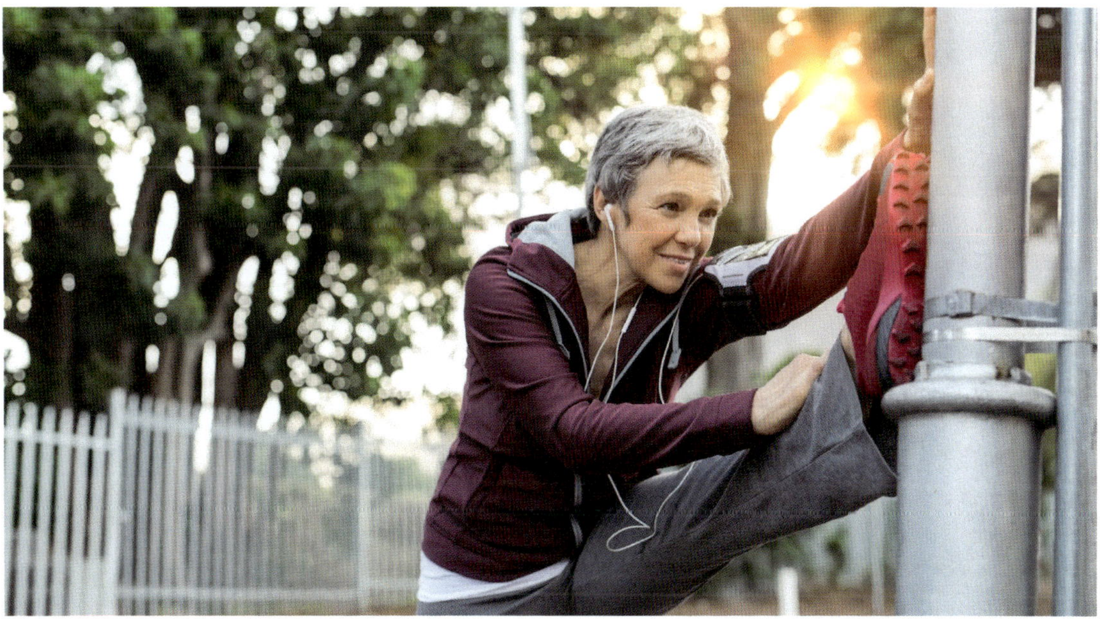

ACTIVITY TIME GUIDELINES: Older people should aim to do flexibility (stretching) exercises at least twice a week, there is no set time given but a sensible target would be at least 15 minutes each time, using sustained stretches for each major muscle group.

Stretching Training Tips

- Before starting stretching training speak with your doctor if you have any health conditions or concerns.
- Before stretching try 10 minutes of gentle exercise, for example, walking on the spot as stretching cold muscles may result in injury.
- Only stretch to the point of mild discomfort.
- Work opposing muscle groups each time you stretch. If you start by stretching the muscles in the back of your thigh, then follow by stretching the muscles at the front.
- Include stretching in your daily routine, for example, before you dress for the day.

Question

Thinking about the last 7-days, how much stretching exercise of blocks of 10 minutes or more have you done?

NONE	30 mins or less	30 - 60 mins	60 - 90 mins	90 - 120 mins	120 - 160 mins	160 mins plus

Question

Thinking about the last 7-days, how many days of the week did you do stretch exercise of blocks of 10 minutes or more?

NONE	1	2	3	4	5	6 or 7

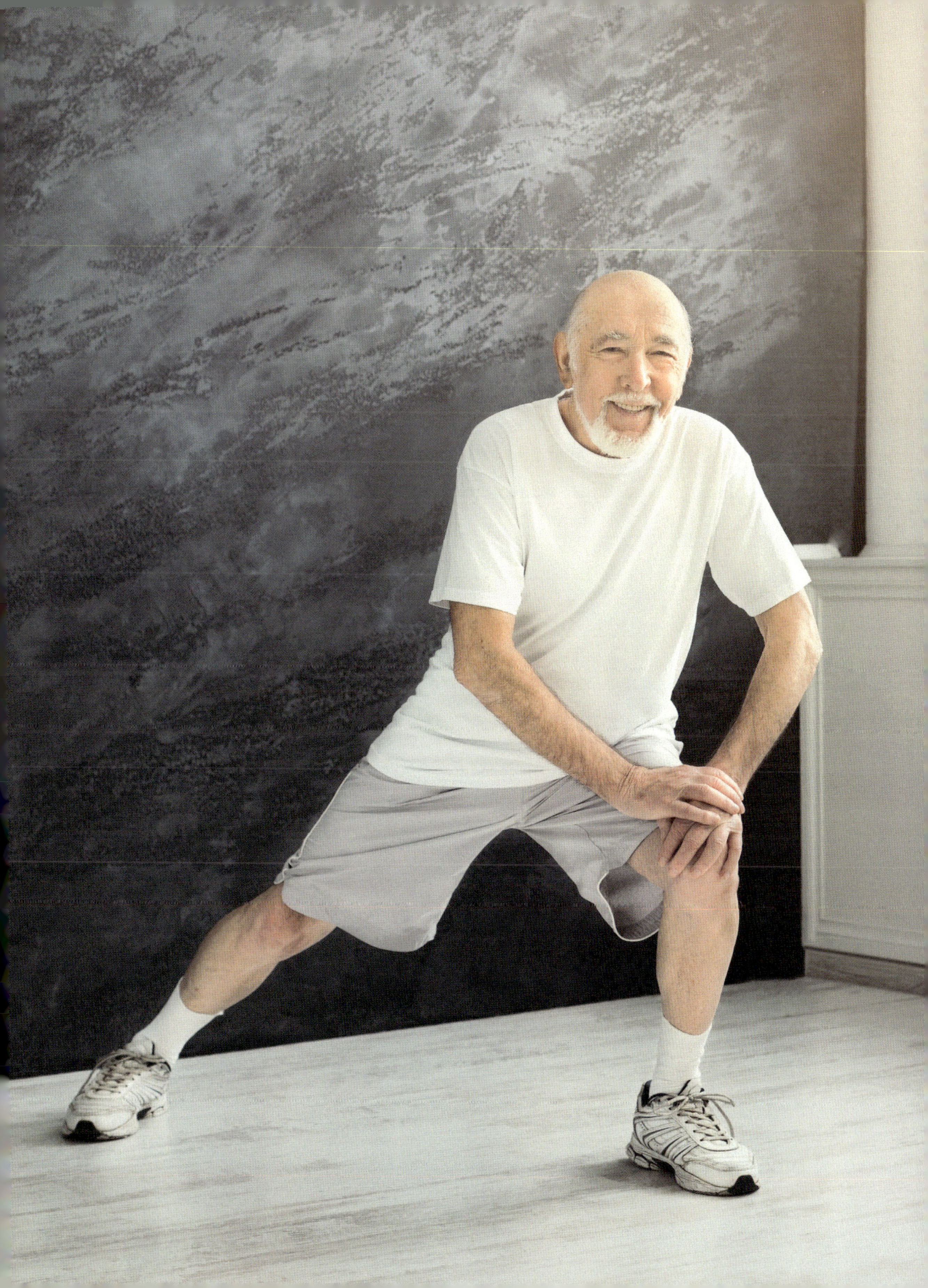

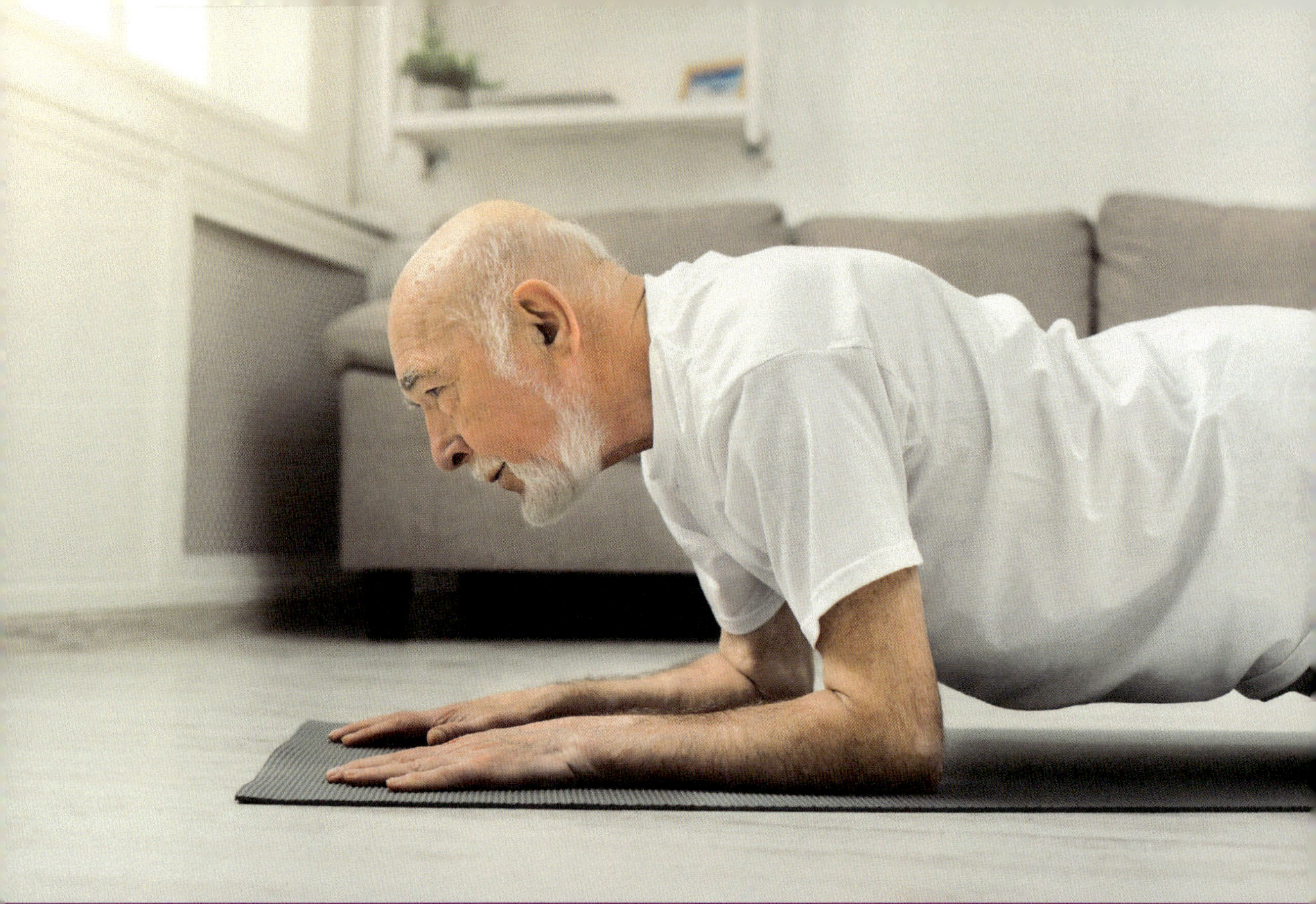

"Don't stop until you're healthy and happy."

CHAPTER 9

How To Get Down & Up Safely From The Floor To Exercise

If you have difficulty getting up from the floor you should not attempt this procedure without seeking advice. For the first few times have someone with you or keep your phone close at hand.

To do this you will need:

- A sturdy chair, ideally with arms, positioned to allow room to lie down.
- You may need some cushions or pillows on the floor until you feel confident performing this procedure as well as for comfort.
- A good quality exercise mat to safely perform your floor- based exercises.

Step-by-step guide

- Start by turning to face your chair, using the chair arms or seat for support if necessary.
- Next slowly lower yourself onto your knees, one leg at a time. This can be achieved more comfortably by using pillows on the floor across the front of the chair and taking them away one at a time, as you become more confident.
- To continue, slide both your hands off the chair and place them onto the floor, step backwards on all fours using your hands and feet one pace to be clear of the chair.
- Now with your hands in front of you, slowly lower your bottom sideways onto the floor, legs to one side.
- Slowly lower yourself completely onto your side.
- From here you can safely roll onto your back or front on your exercise mat in preparation to exercise.
- When getting back up after exercise you simply reverse the instructions above.

View an illustrated guide at 3fspt.co.uk/floorsafety

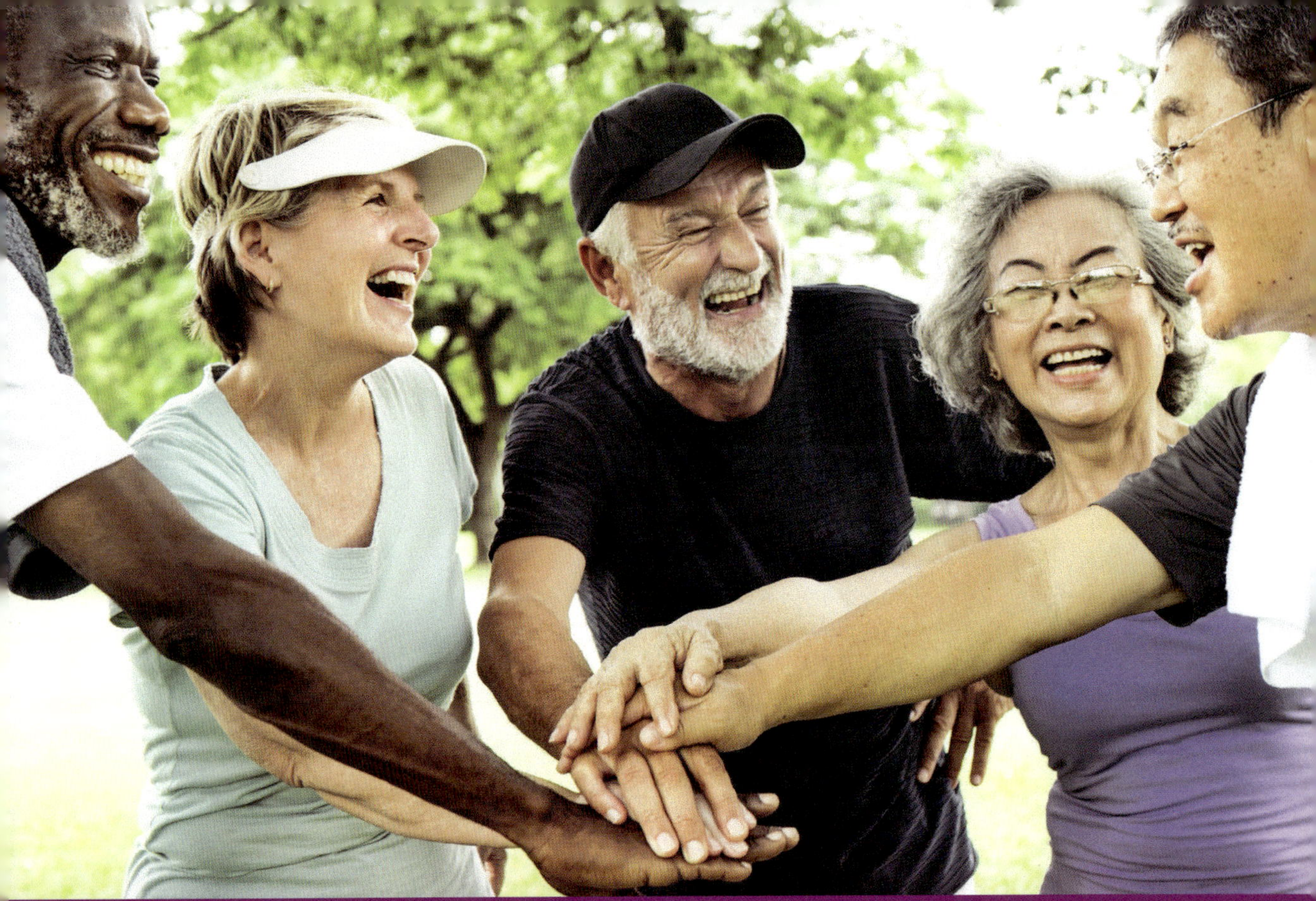

"If you feel like giving up,
just look back to see
how far you've come."

CHAPTER 10

Get Fitter In Just 12-Weeks Challenge

Want to improve your health and fitness and or need to lose some weight? This exercise plan is for you if you've not exercised for an extended period or indeed if you've never really exercised, combining walking and flexibility, balance and strength workouts to get you into the habit of regular exercise in just 12-weeks.

The plan is structured but flexible enough to allow you to fit the exercise sessions around other commitments.

Tips:

- Before starting each week, plot on your 12-week planner what days and times you'll be walking and what days you'll be doing your flexibility, balance and strength routine. This will help you stick to the plan. Don't forget to include 1 or 2 rest days per week on a day of your choosing.
- To get started you don't need any fancy equipment, be sensible though wear comfortable loose-fitting clothing and non-slip footwear. You can treat yourself to trainers if you think it will get you more in the mood for a fitter you.
- Basic exercise equipment for a home workout is a sturdy dining chair, kitchen counter, two tins of food of equal weight, a bottle of water or squash with a firmly fitted top. You can upgrade this equipment to lightweight dumbbells from 0.5kg to 2kg and or a resistance band, these come in various strengths (see chapter 13).
- Walking is a great way to start getting fitter, the weather in the UK can in the Autumn and Winter months pose a hindrance. If you're a fair-weather walker, then consider taking your walk in a nearby Shopping Centre, the often wide walkways with their nice roofs and ambient heating can be a way not to get defeated by the rain, sleet or snow.
- Join the **HOW 2 GET FIT 4 LATER LIFE FACEBOOK GROUP**. I've set this up for everyone who takes up the 12-week challenge to provide peer support, motivation and to share progress. To join the Facebook Group use this link: **www.tiny.cc/H2GF4LL**

Week 1

Day 1: Walk 10 minutes
Day 2: Rest day
Day 3: Walk 10 minutes
Day 4: Rest day
Day 5: Flexibility, Balance & Strength Exercise Routine 10 minutes
Day 6: Rest day
Day 7: Rest day

TOTAL ACTIVITY: 30 Minutes, Target 150 Minutes plus

REWARD: Well done, you're making progress so don't forget to do or have something nice.

Week 2

Day 1: Walk 10 minutes
Day 2: Rest day
Day 3: Walk 10 minutes
Day 4: Flexibility, Balance & Strength Exercise Routine 10 minutes
Day 5: Rest day
Day 6: Rest day
Day 7: Flexibility, Balance & Strength Exercise Routine 10 minutes

TOTAL ACTIVITY: 40 Minutes, Target 150 Minutes plus

REWARD: Well done, you're making progress so don't forget to do or have something nice.

Week 3

Day 1: Walk 10 minutes

Day 2: Rest day

Day 3: Walk 10 minutes

Day 4: Flexibility, Balance & Strength Exercise Routine 15 minutes

Day 5: Rest day

Day 6: Rest day

Day 7: Flexibility, Balance & Strength Exercise Routine 15 minutes

TOTAL ACTIVITY: 50 Minutes, Target 150 Minutes plus

REWARD: Well done, you're making progress so don't forget to do or have something nice.

Week 4

Day 1: Walk 15 minutes

Day 2: Rest day

Day 3: Walk 15 minutes

Day 4: Flexibility, Balance & Strength Exercise Routine 15 minutes

Day 5: Rest day

Day 6: Rest day

Day 7: Flexibility, Balance & Strength Exercise Routine 15 minutes

TOTAL ACTIVITY: 60 Minutes, Target 150 Minutes plus

REWARD: Well done, you're making progress so don't forget to do or have something nice.

Week 5

Day 1: Walk 15 minutes

Day 2: Rest day

Day 3: Walk 15 minutes

Day 4: Flexibility, Balance & Strength Exercise Routine 20 minutes

Day 5: Rest day

Day 6: Rest day

Day 7: Flexibility, Balance & Strength Exercise Routine 20 minutes

TOTAL ACTIVITY: 70 Minutes, Target 150 Minutes plus

REWARD: Well done, you're making progress so don't forget to do or have something nice.

Week 6

Day 1: Walk 15 minutes

Day 2: Rest day

Day 3: Walk 15 minutes

Day 4: Flexibility, Balance & Strength Exercise Routine 20 minutes

Day 5: Rest day

Day 6: Walk 15 minutes

Day 7: Flexibility, Balance & Strength Exercise Routine 20 minutes

TOTAL ACTIVITY: 85 Minutes, Target 150 Minutes plus

REWARD: Well done, you're making progress so don't forget to do or have something nice.

Week 7

Day 1: Walk 15 minutes

Day 2: Rest day

Day 3: Walk 15 minutes

Day 4: Flexibility, Balance & Strength Exercise Routine 25 minutes

Day 5: Rest day

Day 6: Walk 15 minutes

Day 7: Flexibility, Balance & Strength Exercise Routine 25 minutes

TOTAL ACTIVITY: 95 Minutes, Target 150 Minutes plus

REWARD: Well done, you're making progress so don't forget to do or have something nice.

Week 8

Day 1: Walk 15 minutes

Day 2: Rest day

Day 3: Walk 15 minutes

Day 4: Flexibility, Balance & Strength Exercise Routine 30 minutes

Day 5: Rest day

Day 6: Walk 15 minutes

Day 7: Flexibility, Balance & Strength Exercise Routine 30 minutes

TOTAL ACTIVITY: 105 Minutes, Target 150 Minutes plus

REWARD: Well done, you're making progress so don't forget to do or have something nice.

Week 9

Day 1: Walk 20 minutes
Day 2: Rest day
Day 3: Walk 20 minutes
Day 4: Flexibility, Balance & Strength Exercise Routine 30 minutes
Day 5: Rest day
Day 6: Walk 20 minutes
Day 7: Flexibility, Balance & Strength Exercise Routine 30 minutes

TOTAL ACTIVITY: 120 Minutes, Target 150 Minutes plus

REWARD: Well done, you're making progress so don't forget to do or have something nice.

Week 10

Day 1: Walk 20 minutes
Day 2: Rest day
Day 3: Walk 20 minutes
Day 4: Flexibility, Balance & Strength Exercise Routine 35 minutes
Day 5: Rest day
Day 6: Walk 20 minutes
Day 7: Flexibility, Balance & Strength Exercise Routine 35 minutes

TOTAL ACTIVITY: 130 Minutes, Target 150 Minutes plus

REWARD: Well done, you're making progress so don't forget to do or have something nice.

Week 11

Day 1: Walk 20 minutes
Day 2: Rest day
Day 3: Walk 20 minutes
Day 4: Flexibility, Balance & Strength Exercise Routine 40 minutes
Day 5: Rest day
Day 6: Walk 20 minutes
Day 7: Flexibility, Balance & Strength Exercise Routine 40 minutes

TOTAL ACTIVITY: 140 Minutes, Target 150 Minutes plus

REWARD: Well done, you're making progress so don't forget to do or have something nice.

Week 12

Day 1: Walk 20 minutes
Day 2: Rest day
Day 3: Walk 20 minutes
Day 4: Flexibility, Balance & Strength Exercise Routine 45 minutes
Day 5: Rest day
Day 6: Walk 20 minutes
Day 7: Flexibility, Balance & Strength Exercise Routine 45 minutes

TOTAL ACTIVITY: 150 Minutes, Target 150 Minutes plus

REWARD: Success! You're now doing the recommended weekly exercise, don't forget to do or have something nice. KEEP THIS UP!

Flexibility, Balance & Strength Workout Weeks 1 to 3

TIME: 10 to 15 MINUTES

WARM-UP
Neck, Shoulders, Back, Wrists, Hips, Knees & Ankles
Pulse Raiser Knees into Elbows

ARMS
Bicep Curls Seated - 6 to 8 reps

SHOULDERS
Upright Rows Seated - 6 to 8 reps
Lateral Raises Seated - 6 to 8 reps

LEGS
Sit Down Stand Ups - 6 to 8 reps
Leg Extensions - 6 to 8 reps

BALANCE
Single Limb Stance - Aim for a minimum 20 seconds
Side Leg Raises - 6 to 8 reps each leg

END STRETCH
Hamstring Seated
Lower Back Seated
Arms Across Seated
Obliques Reach in Air Stand
Chest Stretch Seated
Shoulders Arms Out
Triceps Seated or Standing
Quads Hold on Chair

Flexibility, Balance & Strength Workout Weeks 4 to 6

TIME: 15 to 20 MINUTES

WARM-UP
Neck, Shoulders, Back, Wrists, Hips, Knees & Ankles
Pulse Raiser Knees into Elbows

ARMS
Bicep Curls Seated - 8 to 10 reps

SHOULDERS
Upright Rows Seated - 8 to 10 reps
Lateral Raises Seated - 8 to 10 reps

LEGS
Sit Down Stand Ups - 8 to 10 reps
Leg Extensions - 8 to 10 reps

NEW: WEIGHTS/ DUMBBELLS
Goblet Squats - 6 to 8 reps
Triceps Extensions - 6 to 8 reps
Figure of Eights - 6 to 8 reps
Lateral Side Bends - 6 to 8 reps

BALANCE
Single Limb Stance - Aim for a minimum 30 seconds
Side Leg Raises - 8 to 10 reps each leg

END STRETCH
Hamstring Seated
Lower Back Seated
Arms Across Seated
Obliques Reach in Air Stand
Chest Stretch Seated
Shoulders Arms Out
Triceps Seated or Standing
Quads Hold on Chair

Flexibility, Balance & Strength Workout Weeks 7 to 9

TIME: 25 to 30 MINUTES

WARM-UP
Neck, Shoulders, Back, Wrists, Hips, Knees & Ankles
Pulse Raiser Knees into Elbows

ARMS
Bicep Curls Seated - 8 to 10 reps

SHOULDERS
Upright Rows Seated - 8 to 10 reps
Lateral Raises Seated - 8 to 10 reps
NEW: Shoulder Press - 8 to 10 reps

LEGS
Sit Down Stand Ups - 8 to 10 reps
Leg Extensions - 8 to 10 reps

WEIGHTS/ DUMBBELLS
Goblet Squats - 8 to 10 reps
Triceps Extensions - 8 to 10 reps
Figure of Eights - 8 to 10 reps
Lateral Side Bends - 8 to 10 reps
NEW: Calf Raises - 10 to 15 reps

BALANCE
Single Limb Stance - Aim for a minimum 40 seconds
Side Leg Raises - 8 to 10 reps each leg
NEW: Walking Heel To Toe - 20 steps each way
NEW: Tiptoe Lifts - 20 reps

END STRETCH
Hamstring Seated
Lower Back Seated
Arms Across Seated
Obliques Reach in Air Stand
Chest Stretch Seated
Shoulders Arms Out
Triceps Seated or Standing
Quads Hold on Chair

Flexibility, Balance & Strength Workout Weeks 10 to 12

TIME: 35 to 45 MINUTES

WARM-UP
Neck, Shoulders, Back, Wrists, Hips, Knees & Ankles
Pulse Raiser Knees into Elbows

ARMS
Bicep Curls Seated - 2 sets of 10 to 12 reps

SHOULDERS
Upright Rows Seated - 2 sets of 10 to 12 reps
Lateral Raises Seated - 2 sets of 10 to 12 reps
Shoulder Press - 2 sets of 10 to 12 reps

LEGS
Sit Down Stand Ups - 2 sets of 10 to 12 reps
Leg Extensions - 2 sets of 10 to 12 reps

WEIGHTS/ DUMBBELLS
Goblet Squats - 2 sets of 10 to 12 reps
Triceps Extensions - 2 sets of 10 to 12 reps
Figure of Eights - 2 sets of 10 to 12 reps
Lateral Side Bends - 2 sets of 10 to 12 reps
Calf Raises - 2 sets of 15 to 20 reps

BALANCE
Single Limb Stance - Aim for a minimum 60 seconds
Side Leg Raises - 10 to 12 reps each leg
Walking Heel To Toe - 20 steps each way x 2 sets
Tiptoe Lifts - 20 reps x 2 sets

END STRETCH
Hamstring Seated
Lower Back Seated
Arms Across Seated
Obliques Reach in Air Stand
Chest Stretch Seated
Shoulders Arms Out
Triceps Seated or Standing
Quads Hold on Chair

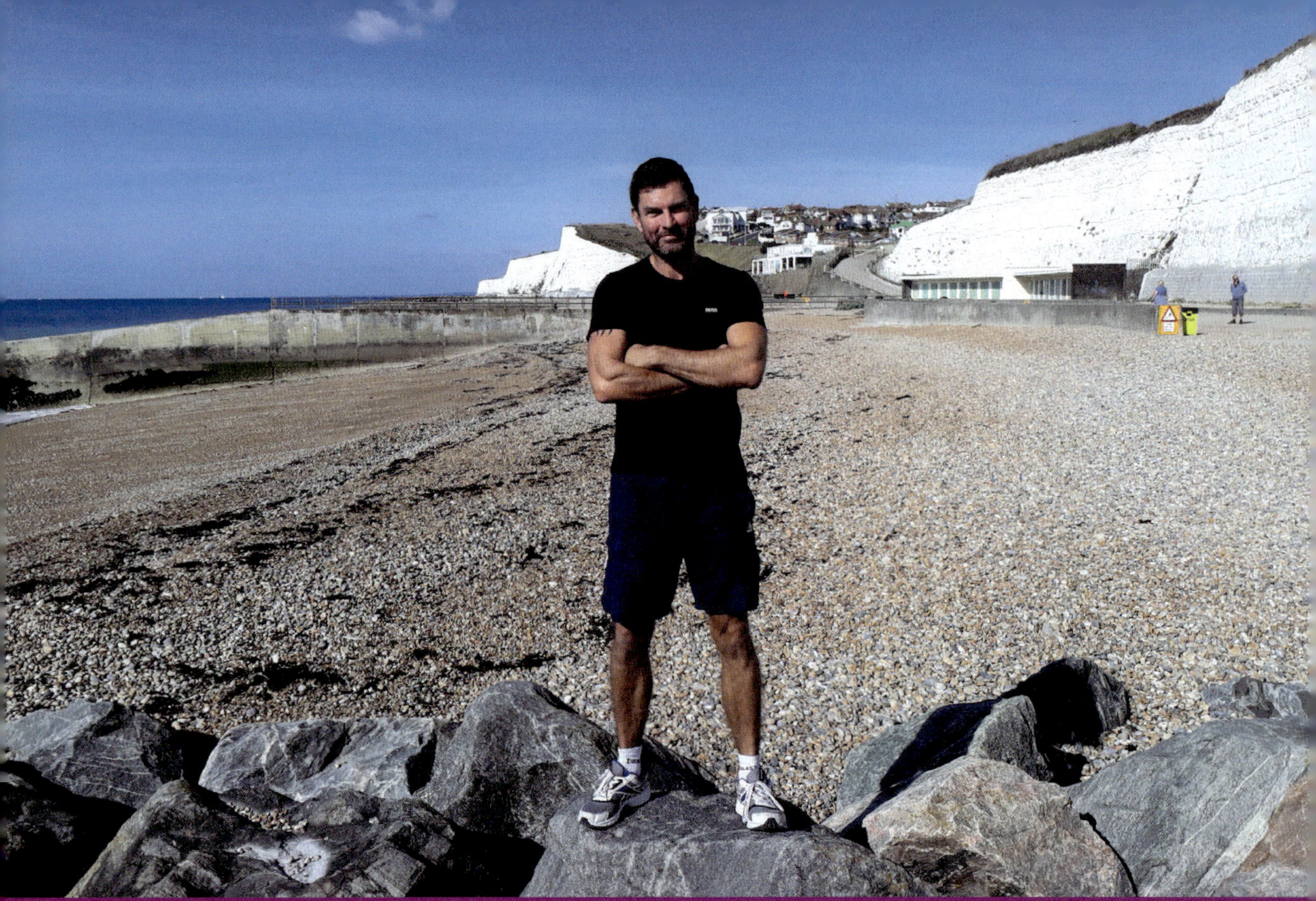

"It's personal,
your health and fitness goal,
is my goal!"

CHAPTER 11

How A Personal Trainer Can Help

As you've purchased this book, you are clearly thinking about making some major changes to your diet and or (re)starting regular exercise. Depending on your level of motivation, you have options on how you approach this.

Option 1: Self-help, and there's a wealth of information in this book for you to start straight away.

Option 2: Consider using a personal trainer like me either to help you kick start your programme of change or to work for a longer period. So if your motivation isn't what you'd like it to be then here are the reasons why a personal trainer like me can help you. You can find a personal trainer by downloading the MY COACH App, you'll find my details on here too.

Education, education, education!

There are two parts to this as your potential new personal trainer:

a. Personal trainers like me have been trained to train you on how to correctly perform a wide range of exercises covering body weight, free weights, cardiovascular as well as resistance machines, the bottom line here is to reduce the risk of injury and increase the effectiveness of your bespoke personal training programme. I tend to work with older adults so keeping you free from injury whilst-progressing you towards your unique health and fitness goal is of paramount importance to me.

b. If you don't know which are the right exercises for your unique health and fitness goal then you are highly unlikely to achieve it. When we meet for the first time, probably via WhatsApp for your health and fitness consultation, I'll drill down to what exactly it is you want to achieve, then based on my fact find I'll develop an exercise programme that aims to achieve your goal within the shortest but most importantly sustainable timeframe. I've helped scores of clients over the years achieve their health and fitness goals.

I will help you execute perfect form

Having me as your personal trainer to show you the correct technique is one of the key benefits. I will ensure that you perform each exercise in your bespoke exercise programme correctly with the right posture to maximise results. If your form is not correct when exercising you will be at increased risk of injury as well as not achieving your health and fitness goal. Nothing kills off a kick-ass exercise plan for change quite like three months of prescribed bed rest from your doctor after trapping a nerve in your lower back.

It's all about you

It may seem obvious but we are all different, and this means your abilities and health and fitness requirements are different than to everyone else. This could be because you've got an old knee injury, or perhaps a health condition such as arthritis or osteoporosis. Perhaps it's that you just hate gyms as you find their environments unfriendly and intimidating. Having a personal trainer with the experience to understand your unique requirements will ensure that you get a bespoke exercise programme that takes account of all your needs and will ultimately deliver your health and fitness goal.

I will help you set realistic health and fitness goals

It's only natural for you to want to achieve your health and fitness goals right away, whether that's dramatic weight loss, six-pack abs, J-Lo butt or Mr Universe strength. However, these are not always achievable, and if you don't hit them quickly then chances are you may feel discouraged, downhearted and then simply give up as yet another attempt to change to a healthier and fitter you, bites the dust.

As your friendly and motivational personal trainer, I will not only help you set realistic SMART goals that you will be able to achieve (on the proviso that you put in the blood, tears and sweat of course) but importantly, I will also keep you on track to hit your health and fitness goal. For example, if your goal is to achieve a size 12 for the summer, it's not just about doing three hours of High-Intensity Interval Training each week for five months. It's also about changing your diet to eat the correct foods with the correct portions based on widely-accepted dietary practices, mixing cardio and weights to work the correct muscles, and setting a realistic timeframe in which your goal can be achieved.

I will help you with specific health and fitness goals

As well as helping 3Fs Personal Training clients set realistic health and fitness goals, I'm the perfect man for the job to help you achieve a specific health and fitness goal. This is ideal for those of you who are training for a specific event such as a 5k run or need to achieve a certain weight before you're able to do something you really want, such as getting fit for an activity and adventure holiday of a lifetime. Hiring me as your personal trainer will put you on the right track and could make the difference whereby you complete your first 5k run in a time that you thought unachievable or paddle furiously through white-water rapids high up in the Rocky Mountains.

I will keep you accountable

Does this sound familiar? You've gone to bed determined that next morning you'll get up an hour early, fix a light healthy breakfast before heading off to the gym you joined ages ago, aiming to work out solidly for an hour before smugly heading off to meet some friends for morning coffee, buzzing from your power workout. At 7am your alarm goes off and you hear the rain beating on the bedroom window. You mutter under your breath several words about the weather before rolling over to hit the snooze button, preferring to stay warm in bed than to hit the gym on a wet grotty morning.

This is where having me as your personal trainer is crucial in ensuring that you commit to your health and fitness goal. If you've made an appointment to meet me for a personal training session in the convenience of your own home, or online given you've paid for this in advance, then you are highly likely to still go ahead than if you are just kidding yourself you that will go to the gym after meeting your friends for coffee, having hit the snooze button first thing in the morning.

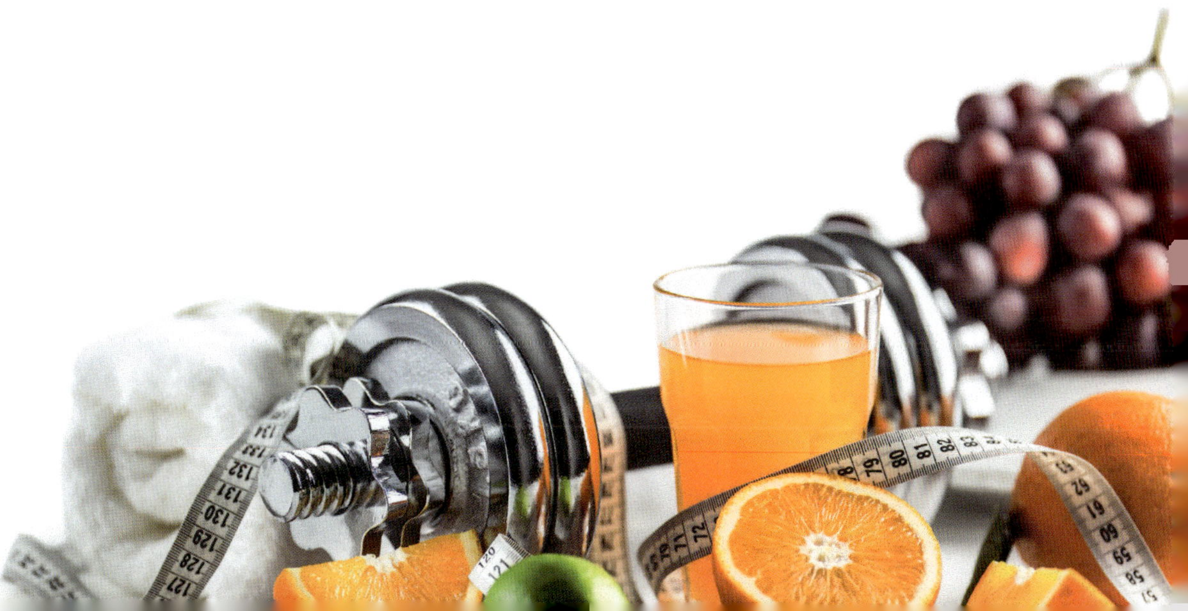

Easily fits around even the most hectic schedule

I offer a mobile as well as a remote video personal training service. I can train you in your home, the office or outdoors in one of the many parks and gardens, even down by the beach is you live in or near Brighton and Hove or via WhatsApp, Skype or Zoom for a remote video workout. I'm available 6-days of the week; Monday to Friday from 6am to 9pm, and Saturday from 9am to 2pm. So no matter how hectic your schedule, I'm sure I can find you a time that suits you.

I will develop a personalised training programme

There are always going to be some exercises that you love to do, some that you're indifferent to and others you simply hate with a passion. For example, just because you can physically do three sets of 12 reps of Goblet Squats using a 10kg kettlebell doesn't mean that you actually want to, but you perhaps love the idea of doing three sets of Burpees instead using a 10kg powerbag. With me as your expert personal trainer, I will tailor your personal training programme to focus on exercises that you enjoy, as well as encouraging you to do the exercises that are best suited to achieving your health and fitness goal.

In addition to this, there is always going to be the odd day when the very last thing you feel like doing is a High-Intensity Interval Training workout, and so having me as your personal trainer means that I can tailor your exercise for that 'off-day' to accommodate your mood while still trying to make the session helpful in terms of achieving your health and fitness goal. I can motivate you to find the energy that you didn't think was there!

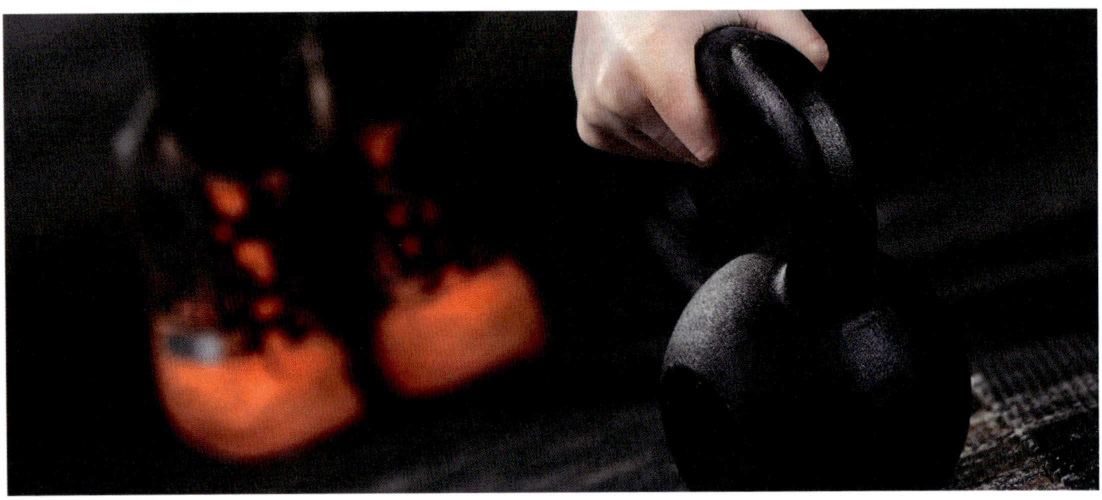

Keeps you and your body constantly challenged

Does this sound familiar? Last year you joined a gym the lovely helpful gym instructor did your induction and gave you great exercise programme. You've been going to the gym three times a week, and religiously have stuck to the routine. In the first few months, you noticed some changes and felt a bit fitter. However, in the last few months, you've felt like you're treading water and are beginning to feel disheartened by the lack of progress. The bad news is you've hit a plateau!

The good news is that hiring me as your personal trainer will make a huge difference, simply by the fact that I will never give you the same workout twice. I strongly believe in mixing it up, keeping your body constantly challenged, and keeping you constantly interested through varying your programme. Above that I'll become your life coach, can advise on nutrition, help you with motivation which when combined will get you to the health and fitness goal that has so far eluded you.

Exercise can help you with mental health

It has long been accepted that moderate-intensity physical exercise can help you with mental health issues such as anxiety and depression. And moderate-intensity physical exercise is recommended as part of treatment by many health professionals. Your doctor may have already mentioned this to you. Having me as your personal trainer could help you with a bespoke exercise programme if you suffer from mental health problems.

I can also help you with motivation as if you've ever suffered from depression, just getting out of bed can be hard, let alone finding the energy and the getup and go to work out for an hour. I will choose the right exercises to release the most endorphins those feel-good chemicals not to mention to offer you a shoulder to lean on. I'm a good listener as well as an excellent personal trainer. Through thick and thin, I'll get you moving forward. You'll find contact details at the end of this book should you be interested in hiring me as your personal trainer.

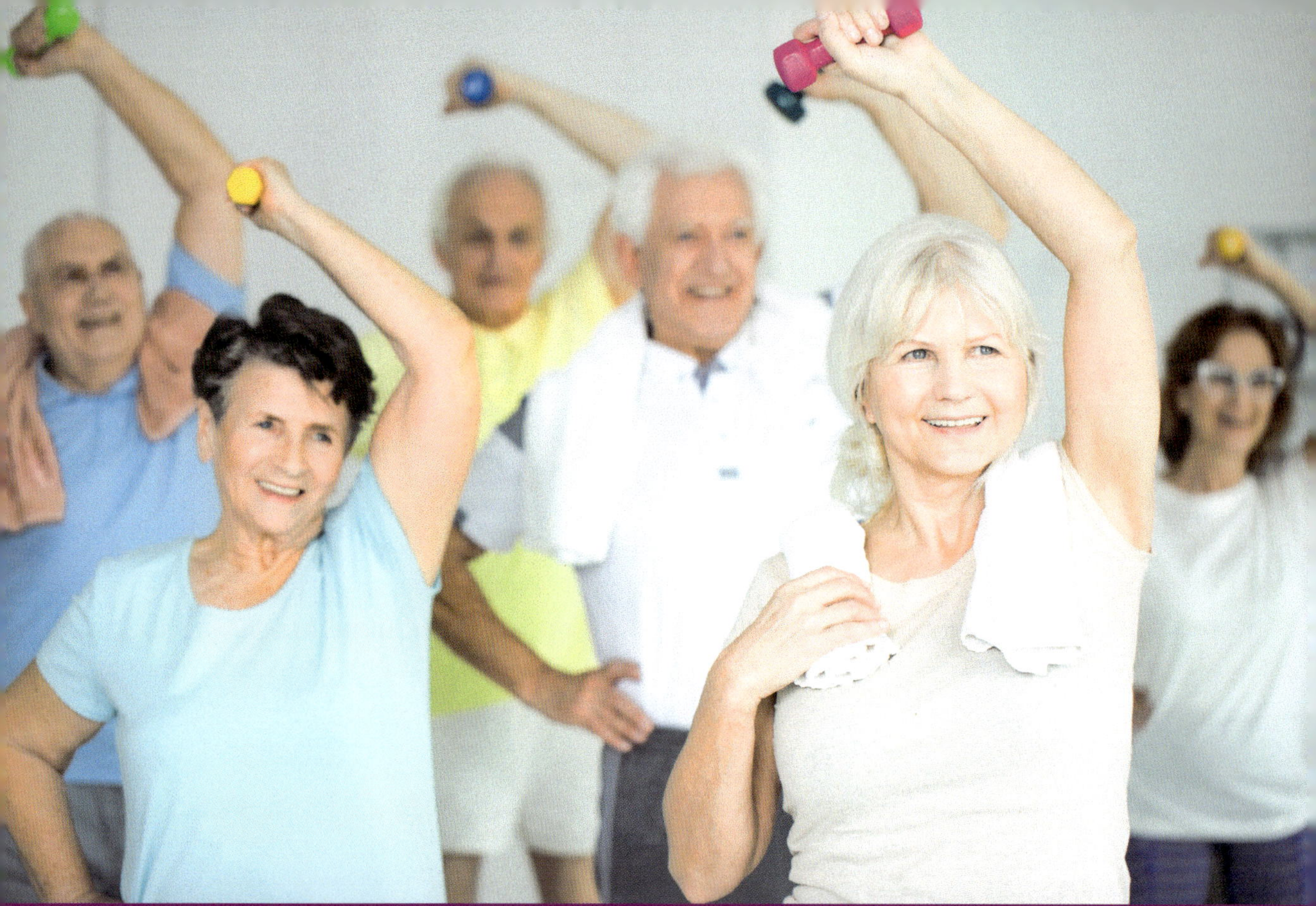

"You are the only one who can limit what you achieve."

CHAPTER 12

How Age-Related Changes Influence Exercise

As a specialist older adult personal trainer, I understand the need to tailor personal training programmes not only to achieve my client's fitness goals but to work them out safely when presented with one or more age-related health conditions.

During the initial health and fitness consultation, I use the Physical Activity Readiness Questionnaire (PAR-Q) to find out about any health conditions and or diseases that will influence how I plan and deliver my client's bespoke exercise programme. Here is an overview of considerations that I take into account for age-related changes and conditions on bones, joints and muscles:

Age-related changes in bones

The main age-related change in bones is the loss of calcium. Calcium loss is unequal between the sexes; loss is more severe in women especially post-menopause than in men. For example, a woman aged 70 her skeleton is likely to have lost approximately 30% or more of its calcium, whereas a man does not tend to lose calcium from his skeleton until after the age of 60.

This equates to an approximate loss of 1% per year for a woman and 0.5% for a man. For a post-menopause woman bone mass losses of 3-5% per year can be expected. The skeleton may also suffer from increased risk of spinal curvatures, brittle bone and fractures.

Osteoporosis is a common age-related bone disease affecting a large percentage of the population and is caused by the decline in osteoblasts activity after the age of 35. Gender is also a significant contributor to age-related osteoporosis being a female greatly increases the risk of this disease. An estimated 3 million people in the UK suffer from osteoporosis. Given that many older adults will suffer from some level of osteoporosis it's important that information on this is gathered using the PAR-Q. In-addition and with the permission of the client, all relevant information will be sought from the client's doctor before engaging in a planned exercise programme to minimise the risk of fractures.

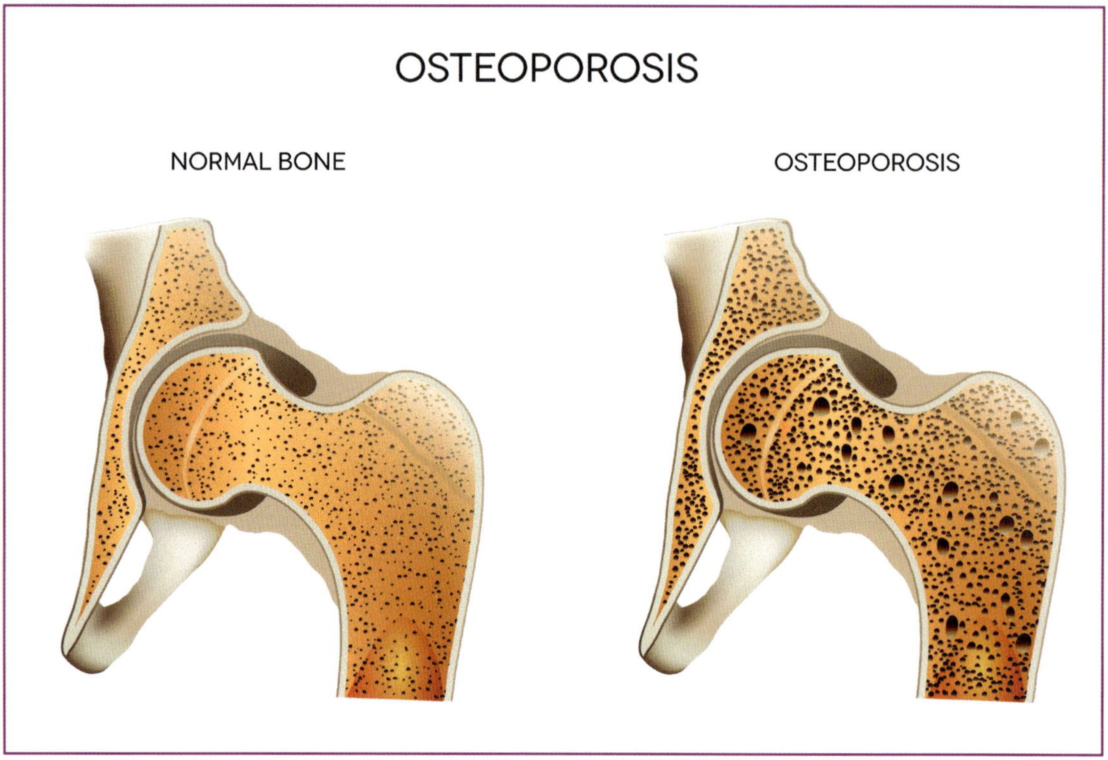

How these changes influence my planning as a personal trainer

Current recommendations when planning an appropriate exercise programme state that a well-balanced approach focusing on both aerobic and strength training activities should be adopted. Vigorous, impact type activities are only suitable for individuals who are not yet classified as severely osteoporotic.

When planning an exercise programme there should be a clear focus on improving balance to reduce the risks of trips and falls and adapting activities of daily living. Strength training should also be included to increase bone mineral density. And a whole-body approach is recommended as changes in bone mineral density are site-specific.

How these changes influence my delivery as a personal trainer

General advice must be given with regards to safe lifting practices, as well as the inclusion of adaptations that avoid positions such as forward flexion and or a combination of forward-flexion and twisting of the spinal column to avoid further risk of fractures. Avoid overstretching or hypermobility, as this could cause pain.

Certain exercises may need to be modified or avoided depending on the severity of osteoporosis, for example, four-point kneeling may not be appropriate especially for those with weak wrists. A whole-body approach is recommended for delivery as changes in bone mineral density are site-specific, therefore increases in bone mineral density will be throughout the skeleton. As for any older adult, a thorough warm-up and post-workout cool down and stretch out will be an essential part of the delivery.

Exercises to avoid

- High-impact exercises that may put too much force on relatively weak bones
- Sports that are associated with a high risk of trips and falls
- Exercises with excessive bending where you bend forward or twist your waist, as these can raise the risk of compression fractures in your spine
- Certain Pilates and yoga moves

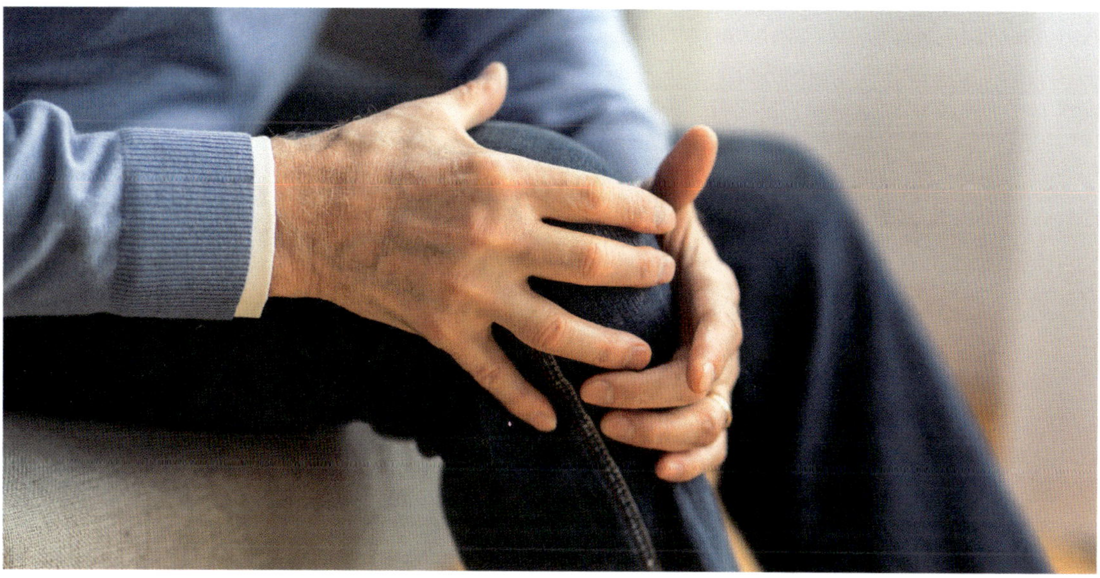

Osteoporosis: Step-By-Step Strength & Balance Exercises

If you are new to exercise, or it's been a while since you have exercised and or you have an underlying medical condition, such as osteoporosis please consult your doctor to see if it's safe for you to start.

A typical osteoporosis strength and balance training exercise routine

- Sit Down Stand-Ups
- Squats
- Standing Calf-Raises
- Side Leg Raises
- Leg Extension
- Wall Press-Up
- Biceps Curls
- Single Limb Stance
- Walking Heel to Toe
- Back Leg Raises
- Side Leg Raises

Sit Down Stand-Ups

- **EQUIPMENT:** Chair
- For this strength exercise, sit towards the front of the chair with your knees bent and both your feet flat on the floor about shoulder-width apart
- Next, lean back slightly with both your hands crossed over your chest, keep your back and your shoulders straight
- Breathe in slowly
- Bring your upper body forward until sitting upright as you breathe out, extend your arms so they are parallel to the floor and slowly stand up pushing up through your heel
- Breathe in as you sit back down slowly under control, this is one rep
- **TARGET:** 2 to 3 sets of 8 to 12 repetitions

Squats

- **EQUIPMENT:** Chair for support (optional)
- For this strength exercise, start by standing up and using the dining chair as support
- Next, bend your knees as much as you can without your knees passing over your toes, then return to the starting position
- Breathe in as you slowly squat down, breathe out as you stand up
- **TARGET:** 2 to 3 sets of 8 to 12 repetitions

Standing Calf-Raises

- **EQUIPMENT:** Bottle of Water or Squash or a Dumbbell
- For this strength exercise, start by standing with your feet quite close together
- Hold the weight in front of you with both hands
- Push upwards through the balls of your feet and raise your heels until you are standing on your toes
- Next, lower slowly back to the start under control, this is one rep
- **TARGET:** 2 to 3 sets of 15 to 20 repetitions

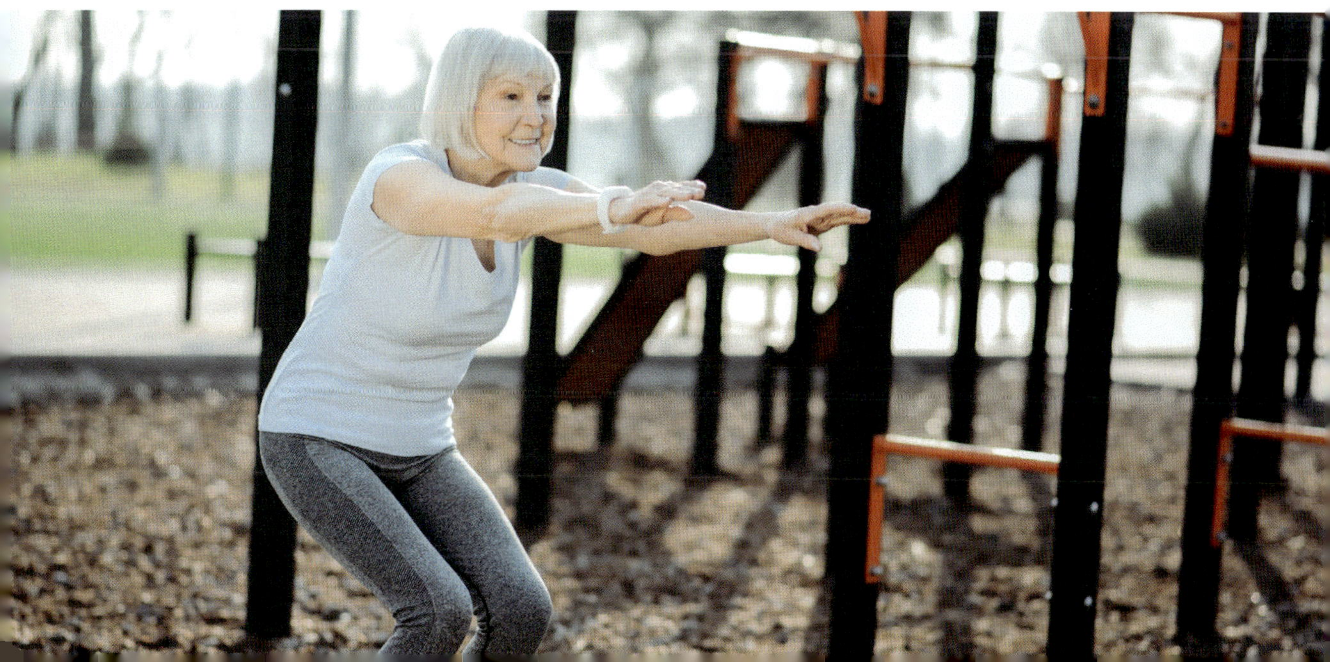

Leg Extension

- **EQUIPMENT:** Chair
- For this strength exercise, sit towards the front of the chair while keeping your left foot on the floor and with your upper body quite still
- Next, extend your right leg until its parallel with the floor and hold it up for the count of two
- Bend knee to lower your right leg back to the starting position, repeat with left leg, this is a complete rep
- Breathe in while lowering legs, breathe out while moving legs up
- **TARGET:** 2 to 3 sets of 8 to 12 repetitions each leg

Wall Press-Up

- **EQUIPMENT:** N/A
- For this strength exercise, stand about an arm's length in front of the wall (for your safety make sure the wall does not have any paintings, decorations, windows or doors)
- Lean forward slightly and put your palms flat on the wall at the same height and slightly wider than your shoulders, keep your feet firmly on the floor as you slowly move your body towards the wall
- Gently push yourself back so that your arms are straight to your starting position, this is one rep
- Take a deep breath while lowering yourself to the wall, breathe out as you push back
- **TARGET:** 2 to 3 sets of 8 to 12 repetitions

Biceps Curls

- **EQUIPMENT:** 2 Tins or 2 Dumbbells or Resistance Band
- For this strength exercise, stand upright with your feet hip-width apart
- Holding a weight in each hand curl slowly upwards to your chest, keep your elbows fixed by your sides
- Lower the tins slowly, this is one complete rep
- Breathe in while lowering weights, breathe out while curling arms up
- This can also be carried out while sitting.
- **TARGET:** 2 to 3 sets of 8 to 12 repetitions

Single Limb Stance

- **EQUIPMENT:** Chair
- For this balance exercise, start by standing behind a sturdy dining room chair and hold firmly on to the back initially using both hands, raise your right foot off of the floor and then balance on your left foot
- Hold the Single Limb Stance position for as long as you can, then change feet and repeat
- Your aim should be to stand in the Single Limb Stance position without holding onto the chair and hold it steady for up to one minute
- Breathe normally

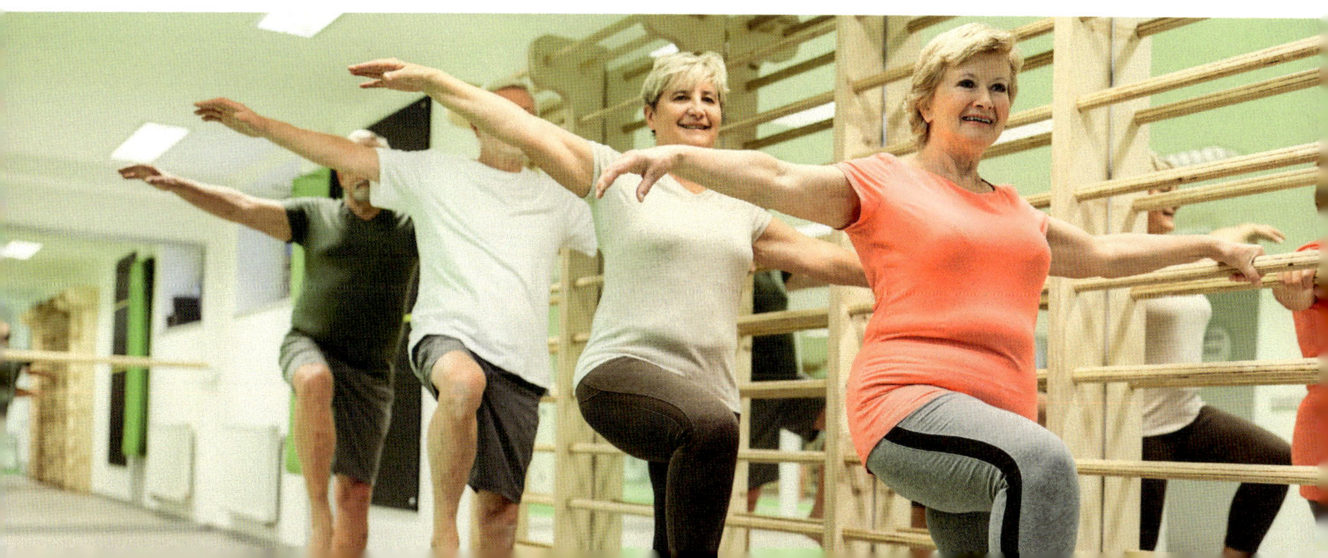

Walking Heel to Toe

- **EQUIPMENT:** N/A
- For this balance exercise, start by placing your right foot in front of left foot so that the heel of the right foot touches the top of the toes of the left foot
- Next, move your left foot in front of your right foot, putting your full weight on the heel, shift weight to your toes
- Repeat the step with the left foot, walk this way for 20 steps, turn around and walk back
- Tip; doing this balance exercise in a hallway with walls either side can make this feel safer, or have someone with you to spot, support you as you Walk Heel to Toe
- Breathe normally

Back Leg Raises

- **EQUIPMENT:** Chair
- For this balance exercise, start by standing behind the dining chair
- Next start lifting your right leg straight backwards, avoid bending at the knees and remain in this balanced position for a couple of seconds before returning the leg back down
- Repeat for the other leg to complete your Back Leg Raises exercises, aim for 8 to 12 reps for each leg
- Breathe normally

Side Leg Raises

- **EQUIPMENT:** Chair
- For this balance exercise, start by standing behind a sturdy dining room chair or kitchen countertop with one or both hands resting on it for support
- Lift your right leg out to the side and then bring it back to the standing position, repeat 10 times for each leg to complete your Side Leg Raises exercise
- Breathe normally

Osteoporosis: Step-By-Step Flexibility Exercises

If you are new to exercise, or it's been a while since you have exercised and or you have an underlying medical condition, such as osteoporosis please consult your doctor to see if it's safe for you to start.

A typical osteoporosis flexibility training exercise routine

- Hamstring Stretch
- Back & Shoulder Stretch
- Obliques Reaching Up Standing Stretch
- Arms Across Body Seated Stretch
- Seated Chest Stretch
- Triceps Stretch
- Quads Leg Stretch

Hamstring Stretch

- **EQUIPMENT:** Chair
- For this stretching exercise, sit on the chair
- Straighten out one leg and place both hands on this bent leg
- Lean gently forwards
- Hold the position for about 10 to 15 seconds and ease further forwards, after about another 10 to 15 seconds ease forward once again
- Repeat with the other leg
- Breathe normally

Back & Shoulder Stretch

- **EQUIPMENT:** Chair
- For this stretching exercise, begin seated clasp both hands together in front with your arms extended out, next drop your head and shoulders forward and then push hands away from your body as far as you can
- Hold for about 10 to 15 seconds
- Breathe normally

Obliques Reaching Up Standing Stretch

- **EQUIPMENT:** N/A
- For this stretching exercise, stand with your feet about hip-distance apart keeping your spine neutral
- Place one hand just below your hip and reach with your other arm up right up above your head
- Next, lean over to one side
- Hold for about 10 to 15 seconds
- Repeat on your other side
- Breathe normally

Arms Across Body Seated Stretch

- **EQUIPMENT:** Chair
- For this stretching exercise, sit on the chair, take one arm and fold it across the front of your body
- Place the palm of the other hand on the back of the upper arm and pull in and hold this position for about 10 to 15 seconds
- Breathe normally

Seated Chest Stretch

- **EQUIPMENT:** Chair
- For this stretching exercise, sit on the chair and place hands on small of your back
- Squeeze your shoulder blades so that they feel as though pinching together
- After about 10 to 15 seconds ease a little further into the stretch
- Breathe normally

Triceps Stretch

- **EQUIPMENT:** Chair
- For this stretching exercise, sit on the chair and place one hand above the head and bend at the elbow, hand touching the back of your shoulder, with your other hand on the back of upper arm apply pressure
- Hold for about 10 to 15 seconds
- Breathe normally

Quads Leg Stretch

- **EQUIPMENT:** Chair (optional)
- For this stretching exercise, stand with feet hip-distance apart, neutral spine
- Hold on to chair or counter if needed, stand on one leg
- Raise one heel towards your bum and hold in your hand, or hold your trouser hem if easier
- After 10 to 15 seconds pull in a little further and hold for another 10 seconds
- Breathe normally

Age-related changes in joints

With the ageing process, there appears to a general decrease in water within the body causing dehydration. Dehydration affects elasticity in the connective tissue in and around the joints. There is evidence that as the body ages the amount of synovial fluid appears to reduce and the fluid itself becomes more viscous leading to a reduction in the overall lubrication within the joint.

Furthermore, the decrease in water content and the increase in calcium salt deposits can affect the cartilage in several ways. As the growth of the cartilage slows down, the possibility of developing microscopic tears is inevitable due to the loss of fluid which reduces the cushioning effect. The cartilage is also prone to becoming hard and brittle.

Due to the decreases in water, the hyaline cartilage is converted to another type of cartilage known as fibro-cartilage, which is relatively sparse compared to its original hyaline formation. These age-related changes can cause pain and discomfort to the individual leading to a decrease in the range of movement, as well as a reduction in joint stability.

The most common age-related conditions to affect the joints is arthritis, of which there are more than 100 types. The most common are; osteoarthritis, rheumatoid arthritis, ankylosing spondylitis and gout. Arthritis describes the inflammation and or degeneration of a joint, making movement painful. Osteoarthritis is the most common age-related condition affecting the joints with some 8.75 million people in the UK suffering from this chronic condition.

NORMAL AND ARTHRITIC JOINTS

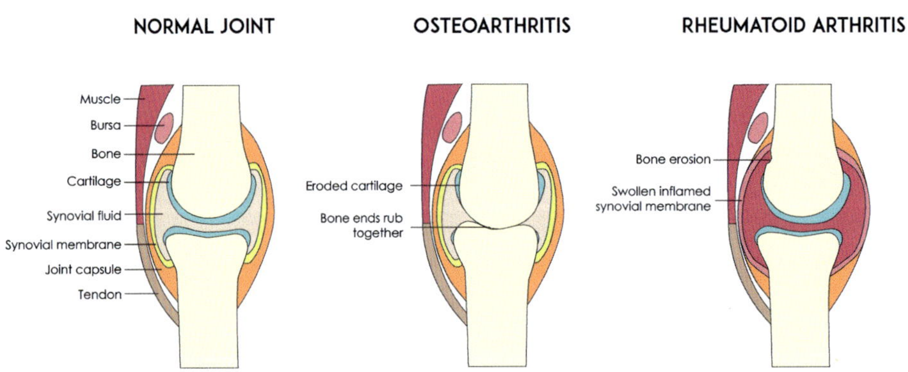

How these changes influence my planning as a personal trainer

For an arthritic client, it is vital that information in relation to this is obtained with the PAR-Q and the PARmed-X offers specific guidance for arthritic conditions. In addition, and with the permission of the client, all relevant information must be sought from the client's doctor, prior to engaging in a planned exercise programme to minimise the risk to the adult living with arthritis.

When planning an exercise programme care must be taken to include a thorough warm-up of joint mobility as the precursor to the main workout regardless of whether the adult is an arthritis sufferer. For sufferers of one of the 100 or so, arthritic conditions exercise plays a vital role in managing the condition. The focus when planning an exercise programme should encompass cardiovascular fitness, muscle strength and endurance training. Recent studies suggest that by incorporating strength training an adult with arthritis can benefit from up to a 43% reduction in pain.

Furthermore, strength training can increase muscle strength, general physical performance as well as decreased disability. Therefore, any planned programme should have a strength training component, as it will also enable the older adult to focus on posture work that is particularly beneficial for functional activities for daily living and decreasing the risk of trips and falls.

At the planning stage, there needs to be thought given to focus on activities that protect the joints rather than encourage further risk of damage. Therefore, joint mobility in the warm-up is extremely important to the arthritic older adult.

When planning an exercise programme, it should be noted that the length of time should not be for too long or curtailed if the client feels a degree of pain.

How these changes influence my delivery as a personal trainer

The type of arthritis will have a bearing on delivery. For example, Osteoarthritis typically affects the weight-bearing joints such as the knees, hips and spine, so particular care and focus should be given to the mobility exercises for these areas. This condition can also affect the fingers. Rheumatoid Arthritis predominantly affects the smaller joints in the body such as the hands, feet, ankles, elbows and wrists, so particular care and focus should be given to the mobility exercises for these areas.

Exercises that can help relieve pain and improve arthritis and joint stiffness

- Walking
- Cycling
- Hand exercises
- Strength training
- Swimming and aqua aerobics

When not to exercise

If you experience any of the following, stop exercising until you see your doctor:

- Increased swelling
- Sharp, stabbing, or constant pain
- Pain that causes you to limp or change your gait
- Joints that feel warm to the touch or are red
- Pain that lasts more than two hours after exercise or worsens at night

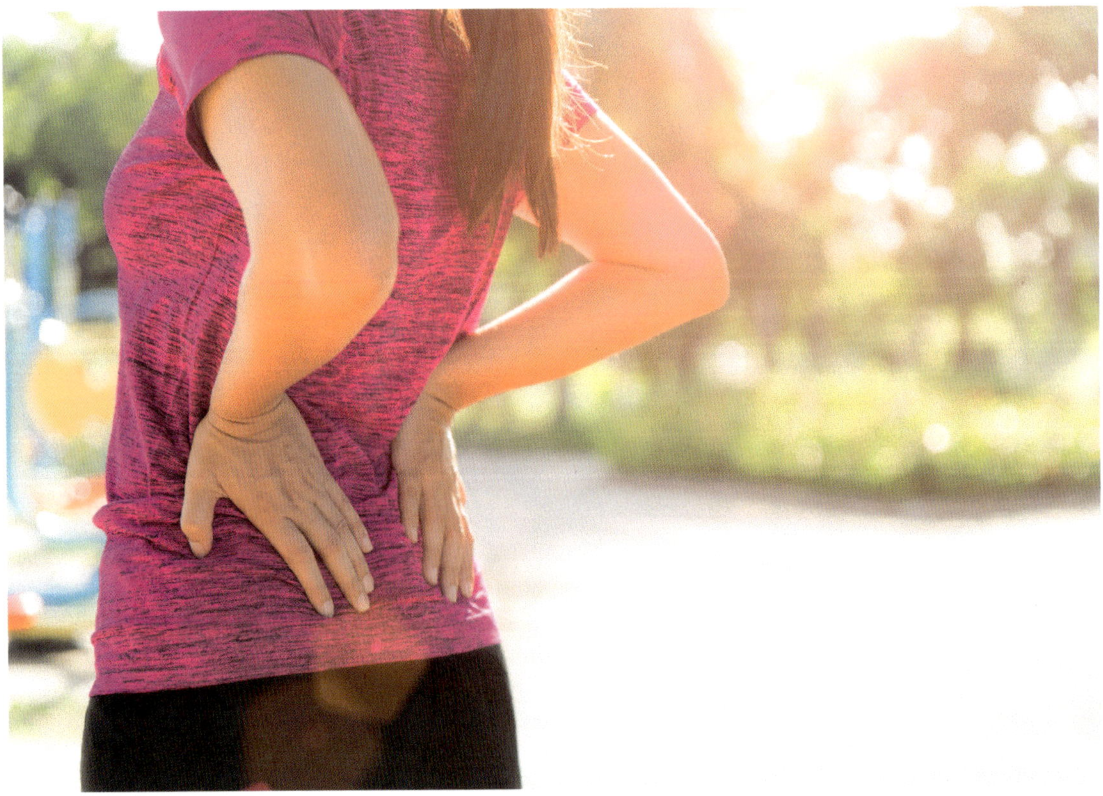

Arthritis:
Step-By-Step Strength & Flexibility Exercises

If you are new to exercise, or it's been a while since you have exercised and or you have an underlying medical condition, such as arthritis please consult your doctor to see if it's safe for you to start.

A typical strength and flexibility training exercise routine targeting arthritis and stiff joints

- Wall Push-ups
- Bicep Curls
- Lateral Raises
- Sit Down Stand-Ups
- Goblet Squats
- Wood Chops
- Hamstring Seated Stretch
- Back & Shoulder Stretch
- Obliques Reaching Up Standing Stretch
- Arms Across Body Seated Stretch
- Seated Chest Stretch
- Triceps Stretch

Wall Push-ups

- **EQUIPMENT:** N/A
- For this strength exercise, stand about an arm's length in front of the wall (for your safety make sure the wall does not have any paintings, decorations, windows or doors)
- Lean forward slightly and put your palms flat on the wall at the same height and slightly wider than your shoulders, keep your feet firmly on the floor as you slowly move your body towards the wall
- Gently push yourself back so that your arms are straight to your starting position, this is one rep
- Take a deep breath while lowering yourself to the wall, breathe out as you push back
- **TARGET:** 2 to 3 sets of 8 to 12 repetitions

Bicep Curls

- **EQUIPMENT:** 2 Tins or 2 Dumbbells or Resistance Band
- For this strength exercise, stand upright with your feet hip-width apart
- Holding a weight in each hand curl slowly upwards to your chest, keep your elbows fixed by your sides
- Lower the tins slowly, this is one complete rep
- Breathe in while lowering weights, breathe out while curling arms up
- **TARGET:** 2 to 3 sets of 8 to 12 repetitions

Lateral Raises

- **EQUIPMENT:** 2 Tins or 2 Dumbbells or Resistance Band
- For this strength exercise, stand upright with your feet hip-width apart
- Ensure that your shoulders are relaxed with your stomach muscles engaged
- Retaining this position, lift the weights out to the sides up to the height of your shoulders
- Pause and then slowly lower the weights back to your starting position, this is one complete rep
- Breathe in while lowering weights, breathe out while moving arms up
- **TARGET:** 2 to 3 sets of 8 to 12 repetitions

Sit Down Stand-Ups

- **EQUIPMENT:** Chair
- For this strength exercise, sit towards the front of the chair with your knees bent and both your feet flat on the floor about shoulder-width apart
- Next, lean back slightly with both your hands crossed over your chest, keep your back and your shoulders straight
- Breathe in slowly
- Bring your upper body forward until sitting upright as you breathe out, extend your arms so they are parallel to the floor and slowly stand up pushing up through your heel
- Breathe in as you sit back down slowly under control, this is one rep
- **TARGET:** 2 to 3 sets of 8 to 12 repetitions

Goblet Squats

- **EQUIPMENT:** Bottle of Water, Squash or a Dumbbell
- For this strength exercise, start by standing with your feet about shoulder-width apart
- Hold the weight with both hands
- Remember to keep your chest up with your heels down throughout
- Perform a standard squat and when on the upward move raise the weight up above your head, this is one rep
- Breathe in as you slowly squat down under control, breathe out as you stand back up
- **TARGET:** 2 to 3 sets of 8 to 12 repetitions

Wood Chops

- **EQUIPMENT:** N/A
- For this core exercise, start the Wood Chop exercise with your feet wider than shoulder-width apart clasping together both hands in front
- Next, pull your arms up to be level with one side of your head
- Squat down while doing a chopping movement with your arms diagonally downwards to the opposite side of your body
- Repeat by performing the chopping action back up towards the top, this is one rep
- Breathe normally
- **TARGET:** 2 to 3 sets of 8 to 12 repetitions each side

Hamstring Seated Stretch

- **EQUIPMENT:** Chair
- For this stretching exercise, sit on the chair
- Straighten out one leg and place both hands on this bent leg
- Lean gently forwards
- Hold the position for about 10 to 15 seconds and ease further forwards, after about another 10 to 15 seconds ease forward once again
- Repeat with the other leg
- Breathe normally

Back & Shoulder Stretch

- **EQUIPMENT:** Chair
- For this stretching exercise, begin seated clasp both hands together in front with your arms extended out, next drop your head and shoulders forward and then push hands away from your body as far as you can
- Hold for about 10 to 15 seconds
- Breathe normally

Obliques Reaching Up Standing Stretch

- **EQUIPMENT:** N/A
- For this stretching exercise, stand with your feet about hip-distance apart keeping your spine neutral
- Place one hand just below your hip and reach with your other arm up right up above your head
- Next, lean over to one side
- Hold for about 10 to 15 seconds
- Repeat on your other side
- Breathe normally

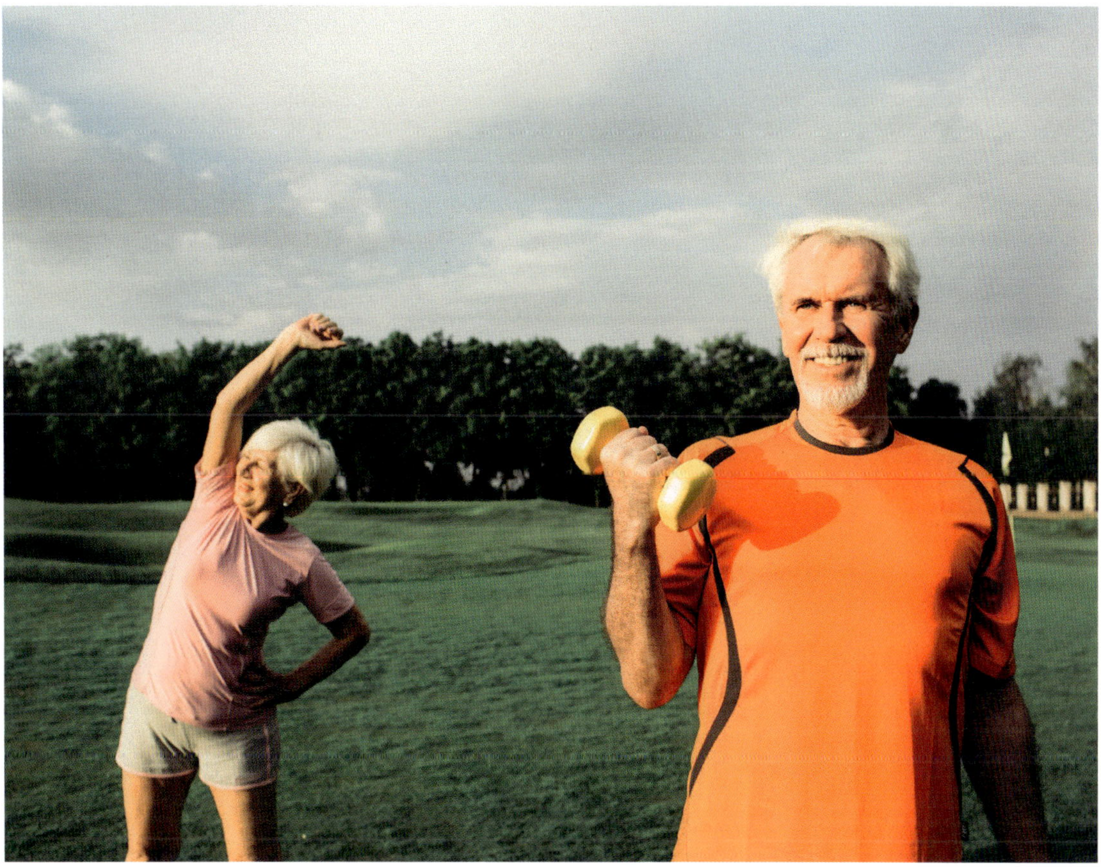

Arms Across Body Seated Stretch

- **EQUIPMENT:** Chair
- For this stretching exercise, sit on the chair, take one arm and fold it across the front of your body
- Place the palm of the other hand on the back of the upper arm and pull in and hold this position for about 10 to 15 seconds
- Breathe normally

Seated Chest Stretch

- **EQUIPMENT:** Chair
- For this stretching exercise, sit on the chair and place hands on small of your back
- Squeeze your shoulder blades so that they feel as though pinching together
- After about 10 to 15 seconds ease a little further into the stretch
- Breathe normally

Triceps Stretch

- **EQUIPMENT:** Chair
- For this stretching exercise, sit on the chair and place one hand above the head and bend at the elbow, hand touching the back of your shoulder, with your other hand on the back of upper arm apply pressure
- Hold for about 10 to 15 seconds
- Breathe normally

Age-Related Changes In Muscles

Peak muscle mass in all muscle tissue is reached around the age of 30, after this, there is a progressive loss of age-related muscle tissue in all areas. On average there is a 30% loss of muscle mass between the ages of 30 and 80. Due to these changes within the muscle tissue, strength and power are affected, with declines in strength at an annual rate of 1.5% and power at 3.5% annually. These losses have a major impact on the functional ability of the older adult.

There are other numerous age-related changes in the muscles:

- Reduced metabolism
- Reduction in capillary density
- Reduction in muscular endurance
- Loss in the number of muscle fibres
- Loss in the number of motor neurons
- Reduction in contractile protein & ATP
- Reduction in elasticity and increases in the overall connective tissue

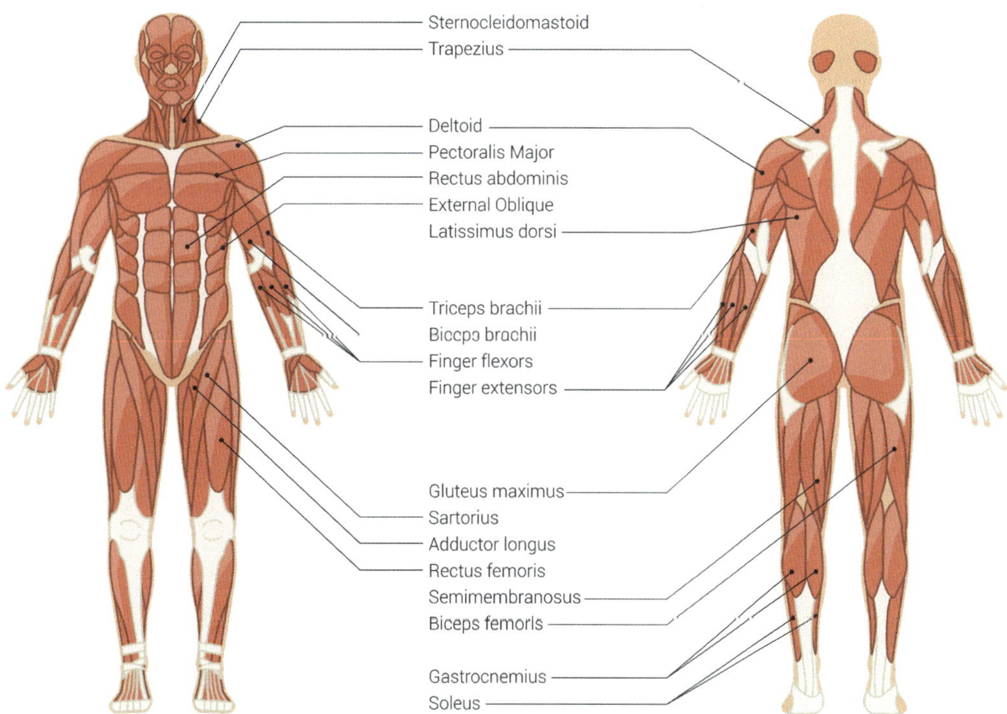

How these changes influence my planning as a personal trainer

When planning an exercise programme for an older adult the emphasis on physical activity, in particular, strength training cannot be ignored. There is scientific evidence reported on numerous occasions that link lean muscle mass with bone mineral density, therefore when planning an exercise programme, an older adult should be encouraged to maintain lean muscle mass through regular exercise.

It should be stressed in the planning stage that a balanced exercise programme should always be adhered to, although it is especially important in ageing to focus on pelvic floor muscles, deep core stabilisers and extension-type activities. Benefits from this approach include:

- Decreased back pain
- Improved self-esteem
- Improved posture and body awareness
- Increased ability to perform functional activities
- Increased resistance to stress incontinence, for example, coughing and sneezing

It is therefore vitally important to include strength training when planning an exercise programme.

How these changes influence my delivery as a personal trainer

Ideally, delivery should focus on a whole-body approach and thought must be given to all muscle groups used in activities for daily living, for example, squats can develop the leg muscles to aid getting up from a chair.

Exercises that can improve muscles

- Cycling
- Walking
- Aerobic training
- Strength training
- Bodyweight training
- Resistance band training

Step-By-Step Strength & Aerobic Exercises

If you are new to exercise, or it's been a while since you have exercised and or you have an underlying medical condition, such as arthritis please consult your doctor to see if it's safe for you to start.

A typical strength and aerobic training exercise routine targeting all major muscle groups

- Knees into Elbows
- Step-Ups
- Wall Push-ups
- Bicep Curls
- Lateral Raises
- Upright Rows
- Sit Down Stand-Ups
- Goblet Squats
- Standing Calf-Raises
- Glute Bridges
- Wood Chops
- Figure of Eights

Knees into Elbows

- **EQUIPMENT:** N/A
- For this aerobic exercise, start by bringing your left knee up and right elbow down towards your knee
- Change sides, bring right knee up and left elbow down
- Continue alternating at a brisk pace
- You can do a variation of this seated
- Breathe normally
- **TARGET:** Aim to build up to 5 - 10 minutes

Step-Ups

- **EQUIPMENT:** Steps
- For this aerobic exercise, start on the bottom step of a set of steps or on your staircase. Step up onto the first step with your left foot and then, and then step up with your right foot, pause briefly
- Next, step back down with your right leg and then with your left leg
- Repeat on the other side
- You can make this a little more challenging by using weights; tins of food or dumbbells in each hand
- Breathe normally
- **TARGET:** Aim to build up to 5 - 10 minutes

Wall Push-ups

- **EQUIPMENT:** N/A
- For this strength exercise, stand about an arm's length in front of the wall (for your safety make sure the wall does not have any paintings, decorations, windows or doors)
- Lean forward slightly and put your palms flat on the wall at the same height and slightly wider than your shoulders, keep your feet firmly on the floor as you slowly move your body towards the wall
- Gently push yourself back so that your arms are straight to your starting position, this is one rep
- Take a deep breath while lowering yourself to the wall, breathe out as you push back
- **TARGET:** 2 to 3 sets of 8 to 12 repetitions

Bicep Curls

- **EQUIPMENT:** 2 Tins or 2 Dumbbells or Resistance Band
- For this strength exercise, stand upright with your feet hip-width apart
- Holding a weight in each hand curl slowly upwards to your chest, keep your elbows fixed by your sides
- Lower the tins slowly, this is one complete rep
- Breathe in while lowering weights, breathe out while curling arms up
- **TARGET:** 2 to 3 sets of 8 to 12 repetitions

Lateral Raises

- **EQUIPMENT:** 2 Tins or 2 Dumbbells or Resistance Band
- For this strength exercise, stand upright with your feet hip-width apart
- Ensure that your shoulders are relaxed with your stomach muscles engaged
- Retaining this position, lift the weights out to the sides up to the height of your shoulders
- Pause and then slowly lower the weights back to your starting position, this is one complete rep
- Breathe in while lowering weights, breathe out while moving arms up
- **TARGET:** 2 to 3 sets of 8 to 12 repetitions

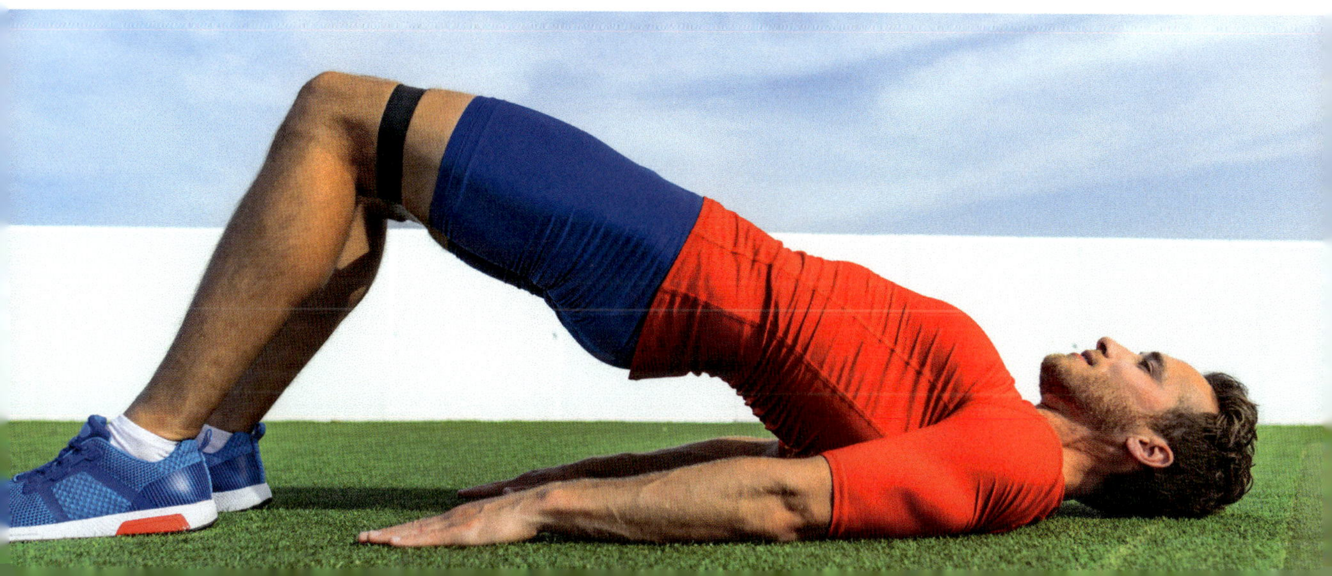

Upright Rows

- **EQUIPMENT:** 2 Tins or 2 Dumbbells or Resistance Band
- For this strength exercise, stand upright with your feet hip-width apart
- Lift the weights by raising your elbows out to the sides until they line up with the height of your shoulders. Your hands should finish up just beneath your chin
- Next, slowly slide the weights down to the starting position, this is one complete rep
- Breathe in while lowering weights, breathe out while moving arms up
- **TARGET:** 2 to 3 sets of 8 to 12 repetitions

Sit Down Stand-Ups

- **EQUIPMENT:** Chair
- For this strength exercise, sit towards the front of the chair with your knees bent and both your feet flat on the floor about shoulder-width apart
- Next, lean back slightly with both your hands crossed over your chest, keep your back and your shoulders straight
- Breathe in slowly
- Bring your upper body forward until sitting upright as you breathe out, extend your arms so they are parallel to the floor and slowly stand up pushing up through your heel
- Breathe in as you sit back down slowly under control, this is one rep
- **TARGET:** 2 to 3 sets of 8 to 12 repetitions

Goblet Squats

- **EQUIPMENT:** Bottle of Water, Squash or a Dumbbell
- For this strength exercise, start by standing with your feet about shoulder-width apart
- Hold the weight with both hands
- Remember to keep your chest up with your heels down throughout
- Perform a standard squat and when on the upward move raise the weight up above your head, this is one rep
- Breathe in as you slowly squat down under control, breathe out as you stand back up
- **TARGET:** 2 to 3 sets of 8 to 12 repetitions

Standing Calf-Raises

- **EQUIPMENT:** Bottle of Water or Squash or a Dumbbell
- For this strength exercise, start by standing with your feet quite close together
- Hold the weight in front of you with both hands
- Push upwards through the balls of your feet and raise your heels until you are standing on your toes
- Next, lower slowly back to the start under control, this is one rep
- **TARGET:** 2 to 3 sets of 15 to 20 repetitions

Glute Bridges

- **EQUIPMENT:** Mat
- For this strength exercise, start by lying down on bed or floor with both your knees bent, your hips are in a neutral position
- Next, lift your bottom as high as you comfortably can off of the floor, pause briefly and then return the body to the starting position and repeat
- Breathe out completely and engage core before upward movement, breathe in during the downward movement
- **TARGET:** 2 to 3 sets of 8 to 12 repetitions

Wood Chops

- **EQUIPMENT:** N/A
- For this core exercise, start the Wood Chop exercise with your feet wider than shoulder-width apart clasping together both hands in front
- Next, pull your arms up to be level with one side of your head
- Squat down while doing a chopping movement with your arms diagonally downwards to the opposite side of your body
- Repeat by performing the chopping action back up towards the top, this is one rep
- Breathe normally
- **TARGET:** 2 to 3 sets of 8 to 12 repetitions each side

Figure of Eights

- **EQUIPMENT:** Bottle of Water, Squash or Dumbbell
- For this core exercise, start seated on the chair with your feet about shoulder-width apart, bracing your stomach muscles, sitting up, holding the weight in both your hands, arms fully extended out
- With your arms fully extended draw big figures of eights, this is one complete rep
- Breathe normally
- **TARGET:** 2 to 3 sets of 8 to 12 repetitions

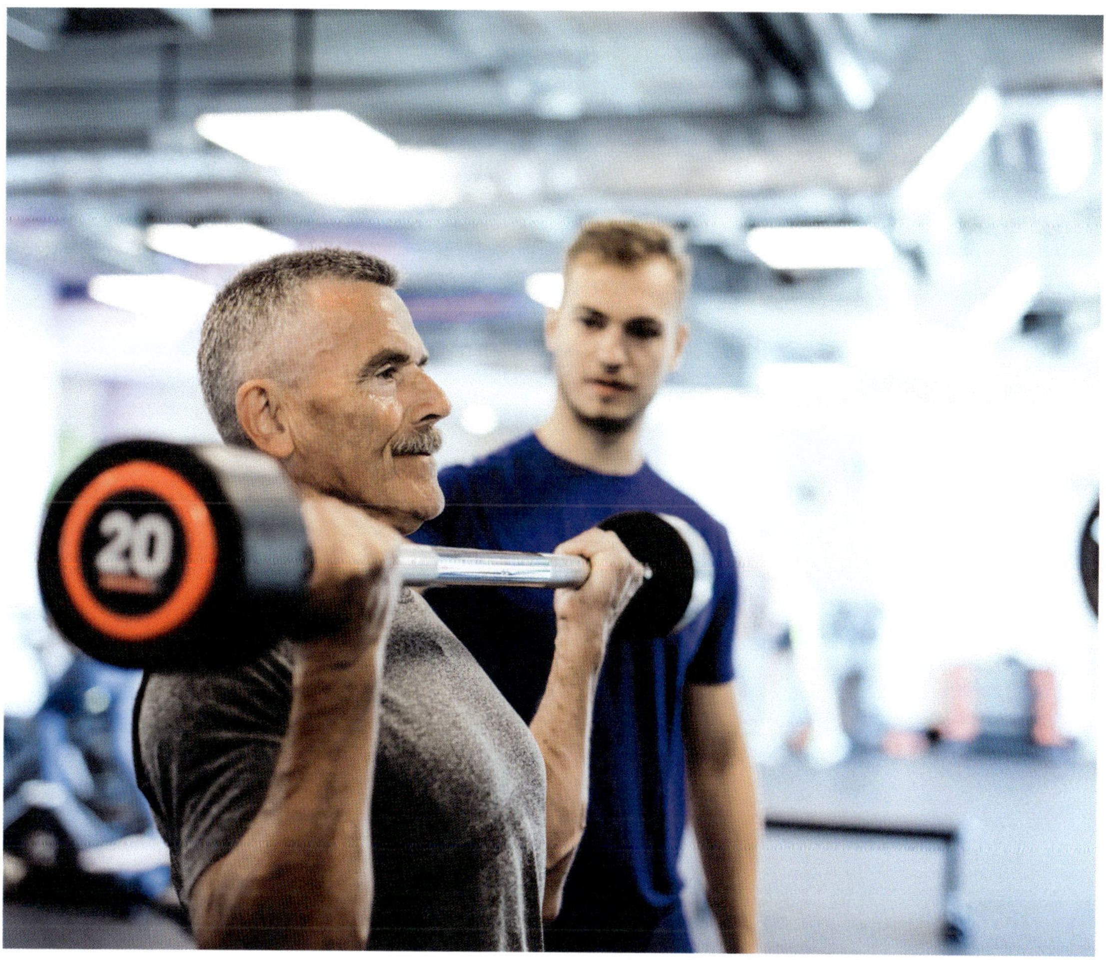

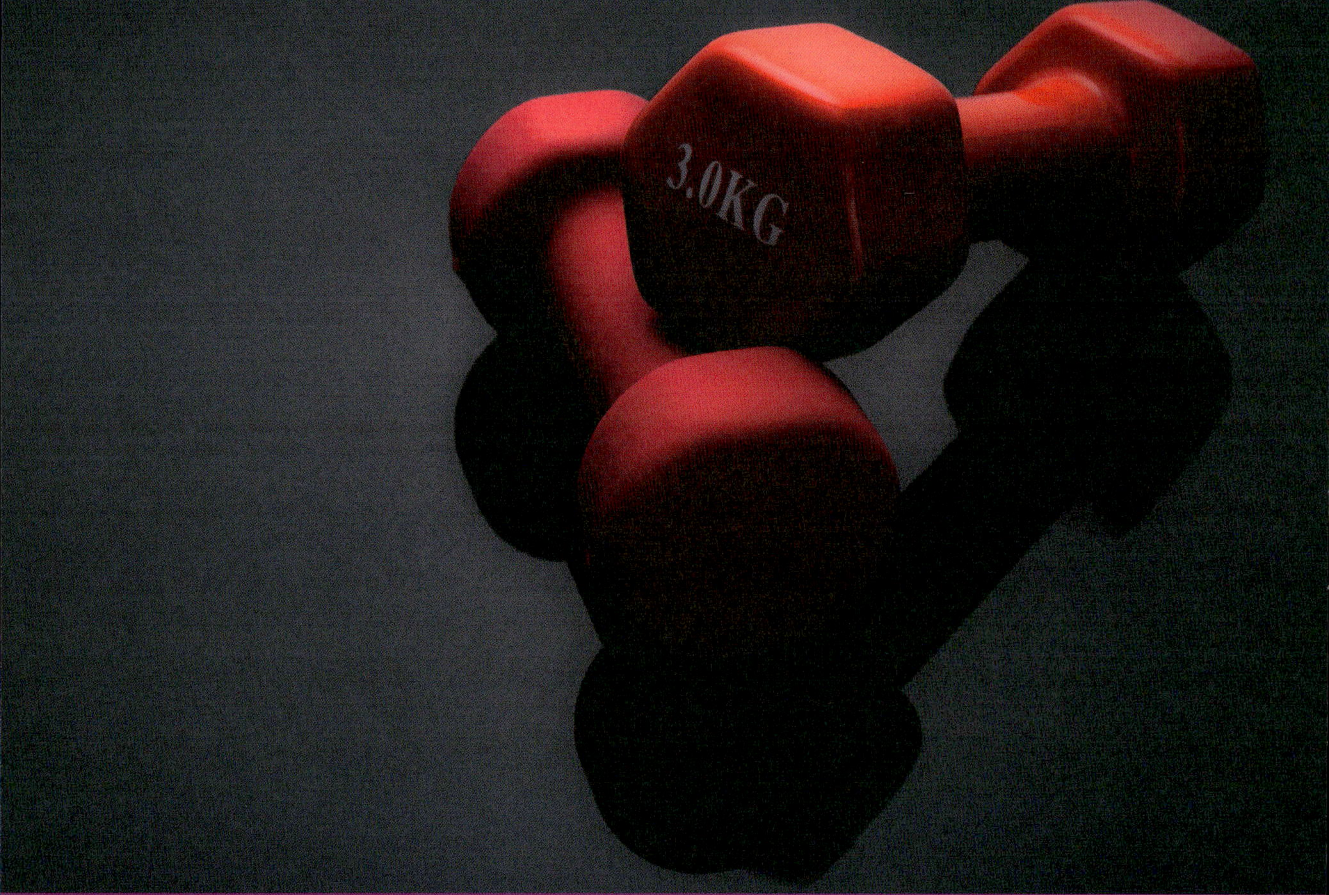

"Motivation gets you started.
Habit keeps you going."

CHAPTER 13

Upgrading Your Exercise Equipment

Once you've got into doing your exercises regularly you may want to upgrade your exercise kit, particularly if you want to progress through increasing the resistance or weight of the exercises. For my older adult clients I use both resistance bands and dumbbells. The resistance bands come in a variety of strengths, and the dumbbells in 0.5kg, 1kg, 1.5kg and 2kg weights. I recommend the following suppliers and I use these in my exercise classes: and with my personal training clients.

Recommended equipment

Dumbbells - DTX Fitness

These are smart with a stylish neoprene coating that I use with my personal training clients.

- 0.5kg - 2kg: Starter Set of 8 Dumbbells £49.99

Visit **www.3fspt.co.uk/shop**

Resistance bands - OMERIL

- Set of 3: £14.99

Visit **www.3fspt.co.uk/shop**

Portable Pedal Exerciser - Drive DeVilbiss Healthcare

I recommend these to my clients who have limited mobility in their legs.

- £24.99

Visit **www.3fspt.co.uk/shop**

Equipment subject to availability and price changes.

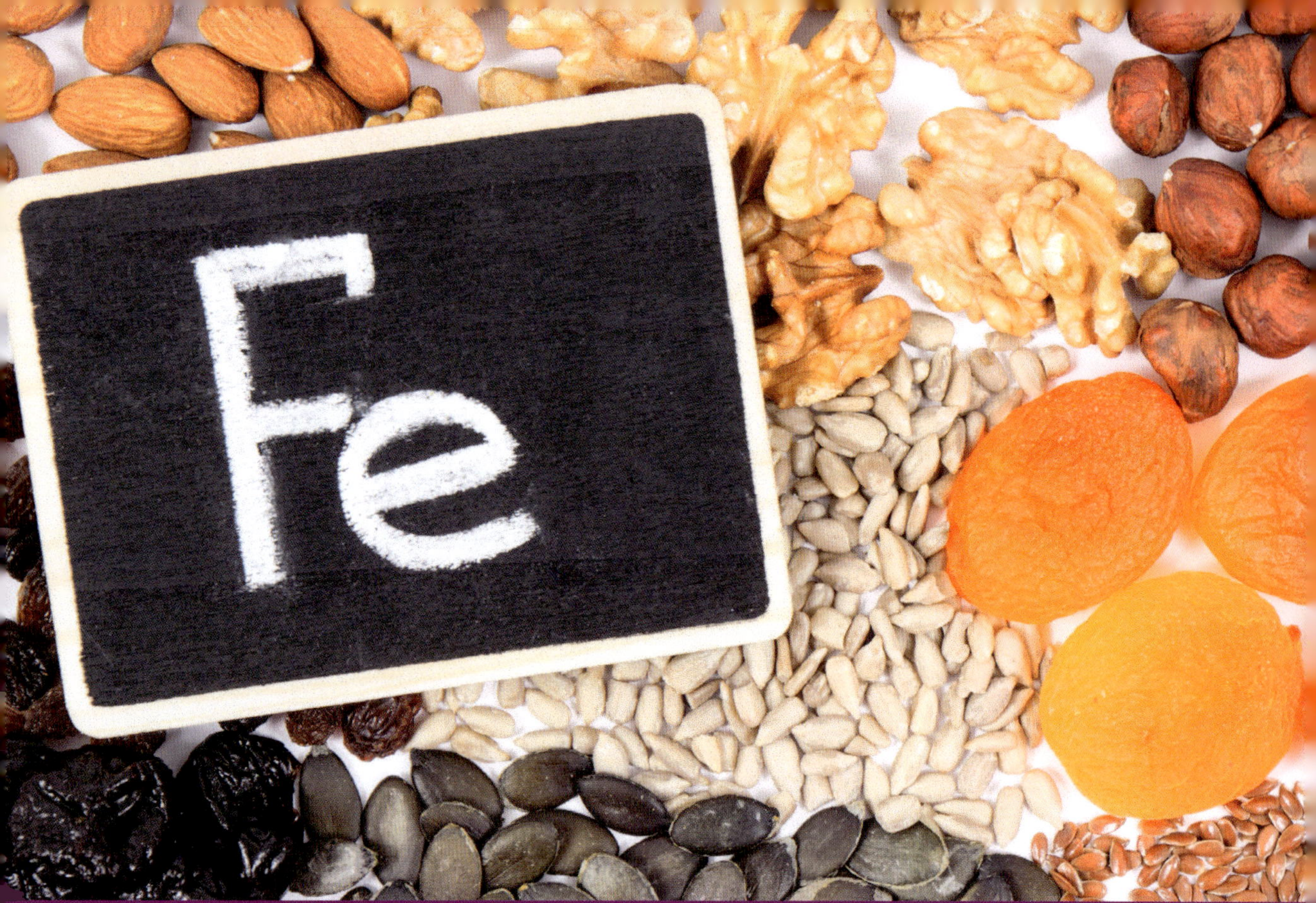

"You will never always be motivated, so learn how to be disciplined."

CHAPTER 14

Why Key Nutrients, Vitamins & Fluid Intake Are Important

Eating right and staying fit are important no matter what your age. However, as we get older our bodies have different needs, so certain nutrients and vitamins become particularly important to maintain good physical health. Doctors are increasingly concerned about boosting the levels of vitamins and minerals that we need as we age.

A worrying common trend is a loss of appetite and as a direct result many people do not take in adequate amounts of vitamins and other nutrients as they did when they were younger. Other factors that can greatly affect appetite and the inadequate uptake of vital nutrients are:

- Diabetes
- Medications
- Certain disabilities
- Changes in the skin
- Age related medical conditions
- Changes in the digestive system

One study estimates that one-third of people aged 60 and above are alarmingly low on important vitamins and minerals. Another study revealed that two thirds of older adults admitted to a hospital are malnourished, resulting in low levels of vital nutrients. When a person is vitamin and mineral deficient, they are more susceptible to illness and infections. It is estimated that deaths due to infections are ten times more likely in people aged 60 and above.

So what is a vitamin and why is it so essential to our bodies?

A vitamin is a molecule that our bodies need to carry out certain biological functions. With only a few exceptions, we have no way to create vitamin molecules ourselves, so these vital building blocks must come in through food that we eat. The human body is known to need at least 13 different vitamins. We are able to store some of these for long periods of time in fat cells or in the liver, for example, vitamin A. However, the majority of vitamins need to be replenished frequently.

Vitamins don't supply us with energy. For energy our bodies require protein, carbohydrates, and fats. What vitamins do is to help the carbohydrates, fats, and proteins release energy. These vital compounds are very important and they are required for all sorts of complex chemical reactions in our bodies. Vitamins are also needed to assist the enzymes that repair tissue and help with the production of cells. Many studies have shown that vitamins and minerals can help or prevent some of the disorders or diseases related to aging.

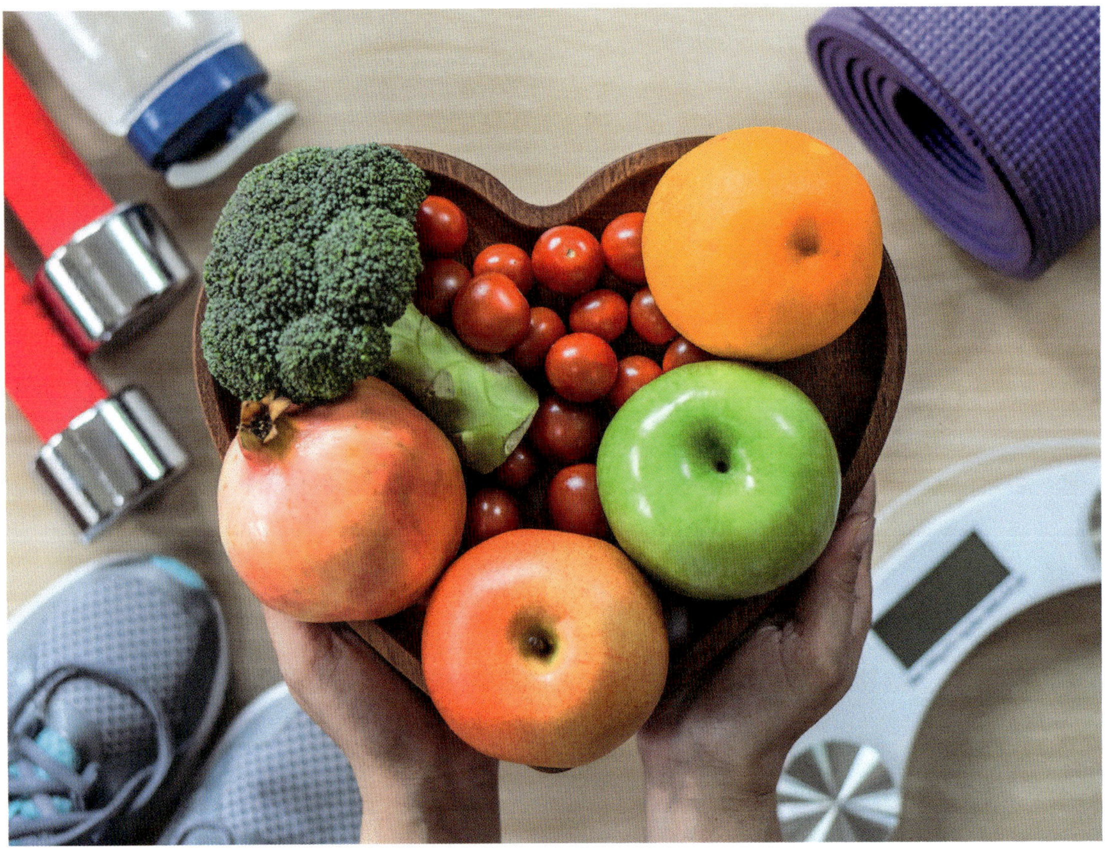

There are two types of vitamins:

- Water soluble
- Fat soluble

Water soluble vitamins are not stored in our body, they pass through us relatively quickly. In order to keep these vital nutrients in our bodies we have to consume them frequently. Water soluble vitamins contribute to our health, energy and stamina. This type of vitamin also helps in the function of over one hundred enzymes and chemical reactions that give our bodies energy.

There are nine water-soluble vitamins found in our diet:

- Vitamin B1 (thiamine)
- Vitamin B2 (riboflavin)
- Vitamin B3 (niacin)
- Vitamin B5 (pantothenic acid)
- Vitamin B6
- Vitamin B7 (biotin)
- Vitamin B9
- Vitamin B12 (cobalamin)
- Vitamin C

Fat soluble vitamins are vitamins that stay in the body and are typically stored in the liver. You can usually receive enough of these compounds by eating a well balanced diet. Any condition that can interfere with the absorption of fat in the body like tuberculosis, cystic fibrosis, hypothyroidism, lactose intolerance, and many other diseases or disorders can cause deficiencies in these vitamins. Before taking the recommended daily allowance (RDA) dose of fat soluble vitamins you must consult your doctor. Taking an overdose of these substances can cause a toxic build-up in the body.

The four fat soluble vitamins found in our diet are:

- Vitamin A
- Vitamin D
- Vitamin E
- Vitamin K

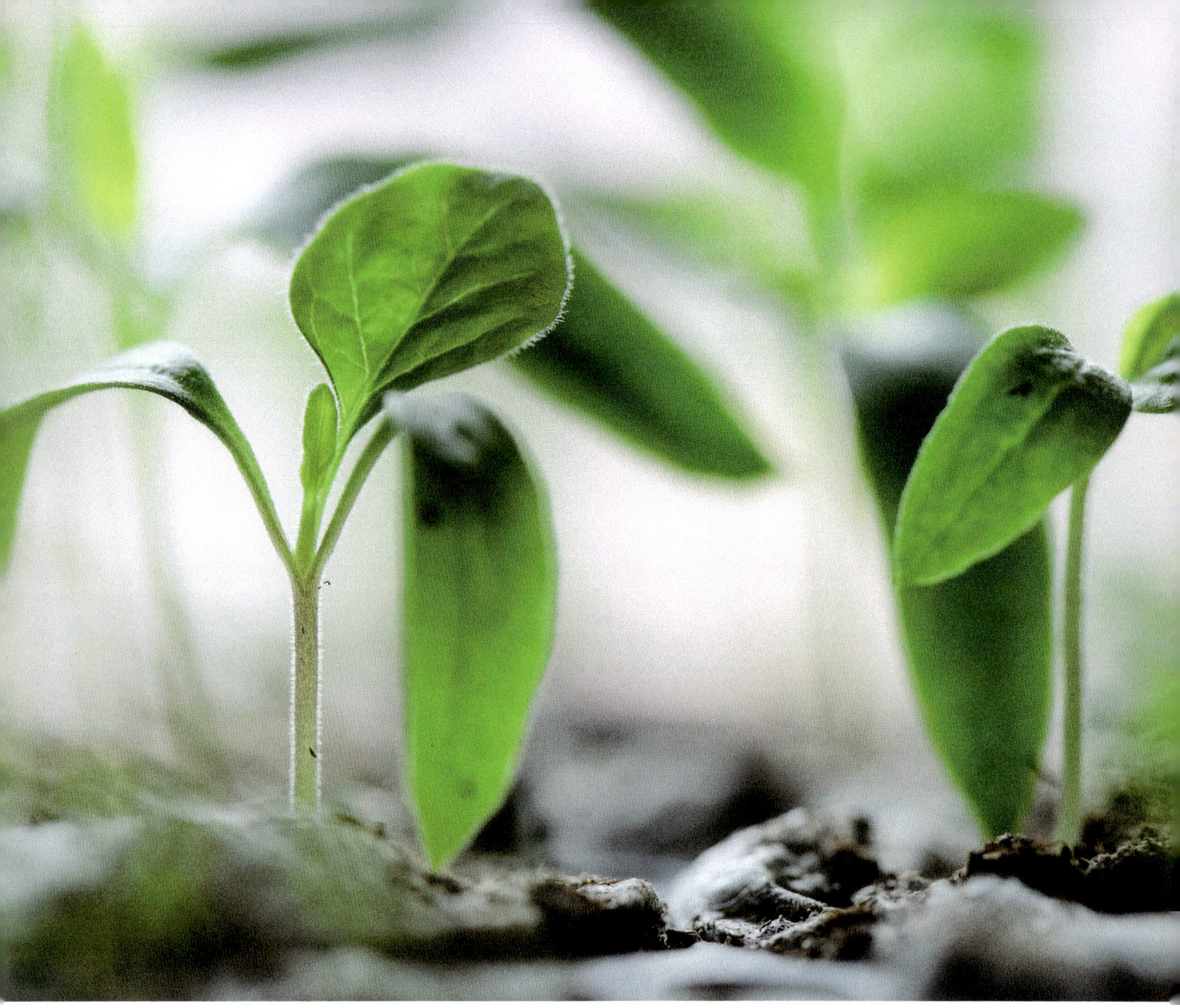

Unlike vitamins, minerals are not manufactured by plants or animals. Minerals form in the earth, and they are absorbed by plants and found in animals that eat the plants.

We use vitamins every day to support the processes our bodies use to maintain life. Ongoing reduced levels of vitamins can make you weak and more vulnerable to disease. Proper nutrition with vitamins and minerals is vital for people aged 60 and above to maintain a healthy lifestyle.

As a general rule, it is always better to get your recommended daily allowance (RDA) by eating a balanced diet. However, if you're concerned that you may not be getting enough of these, speak to your doctor or a qualified nutritionist as they may recommend you take supplements.

The following is a simple overview as to why certain nutrients, vitamins and water are so important:

Calcium

- **What it does:**
  Calcium is essential for healthy bones and helps prevent osteoporosis.
- **How much you need each day:**
  The RDA of calcium in the UK is 700mg a day for adults.
- **Food sources:**
  Milk, cheese and other dairy foods, green leafy vegetables; such as broccoli, cabbage and okra, soya beans, tofu, soya drinks with added calcium, nuts, bread and anything made with fortified flour, fish where you eat the bones such as sardines and pilchards.

Fibre

- **What it does:**
  Fibre helps with bowel movements and prevents constipation. It can also help lower blood cholesterol levels, control blood sugar levels and keep you feeling full for longer which can help with weight control.
- **How much you need each day:**
  The RDA is 30 g for adults. If you haven't been eating much fibre, add fibre slowly and drink more fluids to prevent gas, bloating and diarrhoea.
- **Food sources:**
  Whole grain breakfast cereals, whole wheat pasta, whole grain bread and oats, barley and rye, fruit such as berries, pears, melon and oranges, vegetables such as broccoli, carrots and sweetcorn, peas, beans and pulses, nuts and seeds, potatoes with the skin.

Iron

- **What it does:**
  Iron is a mineral vital to the proper function of haemoglobin, a protein needed to transport oxygen in the blood. Iron also has a role in a variety of other important processes in the body. A shortage of iron in the blood can lead to serious health problems, including iron deficiency anaemia.

- **How much you need each day:**
  Although iron is an essential element for the human body, requirements for iron change with age. The recommended daily allowance for iron for adults over age 60 is 8.7 milligrams per day, regardless of gender.

- **Food sources:**
  Shellfish, spinach, liver and other organ meats, legumes, red meat, pumpkin seeds, quinoa, turkey, broccoli, tofu and dark chocolate.

Potassium

- **What it does:**
  Potassium is one of the most important minerals in the body. It helps regulate fluid balance, muscle contractions and nerve signals. Potassium is good for lowering blood pressure and controlling the balance of fluids in the body. What's more, a high-potassium diet may help protect against stroke and prevent osteoporosis and kidney stones.

- **How much you need each day:**
  The UK RDA of potassium is 3,500 mg.

- **Food sources:**
  Good sources of potassium include fruit (particularly bananas), vegetables, pulses, nuts, seeds, milk, fish, beef, poultry and bread.

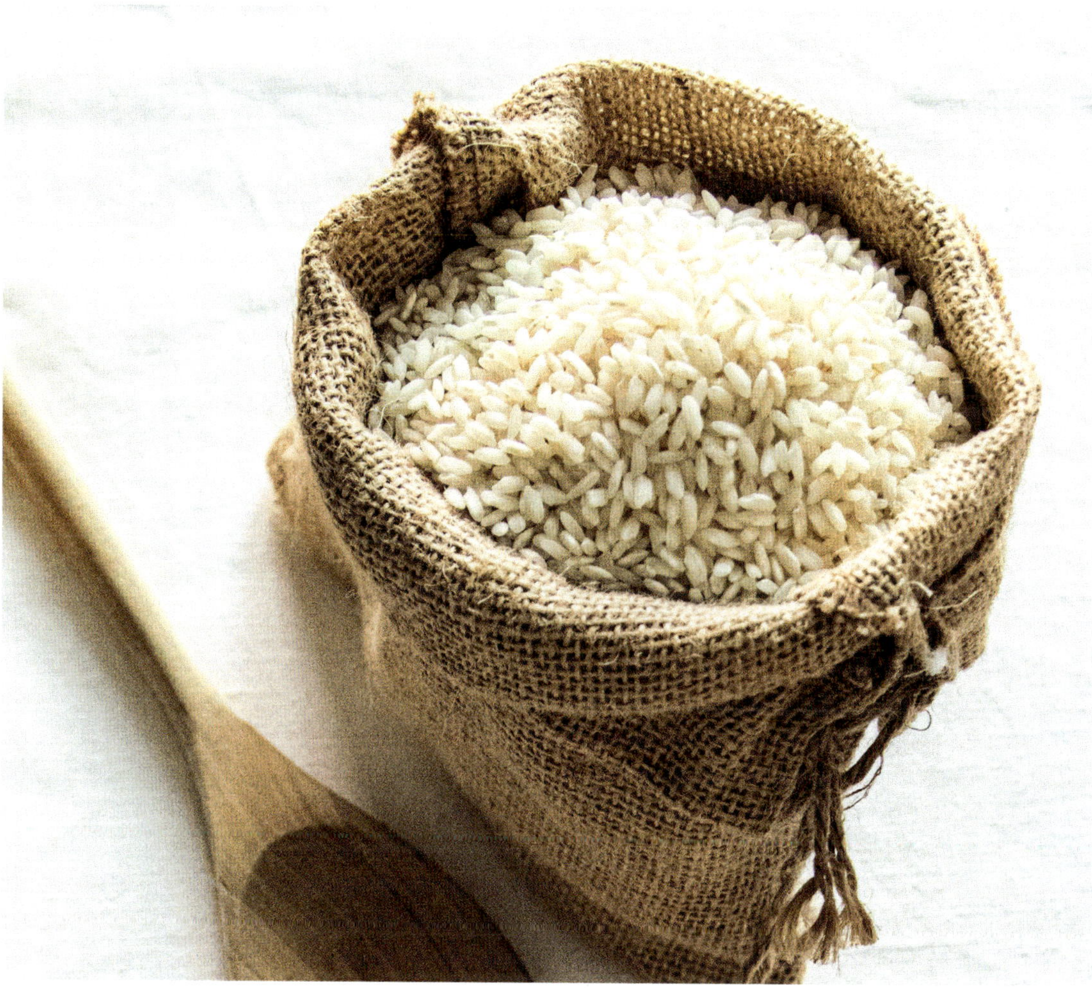

Magnesium

- **What it does:**
  Magnesium is a nutrient that the body needs to stay healthy. Magnesium is important for many processes in the body, including regulating muscle and nerve function, blood sugar levels, and blood pressure and making protein, bone, and DNA
- **How much you need each day:** The UK RDA of magnesium for adults is 270 mg for women and 300 mg for men.
- **Food sources:** Magnesium is found in a wide variety of foods, including green leafy vegetables such as spinach, nuts, brown rice, bread (especially whole grain), fish, meat and dairy foods.

Vitamin B12

- **What it does:**
  Vitamin B12 helps maintain a healthy nervous system and makes red blood cells.

- **How much you need each day:**
  The RDA is 1.5 mcg for adults. Because many adults over age 60 do not absorb vitamin B12 very well, it's recommended you eat foods fortified with B12 or take a multivitamin and mineral supplement that contains B12.

- **Food sources:**
  Foods from an animal such as meat, seafood, milk products, poultry, and eggs; and plant foods with added B12 such as B12 fortified soy beverage and tofu.

Vitamin D

- **What it does:**
  Vitamin D helps your body absorb calcium and balances calcium level for bone health.

- **How much you need each day:**
  Many people are deficient in Vitamin D, with the elderly being particularly at risk. Current UK recommendations say people aged over 65 should take a daily supplement of 10mcg.

- **Food sources:**
  Foods that provide vitamin D include, fatty fish, like tuna, mackerel, and salmon, foods fortified with vitamin D, such as some dairy products, orange juice, soy milk, and cereals, beef liver, cheese, egg yolks.

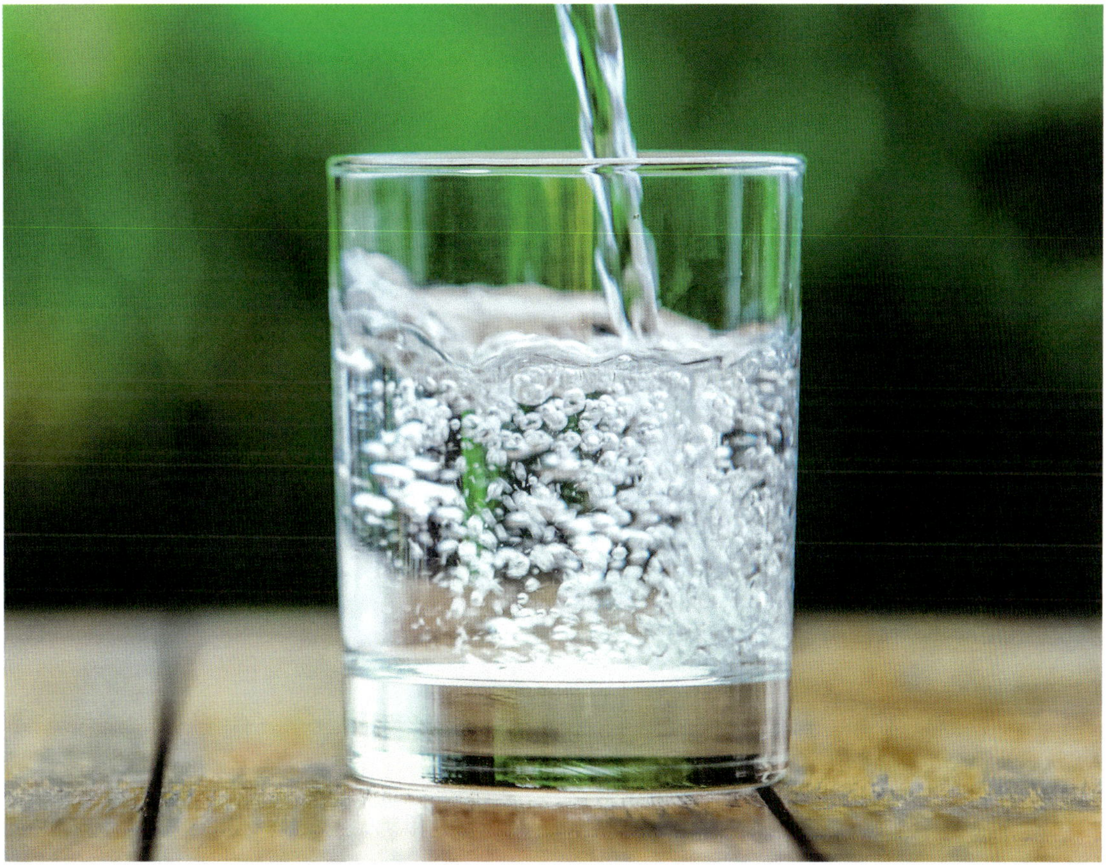

Water

- **What it does:**
  Drinking water helps maintain the balance of body fluids. Your body is composed of about 60% water. The functions of these bodily fluids include digestion, absorption, circulation, creation of saliva, transportation of nutrients, and maintenance of body temperature. Dehydration can be a major problem for older adults.

- **How much you need each day:**
  NHS guidelines recommend that older adults consume at least 6 to 8 glasses per day.

- **Alternative sources to water:**
  If you find drinking water rather boring then you can get water through liquid foods and beverages such as soup, milk, tea, coffee, soda, bottled mineral water and fruit juices, these all count towards your RDA intake.

A – Z Guide to other Vitamins and Minerals

Biotin (vitamin H)

- **What it does:**
  Biotin is good for skin, hair and nails it needs to be eaten daily as your body can't store it.

- **How much you need each day:**
  RDA is 150 micrograms.

- **Food sources:**
  Good sources are liver, eggs, nuts, brewer's yeast and dairy products.

Boron

- **What it does:**
  Boron is said to prevent calcium and magnesium loss from bones and may help with arthritis symptoms. It also helps the body use calcium.

- **How much you need each day:**
  RDA there are no accepted figures. Diets considered to be high in boron provide approximately 3.25 mg of boron per 2,000 kcal per day.

- **Food sources:**
  Boron is found in fresh fruits, for example, apples, pears and grapes; in dried fruits such as apricots and prunes. It is also found in nuts, peas, beans and green leafy vegetables.

Chondroitin

- **What it does:**
  Chondroitin helps keep cartilage healthy by absorbing fluid, particularly water into it and providing the building blocks to produce new cartilage. It has anti-inflammatory actions, controls the formation of new cartilage and improves the production of synovial fluid which is the 'oil' like fluid that lubricates joints.

- **How much you need each day:**
  The recommended dose is 400mg taken three times a day, or 600mg twice a day.

- **Food sources:**
  No food sources. Supplements are the only way to get more Chondroitin into your body.

Chromium

- **What it does:**
  Chromium is an essential trace element required for healthy skin, bone, muscle, hair and blood.

- **How much you need each day:**
  RDA is around 25 micrograms.

- **Food sources:**
  Chromium is found in asparagus, beetroot, black pepper, cheese, chicken, whole grains, eggs, liver, potato skins, vegetables and seafood.

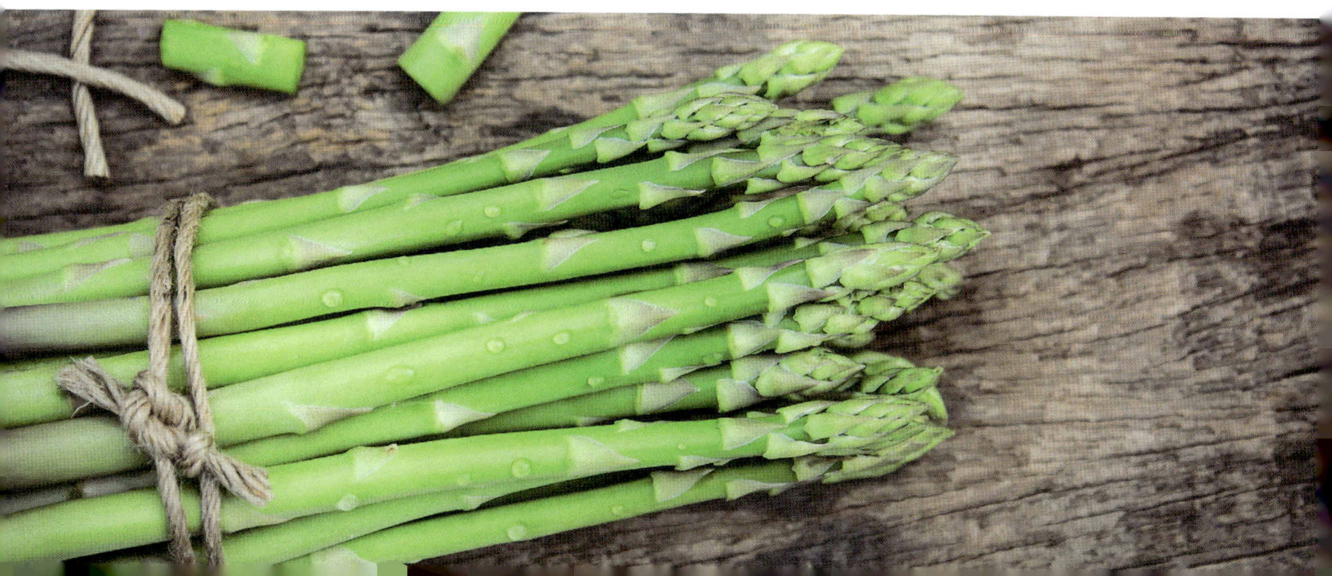

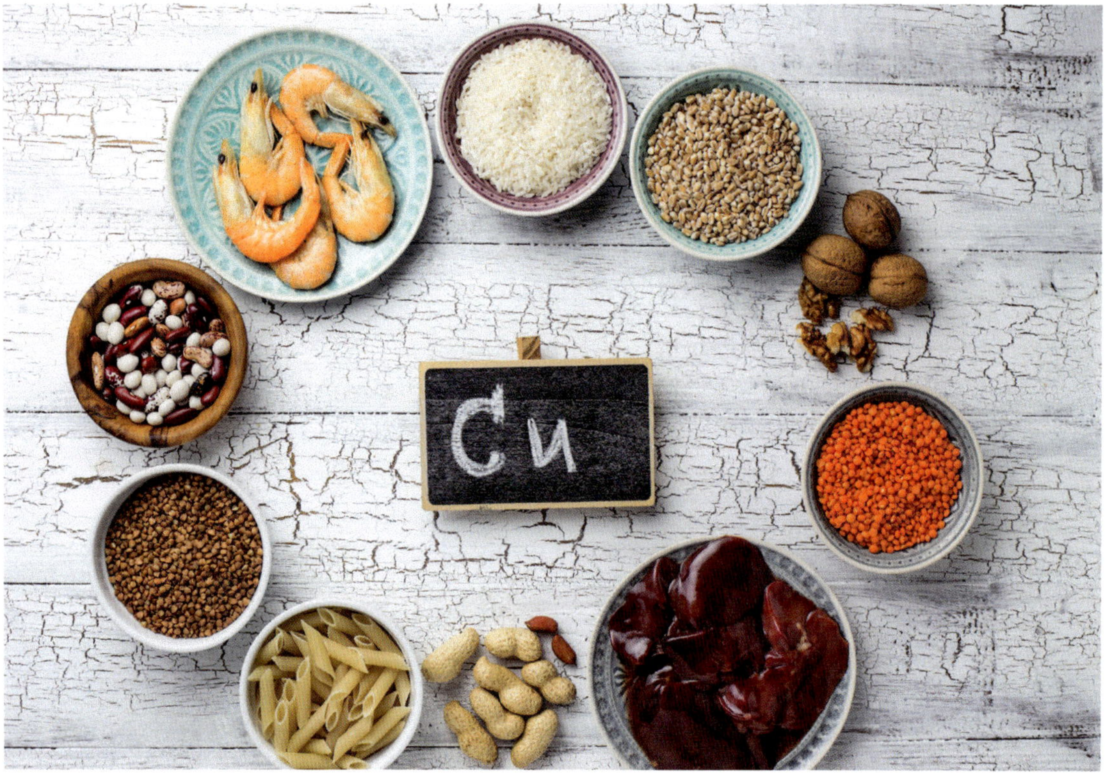

Copper

- **What it does:**
  Copper is needed by the immune system for fighting off infections. It is involved in iron absorption and haemoglobin production; it is also a co-factor in many enzymes. Copper also has a role in nerve transmissions within the brain.

- **How much you need each day:**
  RDA for Copper is 1.2 mg.

- **Food sources:**
  Copper is found in whole grains, seafood, liver, pulses, nuts and potatoes.

Glucosamine

- **What it does:**
  We need glucosamine to keep making synovial fluid, which is the 'oil' like fluid that lubricates joints and keeps cartilage healthy. Ageing cuts down the amount of glucosamine our bodies can make.

- **How much you need each day:**
  A typical dose is 1,500mg per day taken as a single dose or split into two or three separate doses taken through the day.

- **Food sources:**
  No food sources. The only way to increase the amount of glucosamine in your body is to take a suitable supplement.

Iodine

- **What it does:**
  Iodine is needed by the thyroid gland to produce the hormones used all over the body. These hormones help produce energy from fat, control cholesterol levels and keep weight stable. Iodine is also involved in reproduction, nerves and bone and to keep skin, hair, nails and teeth in good condition.

- **How much you need each day:**
  RDA up to 140 micrograms for adults.

- **Food sources:**
  Iodine is found in seafood, kelp and sea salt. It's also found in milk, eggs and meat, depending on the soil conditions and the diet of the animals.

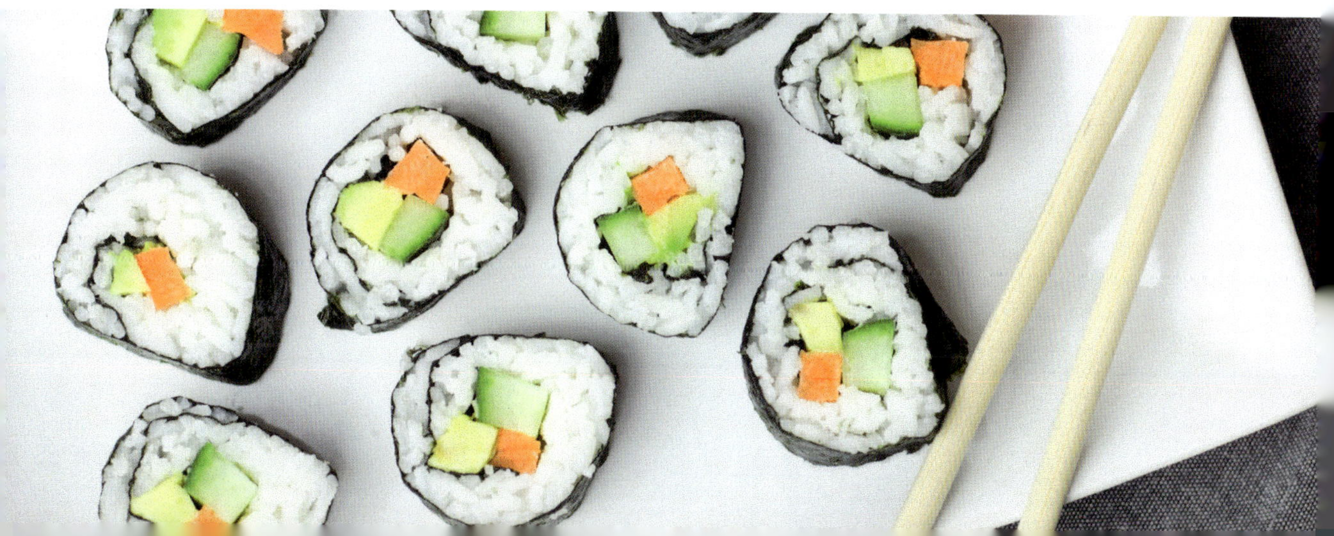

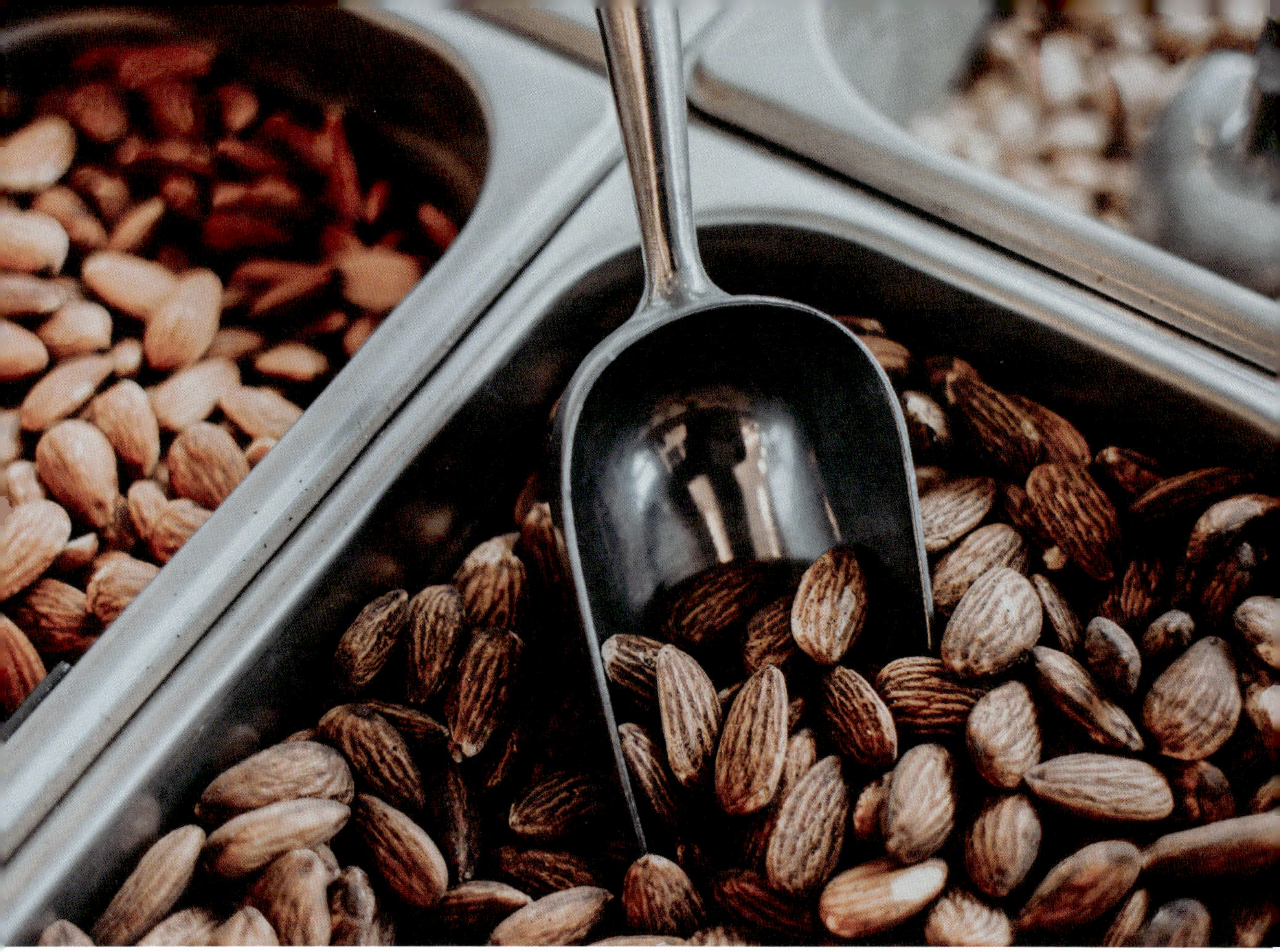

Manganese

- **What it does:**
  It is in at least 20 enzyme systems; is needed for making haemoglobin, bones, cartilage and hormones; it is essential in maintaining blood sugar levels, proper brain function and a healthy nervous system and supports the efficient use of vitamins B1, C, E and biotin.

- **How much you need each day:**
  There are no recommendations on daily intake in the UK, but the World Health Organisation notes a daily intake of 2.5 mg as the absolute minimum requirement.

- **Food sources:**
  Manganese is in a wide variety of plant food, vegetables and salad, pulses, nuts, whole grains, eggs, avocados, pears, bananas, and pineapple. It is also found in tea and coffee.

Molybdenum

- **What it does:**
  It is involved in metabolising food, helps healthy growth and development and aids iron and its uses.
- **How much you need each day:**
  RDA for adult men and women is 45 µg/day.
- **Food sources:**
  Molybdenum is found in whole grains, pulses, sweet potatoes, rice, liver, kidney, chicken, green vegetables, fruit and seafood.

Phosphorus

- **What it does:**
  Phosphorus is vital for energy production and enables the B vitamins to work properly.
- **How much you need each day:**
  RDA for Phosphorus is 550 milligrams.
- **Food sources:**
  Phosphorus is found in meat, poultry, eggs and seeds. Carbonated drinks, for example, colas contain a lot of phosphorus.

Silicon

- **What it does:**
  Silicon is found in trace amounts everywhere in the body, particularly in hair, nails and skin, where it strengthens and keeps cells supple. It also helps keep bones, cartilage, tendons and artery walls strong.
- **How much you need each day:**
  RDA is unknown; estimates vary widely.
- **Food sources:**
  Silicon is found mainly in plant fibres, especially whole grains, for example, wheat, oats, barley and rice. It is also in vegetables such as spinach, kale, onions and beetroot.

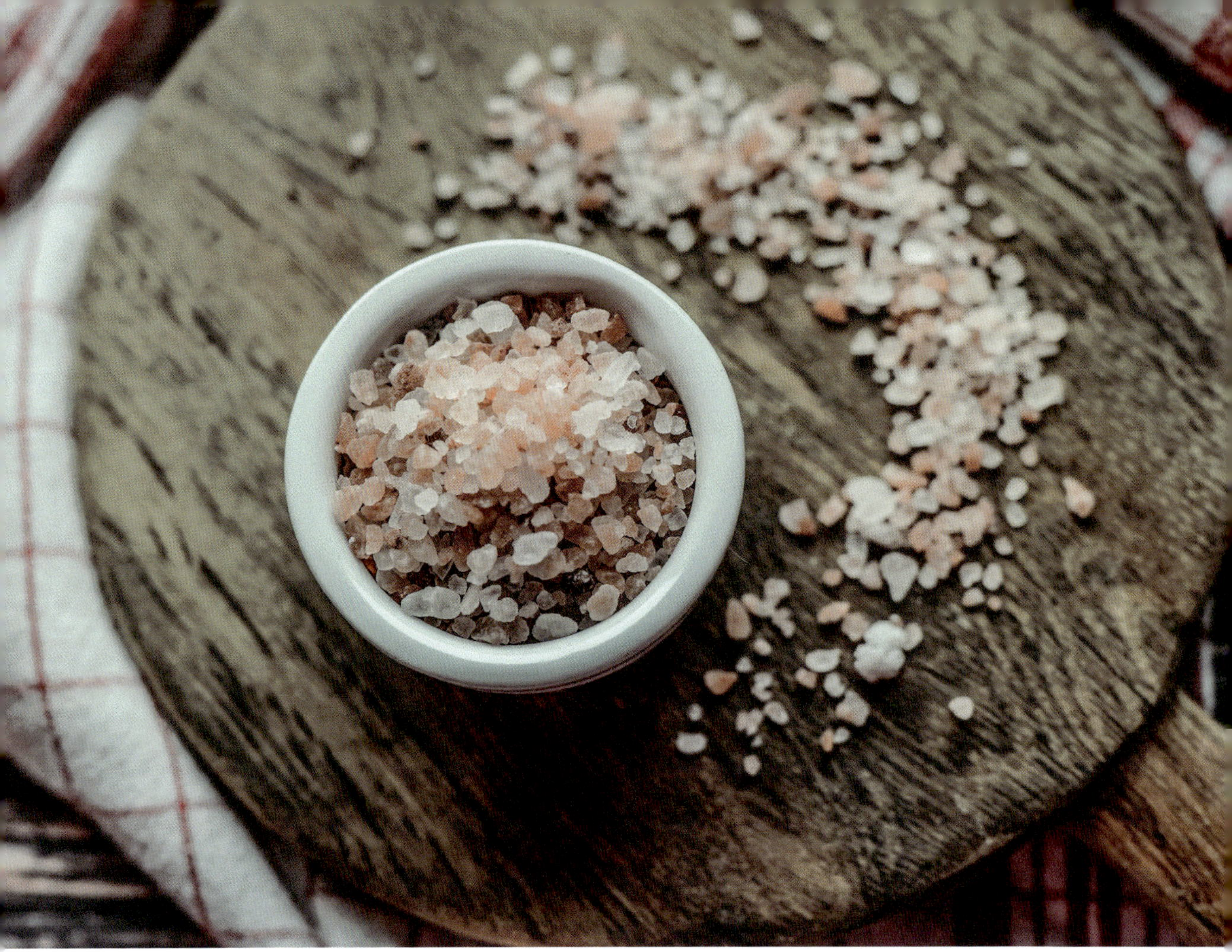

Sodium

- **What it does:**
  Sodium is an essential mineral and nutrient. It is involved in regulating blood pressure and blood volume, helps muscle and nerves work properly, and is concerned in the water balance throughout the body. It regulates the acid and alkali balance along with other minerals such as potassium, calcium and magnesium.

- **How much you need each day:**
  RDA is 2.4g of salt a day.

- **Food sources:**
  In the form of salt or sodium chloride, it is available everywhere. Around 10% naturally comes from root vegetables, milk and dairy products, oatmeal, celery and dried fruits.

Sulphur

- **What it does:**
  Sulphur has been called the 'beauty mineral' as it is found in skin, hair and nails.

- **How much you need each day:**
  There is no RDA for Sulphur.

- **Food sources:**
  Sulphur is found in protein foods such as eggs, meats, shellfish, garlic, lettuce, onions, raspberries, cabbage, turnip, kale and Brussels sprouts.

Vitamin A

- **What it does:**
  It plays a vital role throughout your body. It keeps the eyes in good condition, it boosts the immune system and it is known to reduce the risk of cancer.

- **How much you need each day:**
  RDA is 600 micrograms for women and 700 micrograms for men.

- **Food sources:**
  Vitamin A is obtained from animal foods such as liver, milk and eggs. Carotenoids are in fruit and vegetables, for example, peaches, mangoes, pineapples, apricots, carrots, broccoli and kale.

Vitamin B1

- **What it does:**
  Vitamin B1 is essential for energy; it keeps your nerves in good condition and is also associated with preventing cataracts and the development of arthritis. It is thought to help treat depression and memory loss.

- **How much you need each day:**
  RDA is 1.0 (19-64yrs), 0.9 (65-74yrs), 0.9 (75+yrs) mg for men, and 0.8 (19-64yrs), 0.8 (65-74yrs), 0.7 (75+yrs) mg for women.

- **Food sources:**
  Vitamin B1 is found in whole grains, sunflower seeds, seafood, bacon, beans, potatoes and nuts.

Vitamin B2

- **What it does:**
  Vitamin B2 keeps skin, hair and nails healthy. It is also required for maintaining good eyesight

- **How much you need each day:**
  RDA is 1.3 mg for men and 1.1 mg for women.

- **Food sources:**
  Vitamin B2 is found in many foods, including liver, cheese, eggs, breakfast cereals, milk and green vegetables.

Vitamin B3

- **What it does:**
  Vitamin B3 helps release energy from breaking down the food we eat. It also helps lower cholesterol and works to keep our brain, digestion and skin in good working order.

- **How much you need each day:**
  RDA is 16.5 (19-64yrs), 15.5 (65-74yrs), 15.1 (75+yrs) mg for men, and 13.2 (19-64yrs), 12.6 (65-74yrs), 12.1 (75+yrs) mg for women.

- **Food sources:**
  The main sources for Vitamin B3 are nuts, potatoes, chicken, fish and beans. Fortified breakfast cereals also contain vitamin B3.

Vitamin B5

- **What it does:**
  Vitamin B5 is an anti-stress vitamin and has a role in cholesterol and steroid hormone production. It is also involved in metabolism generally and helps keep skin, muscle and nerves healthy.

- **How much you need each day:**
  The RDA is 5 micrograms.

- **Food sources:**
  Vitamin B5 is found in foods including liver, nuts, wheat germ, pulses, salmon, eggs, raspberries, oranges and broccoli.

Vitamin B6

- **What it does:**
  Vitamin B6 is important as it is involved in many processes in your body. It works to make the chemicals that transmit nerve impulses and in making red blood cells. It also has a role in keeping your immune system in good working order. It plays a part in keeping female hormones in balance and it keeps skin healthy.

- **How much you need each day:**
  RDA is 1.4 mg for men and 1.2 mg for women.

- **Food sources:**
  Sources of vitamin B6 include beef, chicken, eggs, fish, bananas, potatoes and sunflower seeds. Intestinal bacteria can also make some vitamin B6.

Vitamin B9 – Folic acid

- **What it does:**
  Folic acid is important for the growth and division of all cells; blood, skin, hair, nerve, brain cells, everything that makes up your body.

- **How much you need each day:**
  RDA is 200 micrograms.

- **Food sources:**
  Folic Acid is found in spinach, broccoli, Brussels sprouts, lettuce, peas and some fortified foods such as wholemeal bread and cereals.

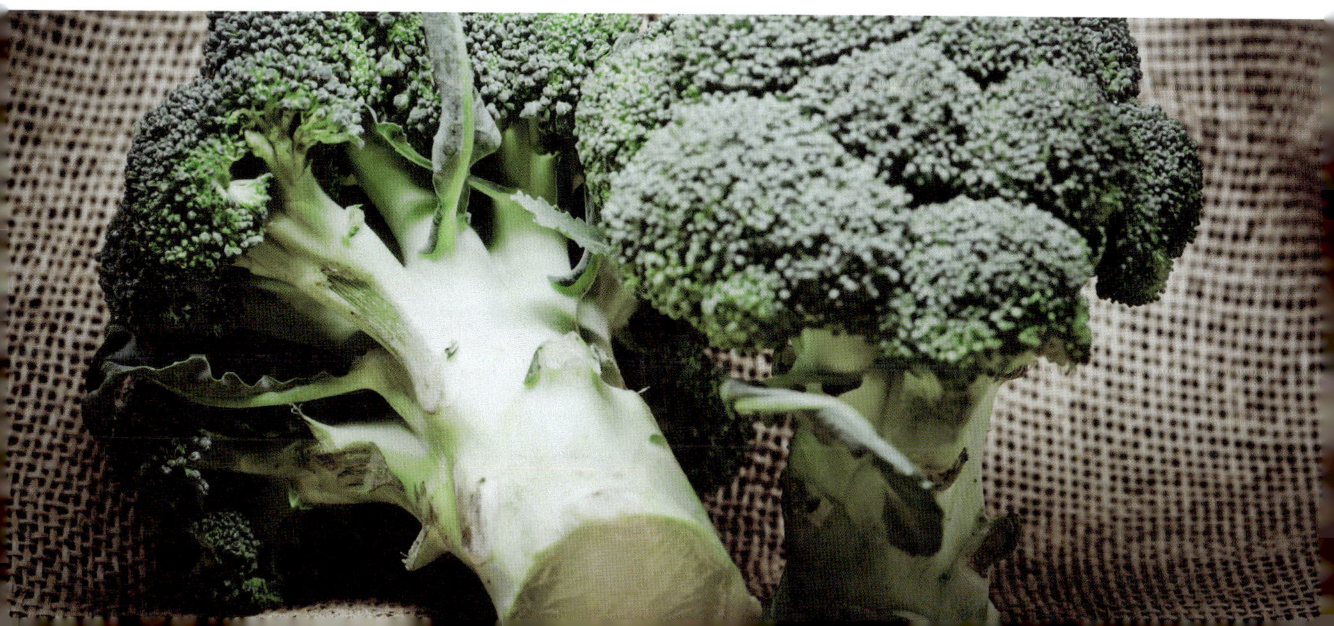

Vitamin C

- **What it does:**
  Vitamin C is necessary for a healthy immune system, to fight colds, infections and illness generally. It is useful in protecting us from strokes and cataracts and helps the healing process of wounds and after surgery.

- **How much you need each day:**
  RDA is 60 mg.

- **Food sources:**
  Vitamin C is found in abundance in fresh fruits such as oranges, grapefruit, blackcurrants, kiwi fruit, lemons and strawberries, as well as in fresh vegetables such as peppers, tomatoes and Brussels sprouts.

Vitamin E

- **What it does:**
  It protects from a wide range of conditions associated with ageing, including heart disease, stroke, arthritis, diabetes, Alzheimer's disease and cancers. It also helps fertility, stamina and endurance as well as boosting your immune system against infections.

- **How much you need each day:**
  RDA is 4 mg a day for men and 3 mg a day for women.

- **Food sources:**
  Vitamin E is found in many foods, such as cod liver oil, sunflower and olive oil, nuts, beans, bananas, apples, lettuce, spinach, onions, Brussels sprouts, prawns and salmon.

Vitamin K

- **What it does:**
  Vitamin K is important for blood to clot properly and for teeth and bones to form correctly.

- **How much you need each day:**
  Adults need approximately 1 microgram a day of vitamin K for each kilogram of their body weight.

- **Food sources:**
  Vitamin K is found in green vegetables, cereals, cheese, liver, eggs and beef.

Zinc

- **What it does:**
  Zinc is required for a healthy immune system, wound healing, maintenance of the senses of taste and smell, for DNA synthesis. It is also necessary for the proper function of many hormones, for example, insulin, growth and sex hormones. Every cell in the body needs zinc to allow it to multiply.
- **How much you need each day:**
  The RDA is 7 mg for women and 9.5 mg for men.
- **Food sources:**
  Most animal foods contain zinc, including shellfish, red meat, eggs, fish, poultry, milk, yogurt and cheese. It is also in shiitake mushrooms, whole grains, nuts, mustard, chilli powder ginger and black pepper.

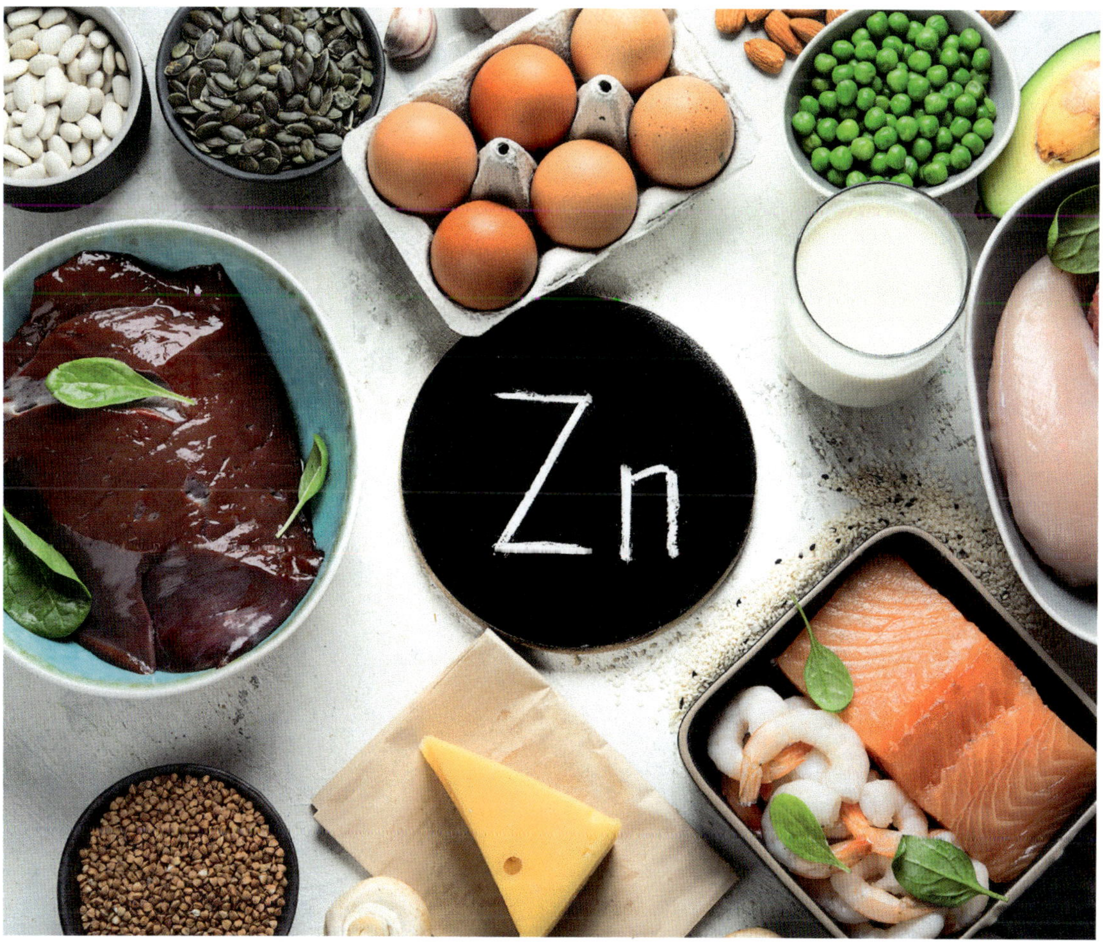

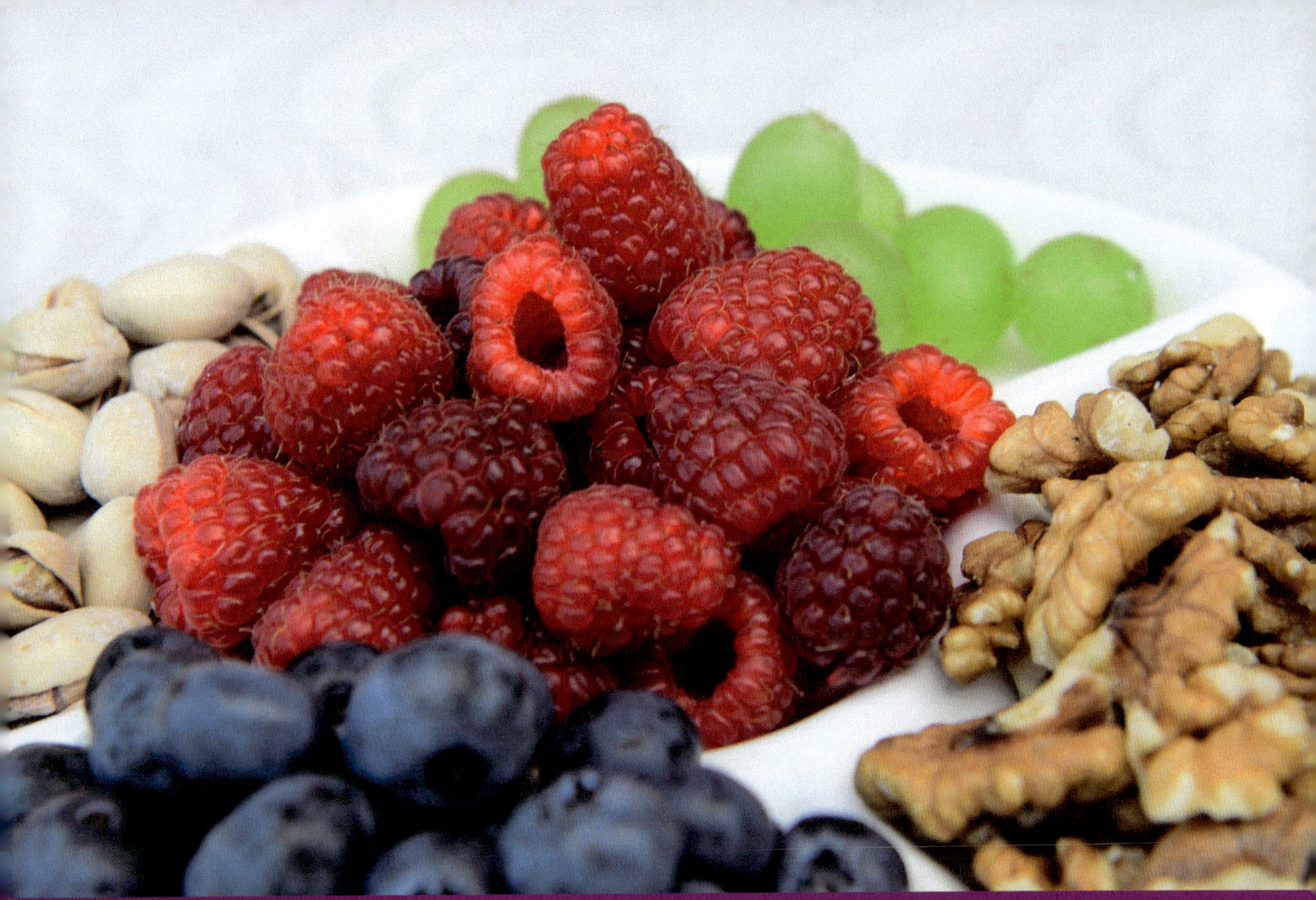

"Exercise and food, what you put in, is what you get back out."

CHAPTER 15

Simple Steps To A Healthy Diet

We all know that we should eat a healthy balanced diet but when you begin to read up on what this means, the sheer volume of information can seem overwhelming. For those that seek a healthier lifestyle, it's a topic that's certainly worth exploring. Here's the thing; basic healthy nutrition is really quite simple. Take these simple steps to a healthier diet.

Step 1 – Make it real food not processed food

Eat real food rather than processed food. What's real food? Real food is fish, meat, vegetables, fruit, nuts, seeds, whole grains, pulses and beans. Try hard to avoid food that is mass-produced ready-made meals, emulsified and with a long-shelf-life. Switching to eating real foods naturally leads you to eat more-nutrient rich food without much thought.

Step 2 – Opt for lean protein

Look life is for living so it's perfectly okay to indulge once in a while in a cooked breakfast and even the occasional hamburger or takeaway. However, on a daily-basis, there is an array of great lean proteins to choose from. Some good meat-free options include peas, quinoa, beans, lentils, tofu, low-fat yogurt and low-fat milk. Fish is another perfect source of protein that can also be rich in healthy omega-3's. When it comes to your weekly shop, cuts of meat that have fillet or loin in the name are usually the leanest and chicken and turkey breast.

Step 3 – Go for complex carbohydrates

When it comes to carbohydrates (carbs) you'll find the more natural and whole they are the better they are for you. Go for complex carbs such as 100% whole grain pasta, brown rice, bread, legumes, starchy vegetables, nuts, seeds, low-fat dairy and decent amounts of fruits and vegetables. Make sure you try to reduce your intake of simple sugars from refined grains and particularly from processed snack foods, sweets and sugar-sweetened hot drinks.

Step 4 – Eat healthy fats

While many people think a healthy diet is a fat-free diet it is important to eat healthy fats as part of a balanced diet. So add avocados, nuts, seeds and oily fatty fish such as tuna and salmon into your weekly diet. And if you cook with oil make sure you choose healthy oils such as olive oil in place of butter or lard. Consider making your own salad dressings with flaxseed oil for a healthy dose of omega-3's.

Step 5 – Eat colourful foods

Include colourful foods into all your meals from dark greens to red berries, yellow peppers and purple onions. Why? Well because the colours in fruits, vegetables and even proteins are associated with important vitamins and minerals. So eating a rainbow of colourful foods, particularly fruits and vegetables, is a brilliant and simple way to get a wide variety of micronutrients in your diet.

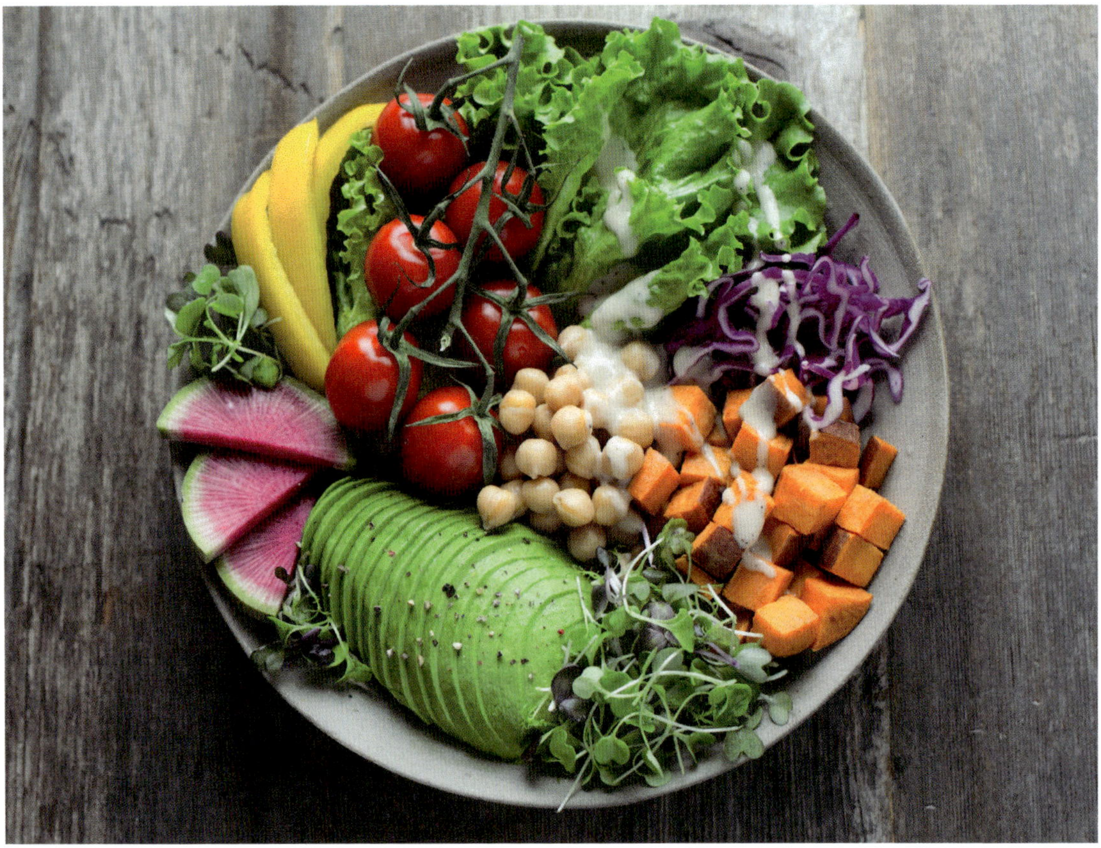

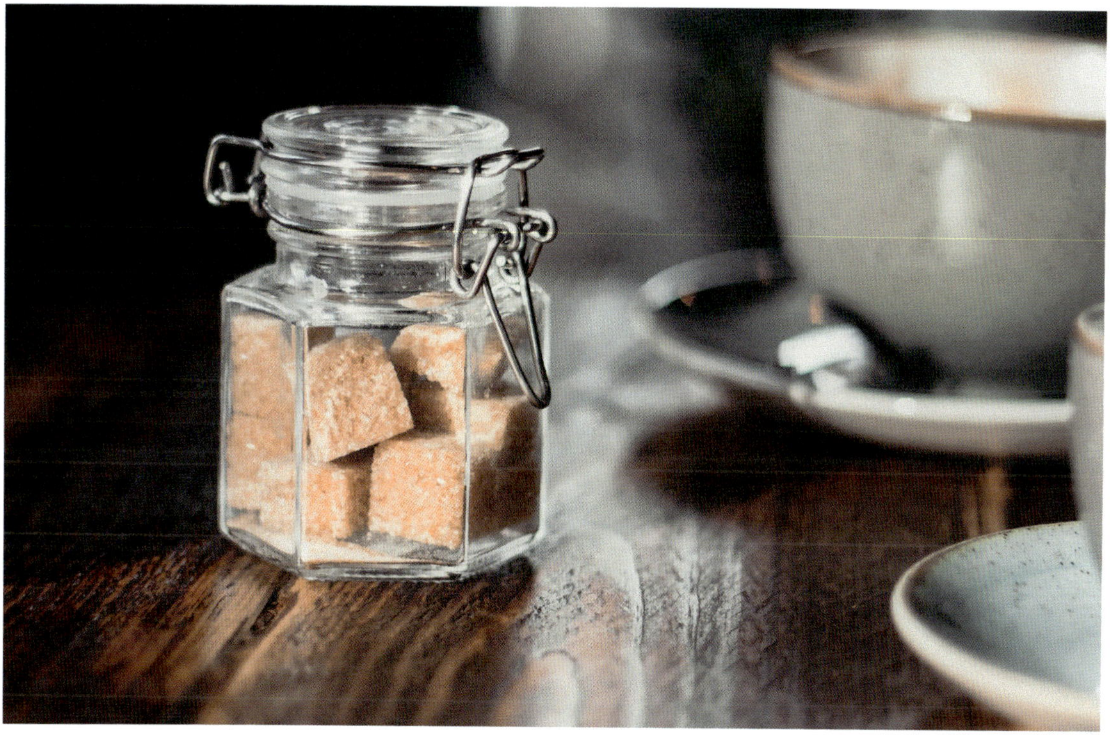

Step 6 – Minimise sugary foods

In its natural unprocessed state sugar is a relatively harmless and even necessary carbohydrate that our wonderful bodies need to function. The natural sugar found in fruits, vegetables and dairy as the compound fructose or lactose is good for you. The problem arises when sugar is added to foods such as ready meals during processing for added flavour, colour and texture. Eating too many of these empty sugary calories has many detrimental health effects, the most obvious being weight gain. Added sugar also drives your insulin levels up, messes around with your metabolism and causes those calories to turn right into belly fat. So keep it natural sugar all the way, and if you can't drink your tea and coffee without it being sweet, then go for a natural sweetener instead.

Step 7 – Balance & control your food portions

Make sure that you eat a balance of proteins, carbohydrates and fats at every meal and choose foods that are rich in fibre, vitamins and minerals. A great way to do this is to fill your plate with three to four different food groups. Eat a combination of protein-rich foods, whole grain, dairy, fruits and vegetables, and add in the food groups that you may have missed at earlier meals.

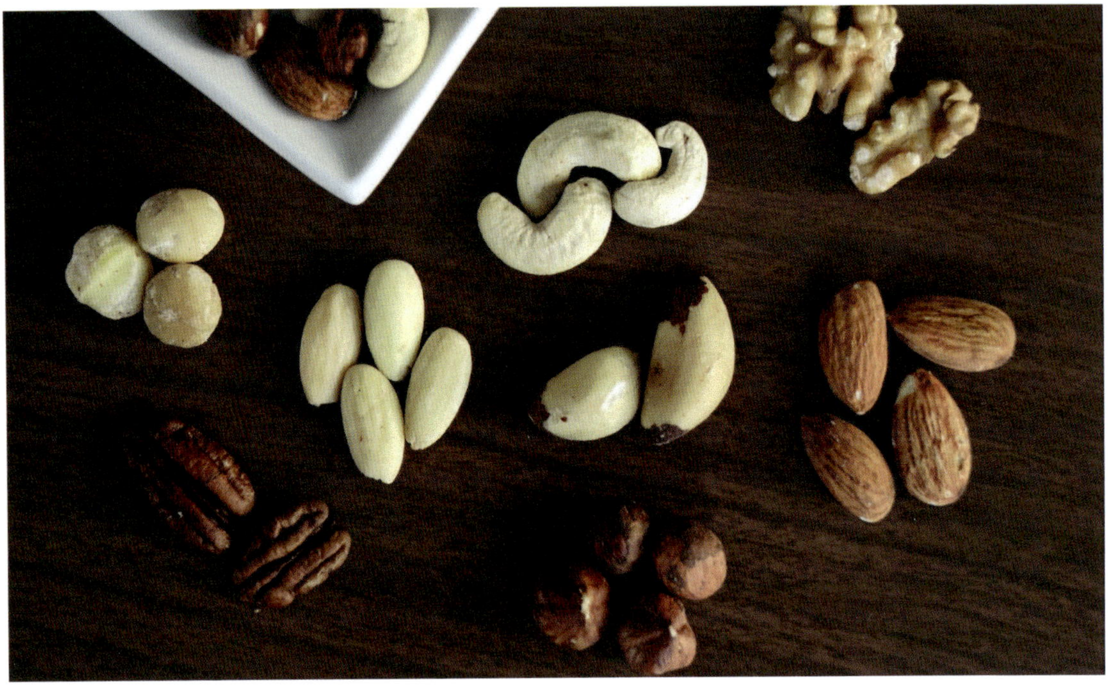

Step 8 – Eat smart snacks

Now as a Brighton and Hove based personal trainer I'll admit I like to snack, I'm always on the go and often the luxury of a lunch-break is not on the menu. However, snack time is when processed foods are the easiest to grab and I'll also admit the odd chocolate bar passes across my lips. However, most of the time I go for a smart snack. So arm yourself with real food snacks that are as minimally processed as possible. So, what exactly is a smart snack? Well take your pick from these tasty treats:

- Fresh fruit, apples, pears, oranges and bananas are my go-to fruits
- Unsweetened dried fruits, think apricots, mango and figs
- Whole grain crackers and rice cakes
- Nuts
- Yogurt
- Dark chocolate, a little is perfectly fine
- Celery sticks
- Carrot sticks
- Pepper sticks
- Mozzarella sticks
- Hard-boiled eggs

These steps will help you make changes to a healthier diet. Any diet must be a balanced diet in order for you to get all the vitamins, minerals and trace elements to main your physical health. I'm an advocate of the NHS Eatwell Plate, which is a simple guide to how to eat and keep to a balanced diet. You do not need to achieve this balance with every meal, but it is sensible to try and get the balance right over a day or over a week.

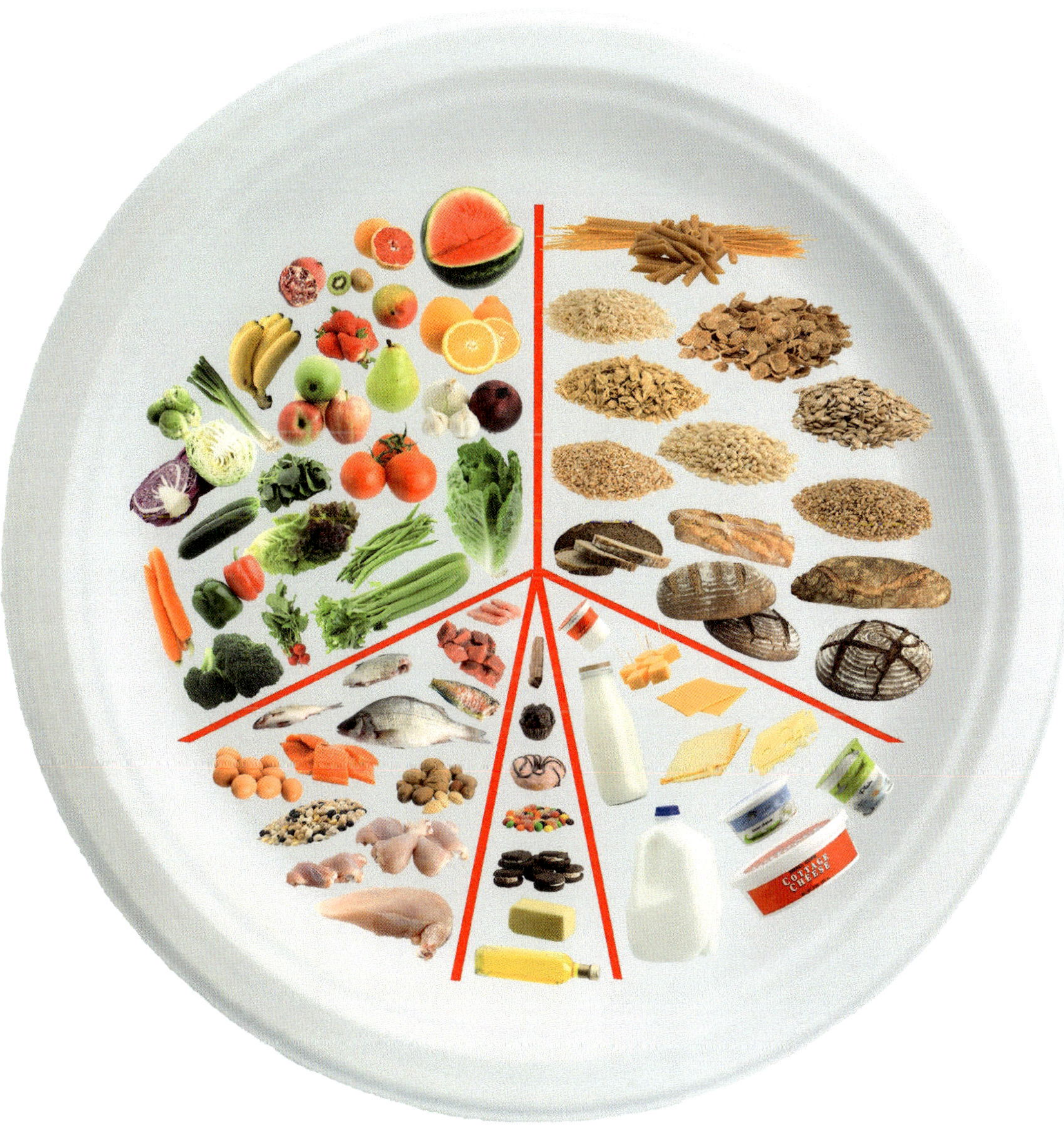

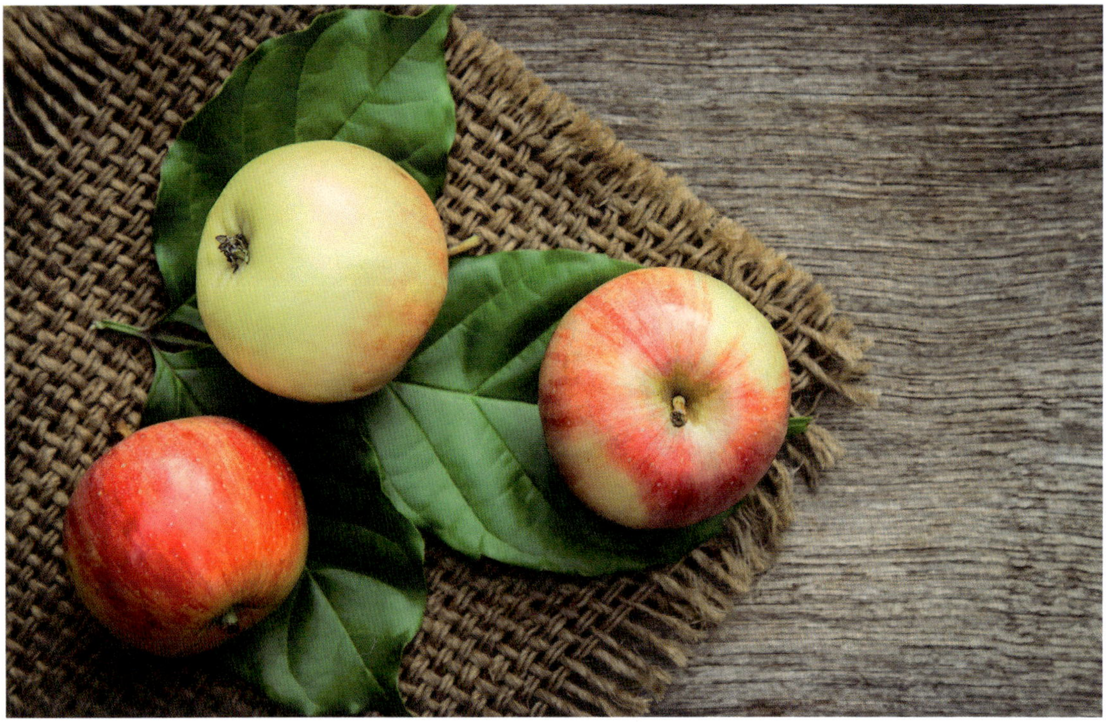

Fruit & Vegetables

- Eat at least 5 portions of a variety of fruit and vegetables every day. Most of us still are not eating enough fruit and vegetables. They should make up over a third of the food we eat each day. Fruit juice and smoothies should be limited to no more than a combined total of 160ml a day.
- Fruit and vegetables are also a great source of vitamins, minerals and fibre.

Potatoes, bread, rice, pasta and other starchy carbohydrates

- Choose whole grain or higher fibre versions of these foods with less added fat, salt and sugar.
- Base meals on potatoes, bread, rice, pasta or other starchy carbohydrates.
- Starchy food should make up just over a third of the food we eat. Choose higher fibre whole grain varieties, such as whole wheat pasta and brown rice, or simply leave skins on potatoes. There are also higher fibre versions of white bread and pasta. Starchy foods are a good source of energy and the main source of a range of nutrients in our diet.

Oils and spreads

- Choose unsaturated oils and use in small amounts.
- Eat these in small amounts. Unsaturated fats are healthier fats and include vegetable, rapeseed, olive and sunflower oils. Remember all types of fat are high in energy and should be eaten sparingly.

Dairy and alternatives

- Choose lower fat and lower sugar options. Have some dairy or dairy alternatives, for example, soya drinks and yogurts.
- Milk, cheese, yogurt and fromage frais are good sources of protein and some vitamins, and they're also an important source of calcium, which helps keep your bones strong. Try to go for lower fat and lower sugar products where possible, like 1% fat milk, reduced-fat cheese or plain low-fat yogurt.

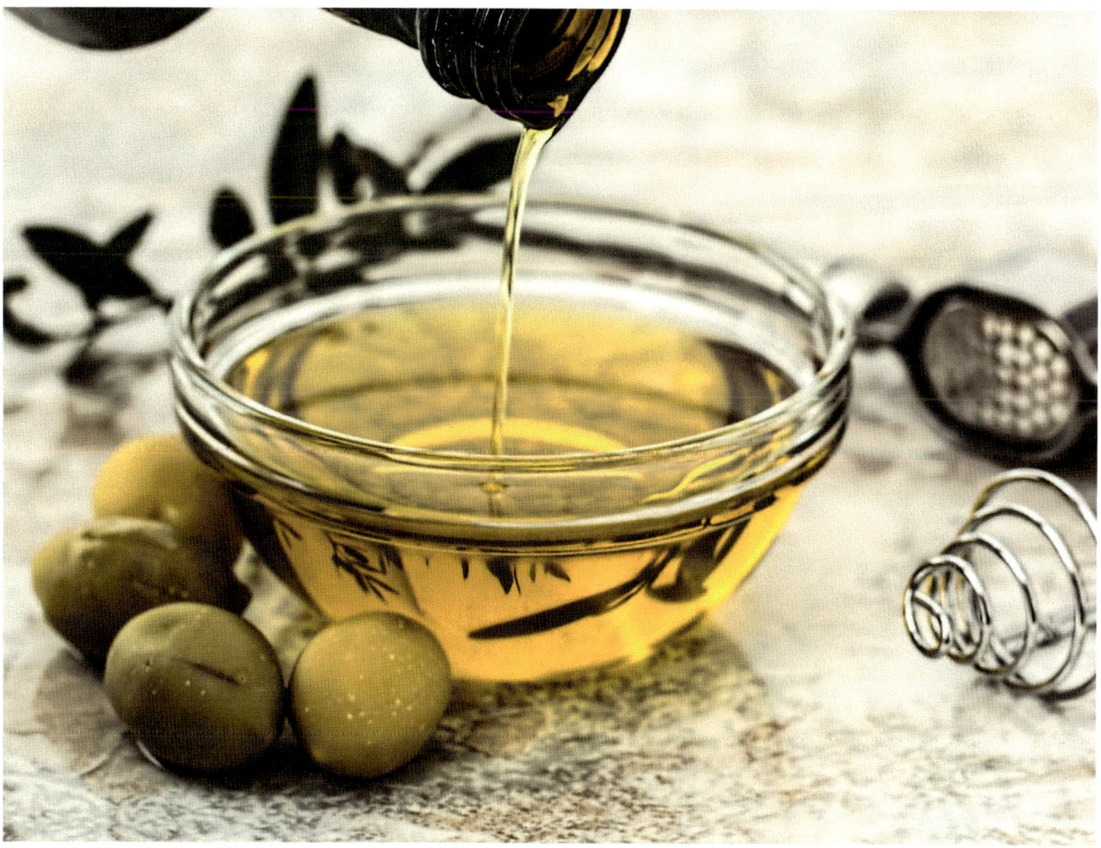

Beans, pulses, fish, eggs, meat and other proteins

- Eat more beans and pulses, 2 portions of sustainably sourced fish per week, one of which is oily. Eat less red and processed meat.
- These foods are good sources of protein, vitamins and minerals. Pulses, such as beans, peas and lentils, are good alternatives to meat because they're lower in fat and higher in fibre and protein, too.
- Choose lean cuts of meat and mince, and eat less red and processed meat like bacon, ham and sausages. Aim for at least 2 portions of fish every week, 1 of which should be oily, such as tuna, salmon or mackerel. Tinned tuna, sardines, salmon and other oily fish is also a good choice, if fresh oily fish is not easy to find.

Fluids, water, tea, coffee, fruit juices and squash

- Drink plenty of fluids the government recommends 6 to 8 cups or glasses a day.
- Water, lower-fat milk and lower sugar or sugar-free drinks, including tea and coffee, all count. Limit smoothies and fruit juice to 160ml each day.

Recommended daily calorie intake

- Men: 2,600kcal
- Women: 2,000kcal

Source: NHS

For more information visit:
www.nhs.uk/live-well/eat-well/the-eatwell-guide/

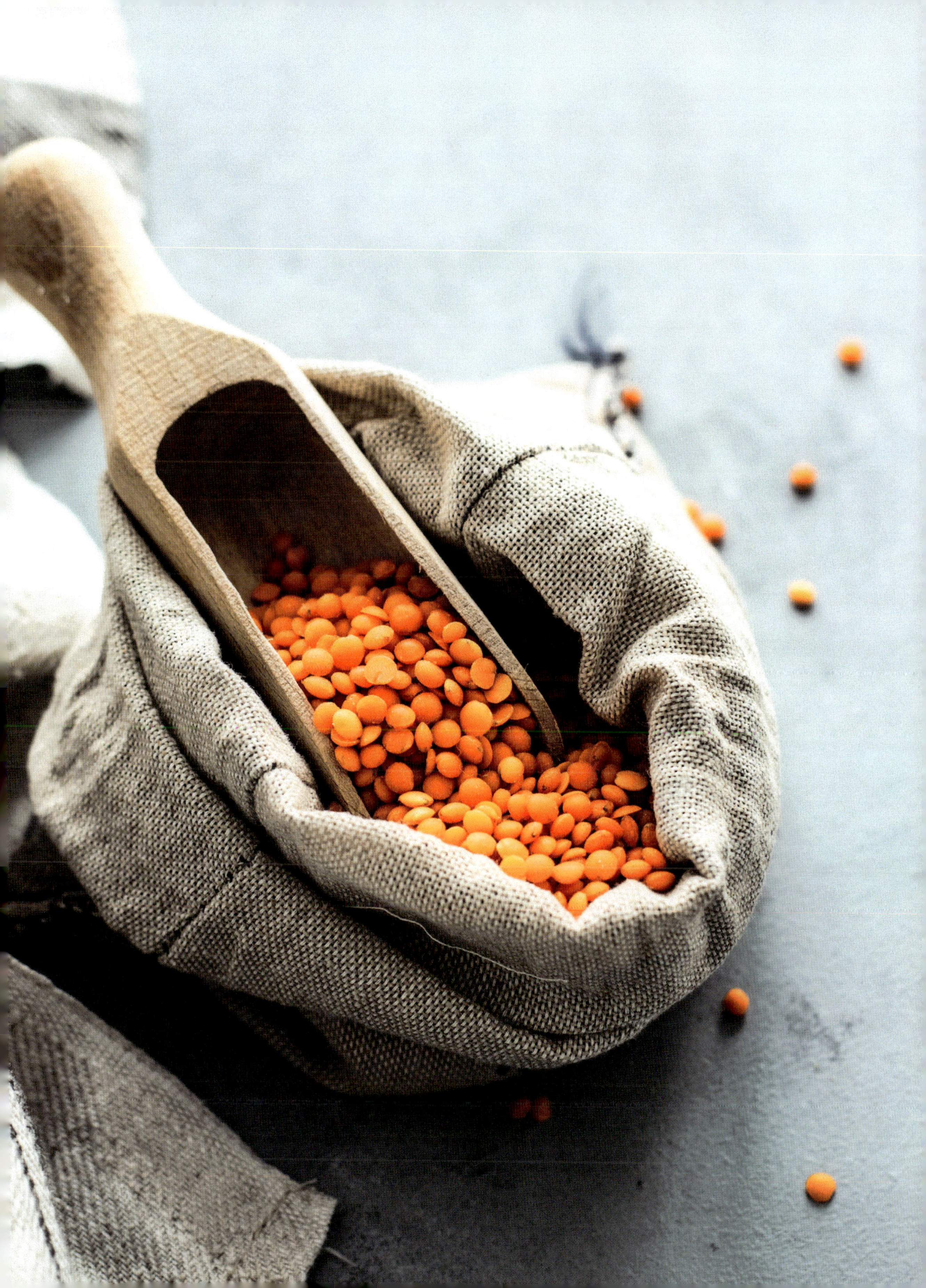

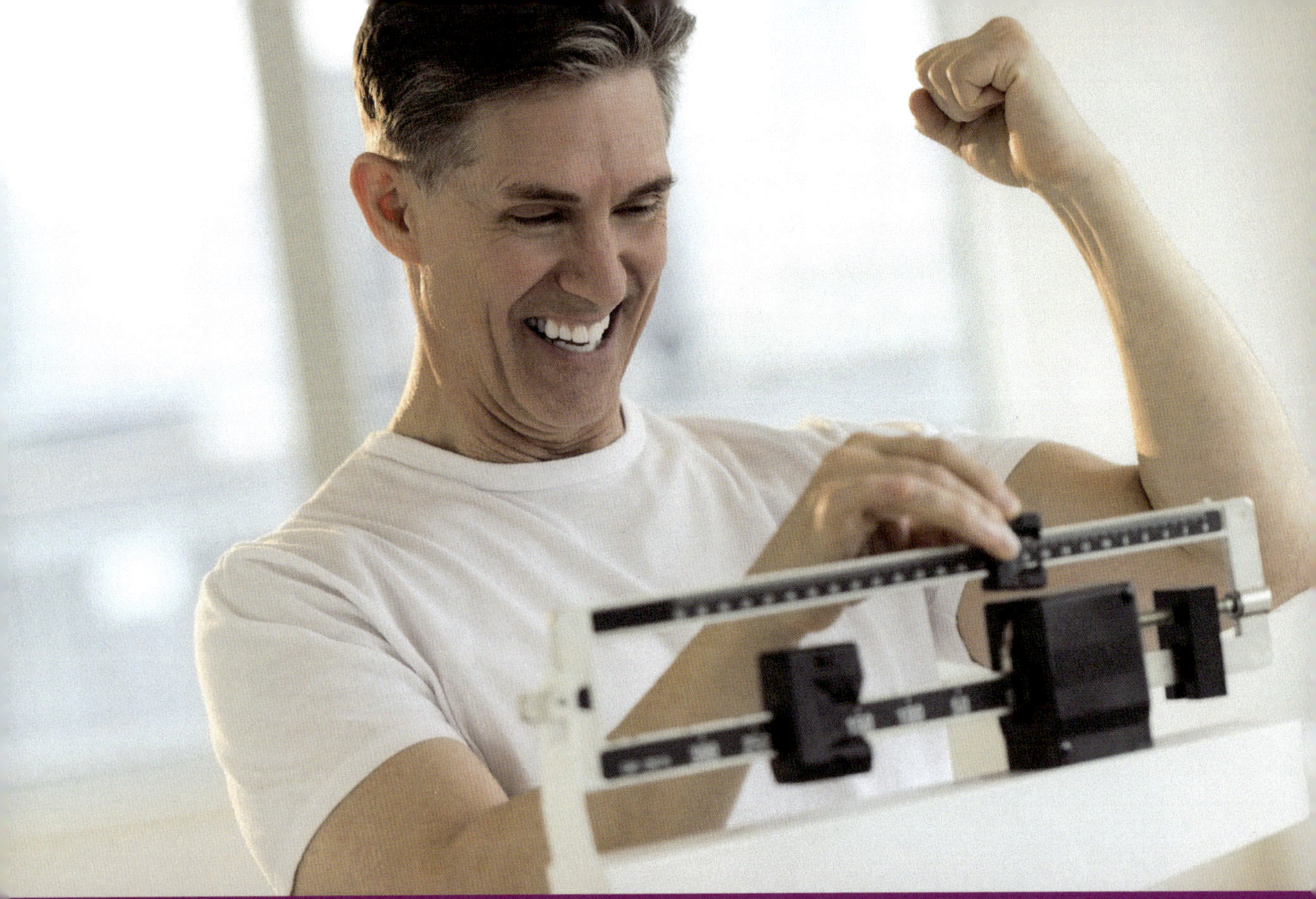

"Don't wish exercising and dieting was easier. Wish that you were fitter and healthier."

CHAPTER 16

How Knowing Your Body Mass Index & Basal Metabolic Rate Can Help Dieting

What is Basal Metabolic Rate?

Basal Metabolic Rate, also known as BMR, is the amount of energy your body burns at rest daily. In other words, it is the number of calories required to keep your body functioning while you are not doing any physical activities.

A deeper understanding of Basal Metabolic Rate

Even when you are resting your body is using energy to function effectively. Your body is making your heart pump blood through your veins, for example. Or your stomach is processing the food you just ate. This process is better known as your Basal Metabolic Rate. Your body consumes almost 70% of the calories to function effectively. Calories are also the first metric for you to take into consideration when losing weight. Here your BMR comes into play. Increasing your muscle mass helps your BMR. By gaining more muscles the number of calories you burn increases and this will help you to decrease body fat. Your BMR measurement can be used as a baseline for a diet programme. Extra calories can be included depending on your level of activity. The more active you are the more calories you will burn. Next to this, you'll build more muscle mass. This means that you need to keep a close eye on the number of calories you consume to keep your body fit and healthy.

How do you calculate your Basal Metabolic Rate?

The maths behind this is a little complicated, fear not, there are several free online calculations to use. There are four bits of data to enter; your age, gender, height in centimetres and weight in kilos. There are some slight variations to calculate your BMR, I use the one attributed to Harris-Benedict. You'll see this as an option on the online calculator.

I use **www.calculator.net/bmr-calculator.html**

If you want to do the maths yourself the Revised Harris-Benedict Equation is:

For men:
BMR = 13.397 x Weight kg + 4.799 x Height cm - 5.677 x Age + 88.362

For women:
BMR = 9.247 x Weight kg + 3.098 x Height cm - 4.330 x Age + 447.593

Example:
Using my details: Weight 87 kg, Height 189 cm, Age 53
BMR = **1,860** Calories per day

Activity Level	Calorie
Sedentary: little or no exercise	2,232
Exercise 1-3 times/week	2,558
Exercise 4-5 times/week	2,725
Daily exercise or intense exercise 3-4 times/week	2,883
Intense exercise 6-7 times/week	3,209
Very intense exercise daily, or physical job	3,534

As a personal trainer I exercise daily, therefore adjusting my BMR for the level of my physical activity shows that I need to consume 2,883 calories per day to keep my body functioning.

Now if I wanted to diet, aiming to lose 0.5 kg to 1.0 kg (1 to 2 pounds) per week, then I would simply take my BMR result and subtract 500 calories per day:

2,883 - 500 = 2,383 calories per day

Question

Using the BMR Calculator above, what is your BMR result?

Body Mass Index (BMI)

What is your Body Mass Index?

Your BMI is a measurement that is a ratio of your weight and height. It's a good way to gauge whether your weight is in healthy proportion to your height. In fact, knowing your BMI can help you and your doctor determine any health risks you may face if it's outside of the healthy range.

Being **overweight** can lead to a range of chronic conditions including:

- Type 2 diabetes
- High blood pressure
- Cardiovascular disease
- Musculoskeletal problems
- Heart or blood vessel problems

Being **underweight** can result in other health issues like:

- Anaemia
- Osteoporosis
- Risk of malnutrition

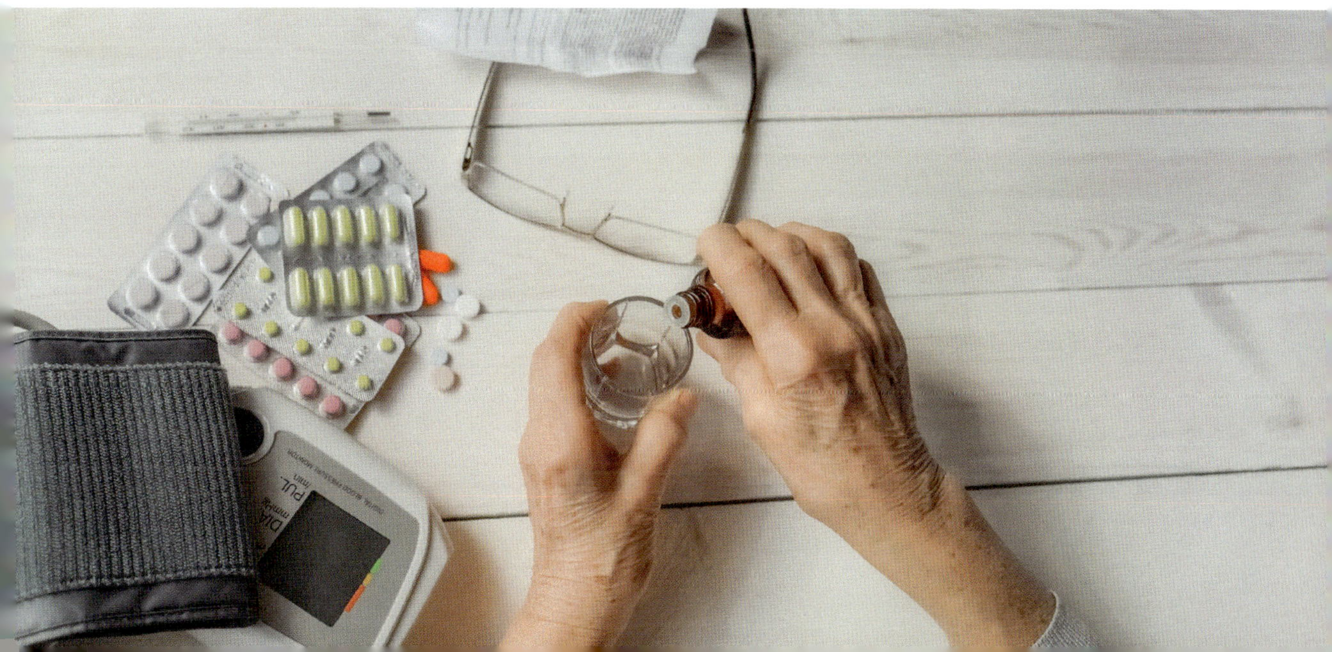

How to calculate your Body Mass Index

Simply divide your weight in kilograms by your height in metres squared. As with calculating your BMR, there are several online BMI calculators. I use the NHS one: **www.nhs.uk/live-well/healthy-weight/bmi-calculator/** For example, if you weigh 70kg and you are 185cm tall your BMI calculation will look like this:

$$BMI = \frac{70}{1.85^2} = 20.4$$

The BMI scale

18.5 to 24.9 = healthy
25 to 29.9 = overweight
30 and above = obese
18.4 and under = underweight

BMI is a good measure of your health, but it's not perfect

While it may be a great guide to establishing the amount of body fat you carry, your BMI doesn't take into consideration your age, sex, ethnicity, or even muscle mass. There have also been some suggestions by health experts that for older adults a BMI of 25 to 27 is more appropriate. Nonetheless, it's useful to know what your BMI before you start a calorie-controlled diet. Chat through with your doctor as he or she may offer guidance on what BMI you should aim for.

Question

Using the NHS BMI Calculator above, what is your BMI result?

Question

Thinking about your current diet, how many calories do you eat on a daily basis?

If you don't know, use the 3-Day Food Diary sheet in the **GET FIT TOOL KIT** to record what you eat over a typical three days. Please don't change your diet to do this. Then by using the **A-Z CALORIE COUNTS FOR POPULAR FOOD LISTS** also found in the **GET FIT TOOL KIT**, work out how many calories you ate for each day. Compare these to your BMR result. This will help you decide whether you're eating too many, too little or just about the right number of calories.

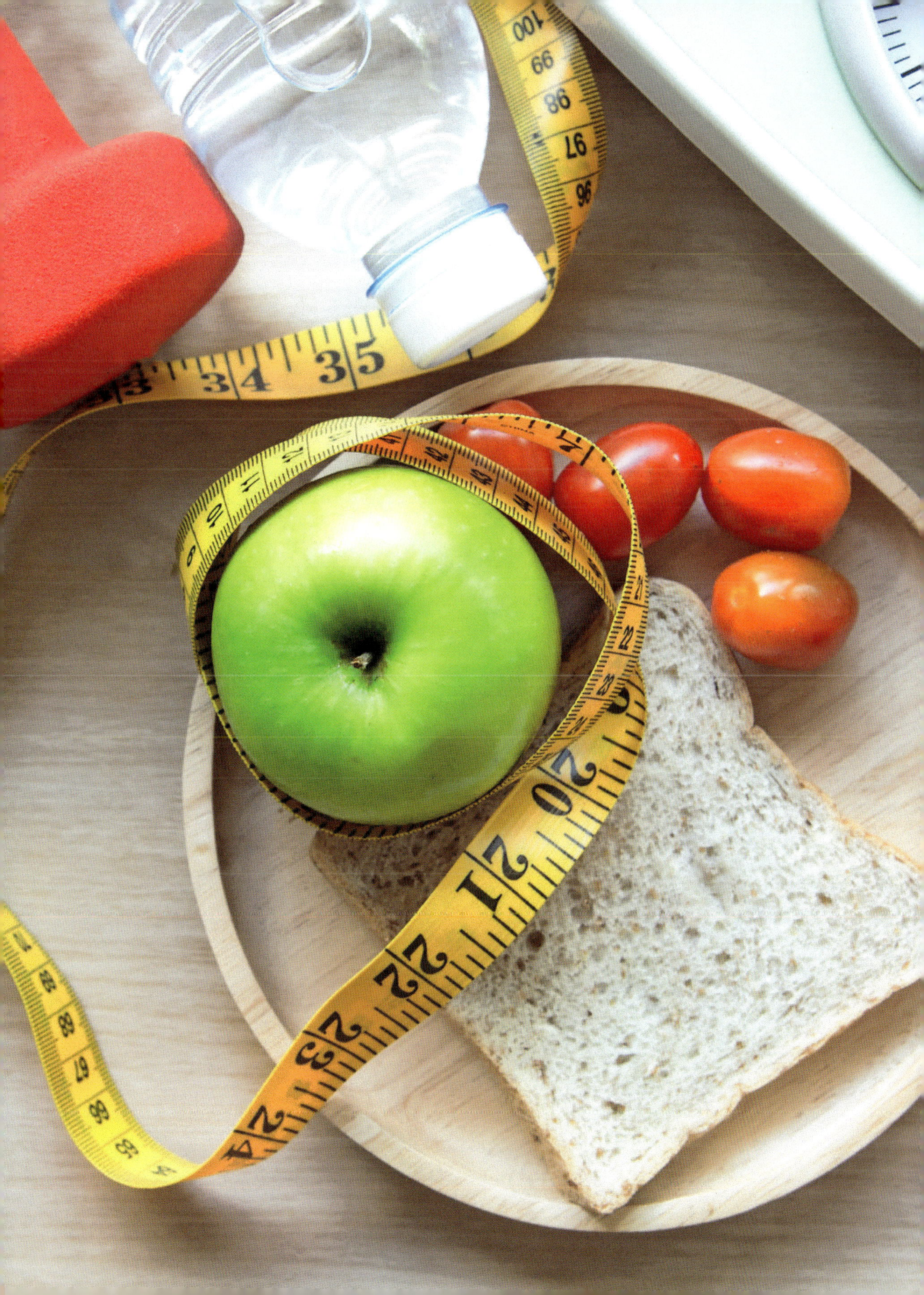

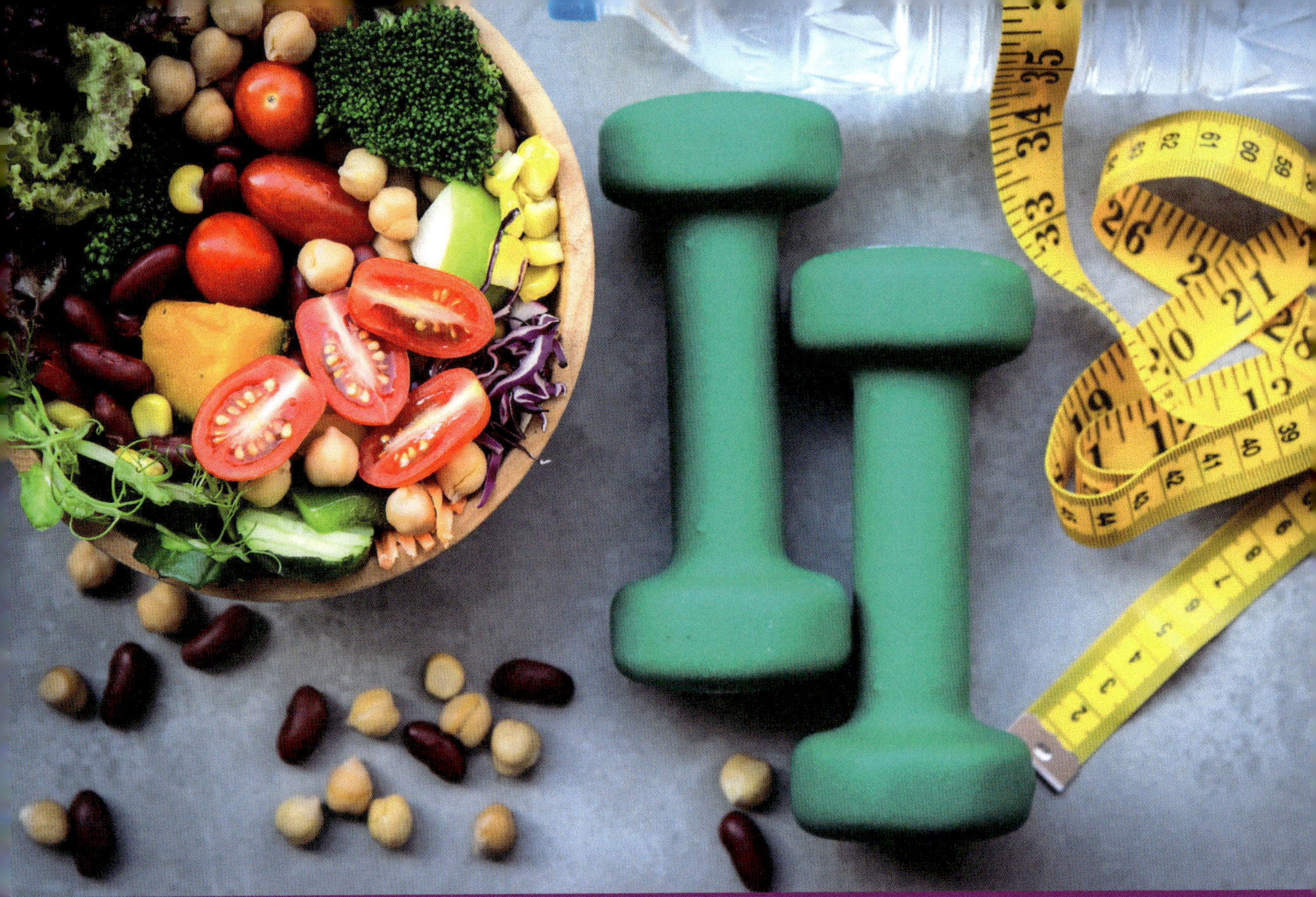

"Exercise is to have fun and be healthy, not punishment for what you just ate."

CHAPTER 17

Tips For Getting & Staying Motivated When Dieting

Set small, measurable goals that will help you get to your overall large goal. For example, I will eat 5 servings of fruit and vegetables a day, incorporate leafy green vegetables into 2 meals a day and drink at least 6 glasses of water daily.

Keep a food and exercise journal. This is extremely helpful to track how much you're eating, sometimes you don't realise how many small bites here and there add up in terms of calories. You can do a hand-written journal or go digital and log your food and fitness from the computer or your Smartphone. MyFitnessPal is a popular choice for this.

Enlist support from your friends and family. Moral support and encouragement from friends and family can really make a difference.

Crowd processed junk food out of your diet by adding in more nutritious whole foods.

Skip the food cupboard and head to the fridge. No one really keeps a lot of processed foods in their fridge because they're usually self-stable. When looking for an afternoon snack I tend to stick with something from the fridge; non-fat Greek yogurt and fruit.

Try new foods. Look for new healthy recipes online, in cookbooks or magazines so you don't get bored with eating healthy foods.

Keep nutritious foods on hand and ready to eat. Preparation is the key to eating healthy! Having fresh vegetables and fruits, lean protein, healthy fats and smart carbohydrates each week is helpful for staying on track.

Team up with a friend and hold each other accountable for healthy eating.

Keep tempting foods that trigger you to overeat out of the house. If it's not in the food cupboard and or fridge, you can't eat it. I have a weakness for biscuits, with little power to resist eating only one or two at a time. To avoid eating an entire packet in one sitting I simply don't buy them in the first place.

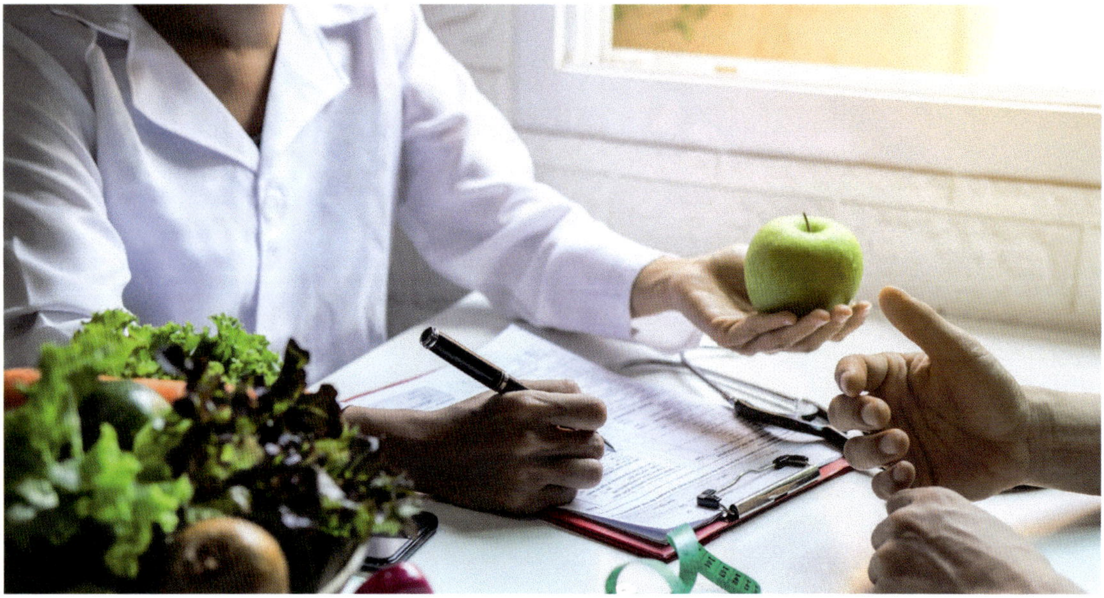

Eat something every 2-3 hours. This keeps your metabolism running and also makes sure you don't get ravenous and end up eating whatever is in sight to satisfy your hunger.

Always take a healthy snack with you when you leave the house for more than a couple hours. Apples, bananas or indeed any fruit, nut bars and carrots are perfect to pop into your bag.

When going out to eat, look at the menu for the restaurant online. Deciding beforehand what healthy option you're going to get can be helpful so you're not tempted by unhealthy options once you're there, seasonal fruit salad rather than sticky toffee pudding.

Eat and enjoy your favourite foods in moderation. Deprivation tends to backfire so if you really want a treat, then eat and enjoy it. I do have to watch my weight even with the amount of exercise I do, so I tend to aim to be really good 5-days of the week, for the other 2, if I fancy it, I eat it!

Don't let one set-back keep you from working toward your goal. Don't get down on yourself if you slip-up, just make sure your next meal is a healthy one.

Consider joining Weightwatchers, Slimming World or similar. There is something to be said for the sociability of a club, lots of different people uniting around a shared goal. Wins hands-down for providing structure and moral support.

Use the NHS 12-Week Diet Plan. You'll find some really good information about healthy eating and dieting on the NHS website. You can download a great 12-week diet plan to help you achieve your weight loss goal. Use the link below: **www.nhs.uk/live-well/healthy-weight/start-the-nhs-weight-loss-plan/**

For optimal results. Combine your 12-week diet plan with the 12-week exercise plan and you'll be well on the way to a slimmer, healthier and fitter you. Always consult with your doctor before embarking on any new diet and exercise plan.

Facebook Group: Join the **HOW 2 GET FIT 4 LATER LIFE FACEBOOK GROUP**. I've set this up for everyone who takes up the 12-week challenge to provide peer support, motivation and to share progress. I also want to encourage your friends and family members to join, so that they can lend their support in your quest for a healthier and fitter you. To join the Facebook Group use this link: **www.tiny.cc/H2GF4LL**

Hopefully, this list of tips helps give you some ideas on how to stay motivated to eat more healthily.

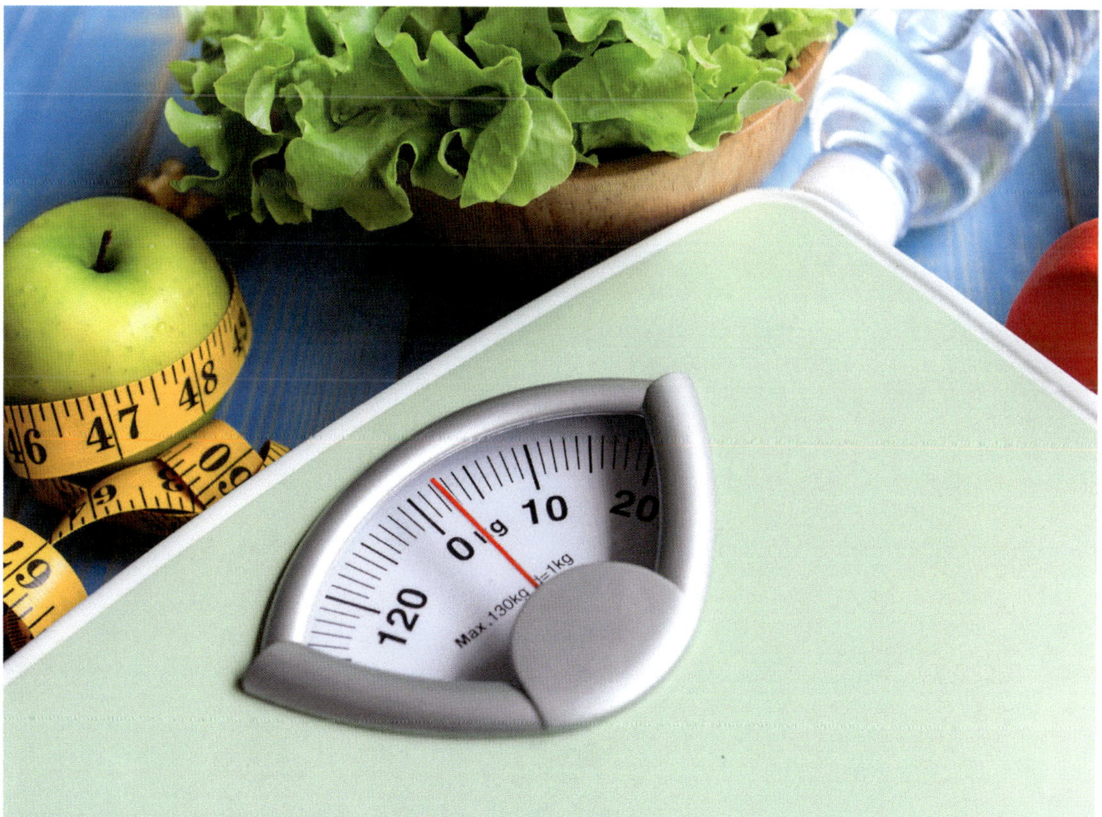

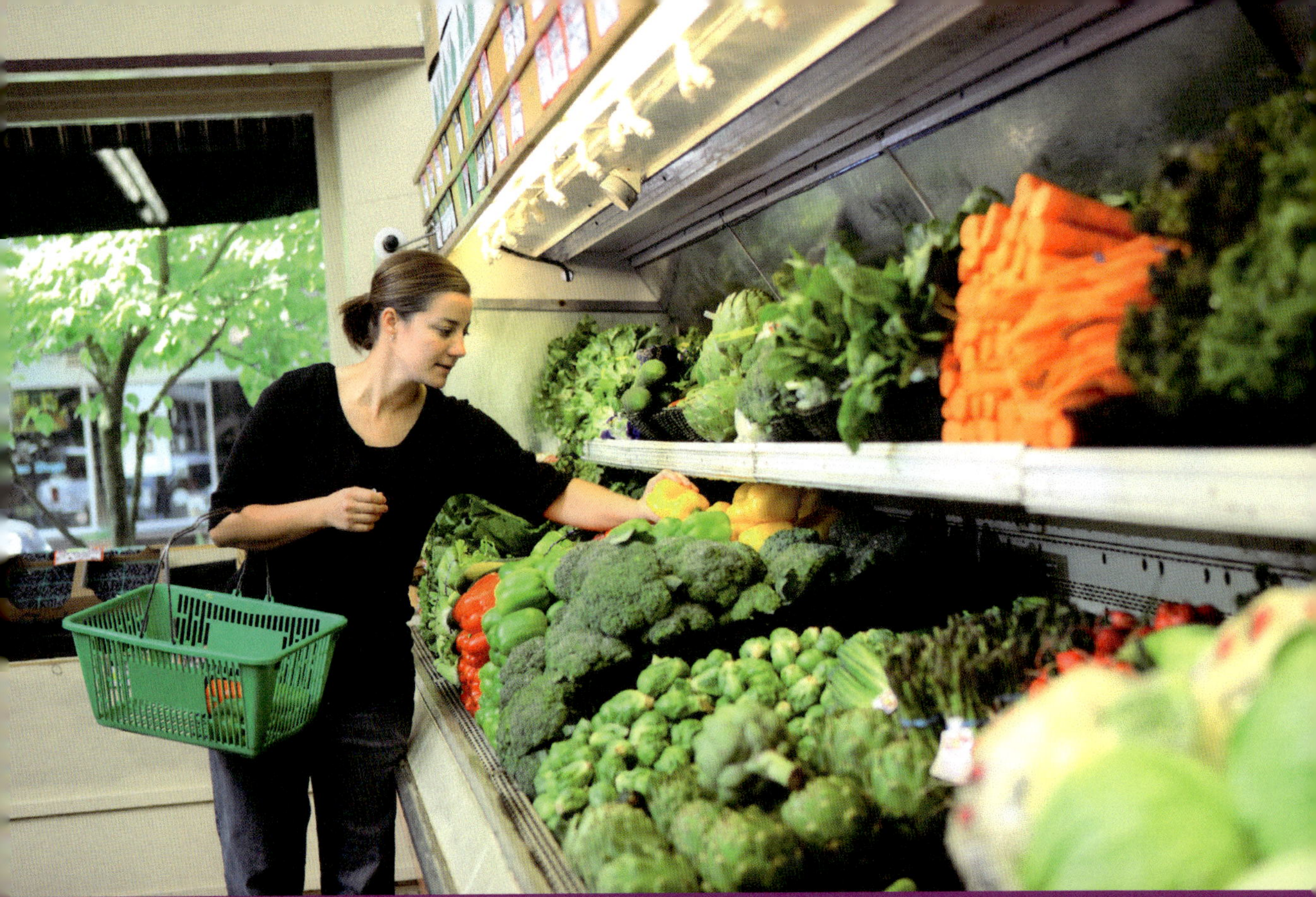

"It doesn't matter if progress is slow, so long as it never stops."

CHAPTER 18

Tips For Making Healthy Choices While Food Shopping

Healthy eating starts at the supermarket and your local shops, so it's important to make good choices. Here are some tips to help you shop smart. Use the food traffic light label to compare foods and find what's right for you. Choose items higher in dietary fibre, vitamins, minerals and lower in fats, saturated fat, sugars and salt.

Food in the UK is labelled with the traffic light and reference intake system. There is a separate section on this.

- Check the serving size when comparing calories and nutrients in different food products. The nutrition information listed on the food traffic light label and reference intake label and is based on the serving size listed on the label, which is usually one serving.
- Balance calories in and out. A total intake of 2,000 calories a day is used as a general guide for nutritional advice. Your caloric needs may be higher or lower and vary depending on your age, sex, and level of physical activity.
- Look at the % recommended intake label to choose products that are higher in nutrients you want to get more of such as dietary fibre, vitamin B12, vitamin D, calcium, iron, magnesium and potassium, and lower in nutrients you want to get less of, such as fats, saturated fat, added sugars and salt.
- Eat before you shop. Food shopping hungry can lead to impulse buying and or unhealthy food choices.
- Use fresh fruits and vegetables that are in season. They are generally easy to get, have more flavour and are usually less expensive than out of season fruit and vegetables.
- Try canned or frozen fruits and vegetables. Canned and frozen items may be less expensive than fresh. For canned items, choose fruit canned in 100% fruit juice without added sugars and vegetables with low salt or no added salt on the label. For frozen items, look for vegetables without sauce or seasoning, which can contain added sodium and added sugars.

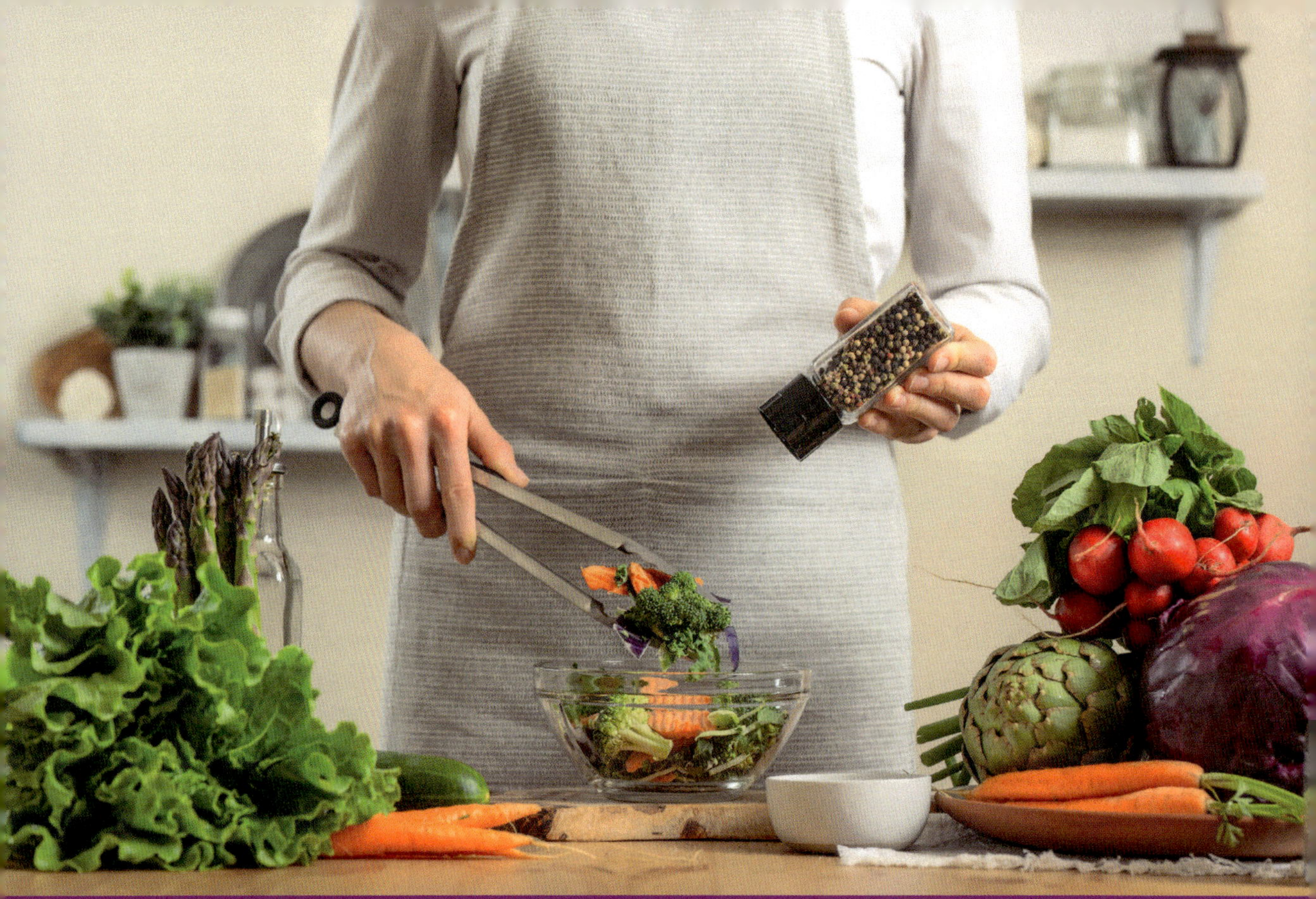

"You have to be at your strongest, when you feel at your weakest."

CHAPTER 19

Tips For Bringing More Nutrition Into Your Home

If you've generally relied on readymade meals and other processed foods for a large part of your diet, then here are some tips to help you prepare healthier meals. You don't need to be a celebrity chef, so try these tips:

- If possible, prepare ingredients in advance of cooking. For example, chop vegetables and refrigerate them until you are ready to use them.
- Buy frozen (without butter, sauce, or added seasoning) and low-sodium or no-salt-added canned vegetables to ensure that you always have some basic ingredients on hand.
- Try baking, boiling, grilling, or steaming instead of frying.
- Cook with herbs, spices, lemon juice, or no-salt seasonings, which add flavour without adding sodium.
- Prepare extra servings of a favourite, healthy dish to eat throughout the week. Making leftovers part of your plan can save time.
- Start collecting simple, healthy recipes from your local supermarket, you'll also find lots of recipes to download online. Organise them online or in a file box or binder.
- If you still want the occasional ready meal, choose healthier options, Weightwatchers or Sainsbury's Be Good To Yourself range of meals, for example.

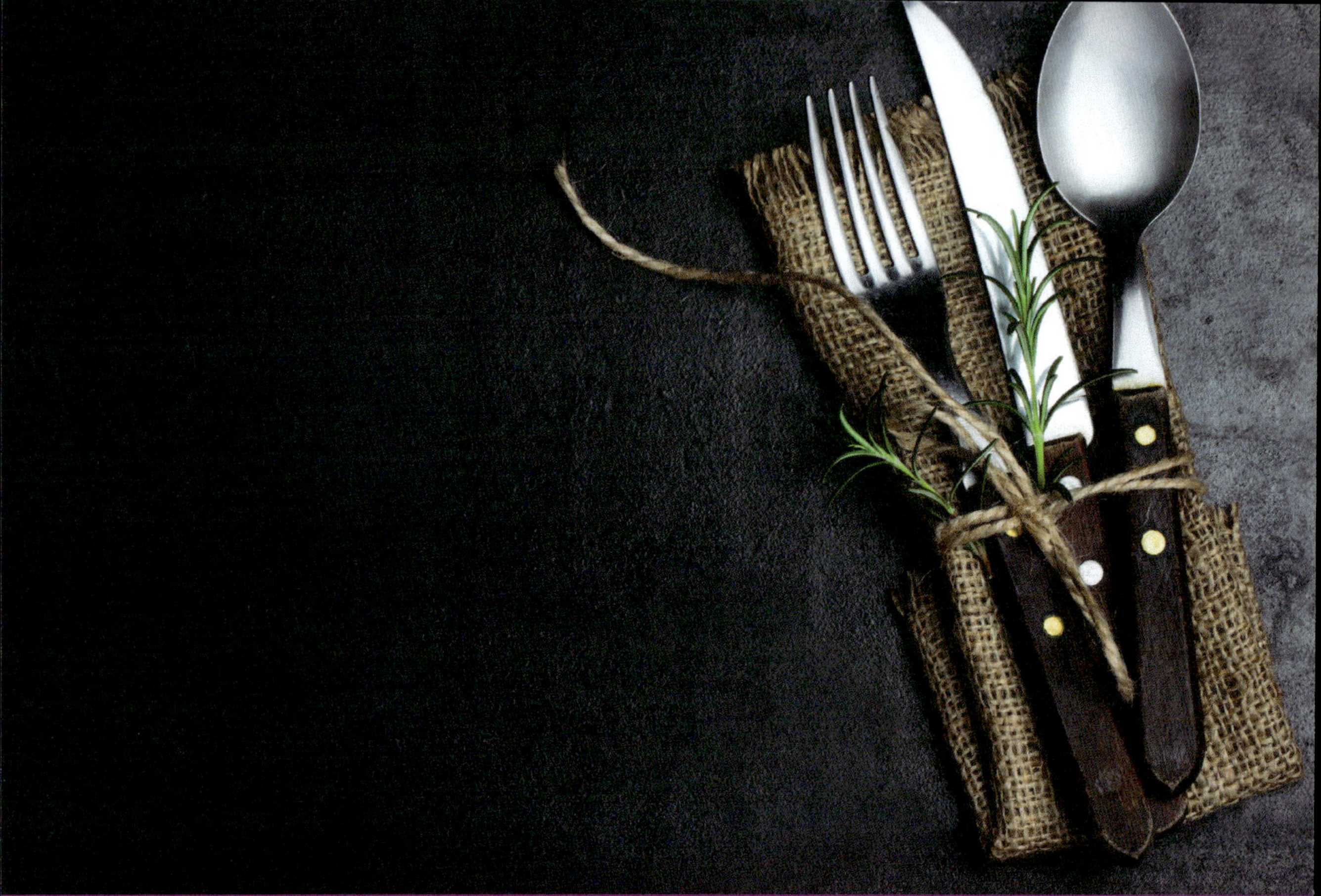

"It's not about being perfect, it's about giving 100%-effort."

CHAPTER 20

Tips For Making Healthy Choices When Eating Out

Find out YOUR calorie needs are. A total intake of 2,000 calories a day is used for general nutritional advice. However, your calorie needs may be higher or lower and vary according to age, sex, and physical activity. See Chapter 16 to calculate your daily caloric needs. In today's busy world of convenience foods, takeaways and fast-food restaurants it has become all too easy to eat high calorie, low-quality foods, often without even realising it. Here are tips for making eating out choices that are healthy as they are delicious.

- Look for calorie and nutrition information. Calorie information can be found on menus or menu boards of restaurants and other food establishments that are part of a chain and additional nutrition information is also available upon request. Many chain restaurants also include nutrition information online, so you can also check restaurant websites for nutrition information before going out. Make the best choice for you. Comparing calorie and nutritional information can help you make better decisions before you order.
- Side dishes can add many calories to a meal. Steamed, grilled, or boiled vegetables and fruit are often lower-calorie options. Armed with caloric information, you can make the best choice for you.
- Calorie information can help you decide how much to enjoy now and how much to save for later.
- Foods described with words like creamy, fried, breaded, battered, or buttered are typically higher in calories than foods described as baked, roasted, steamed, grilled, or boiled. Use the calorie information to help you make the choice that is right for you. Remember that 600 calories will take about two hours to exercise off.
- Calories from beverages and alcohol add up quickly. With calorie information, you can find lower-calorie options.
- Sauces and salad dressings can be particularly high in calories, ask for them to be served on the side or even without.

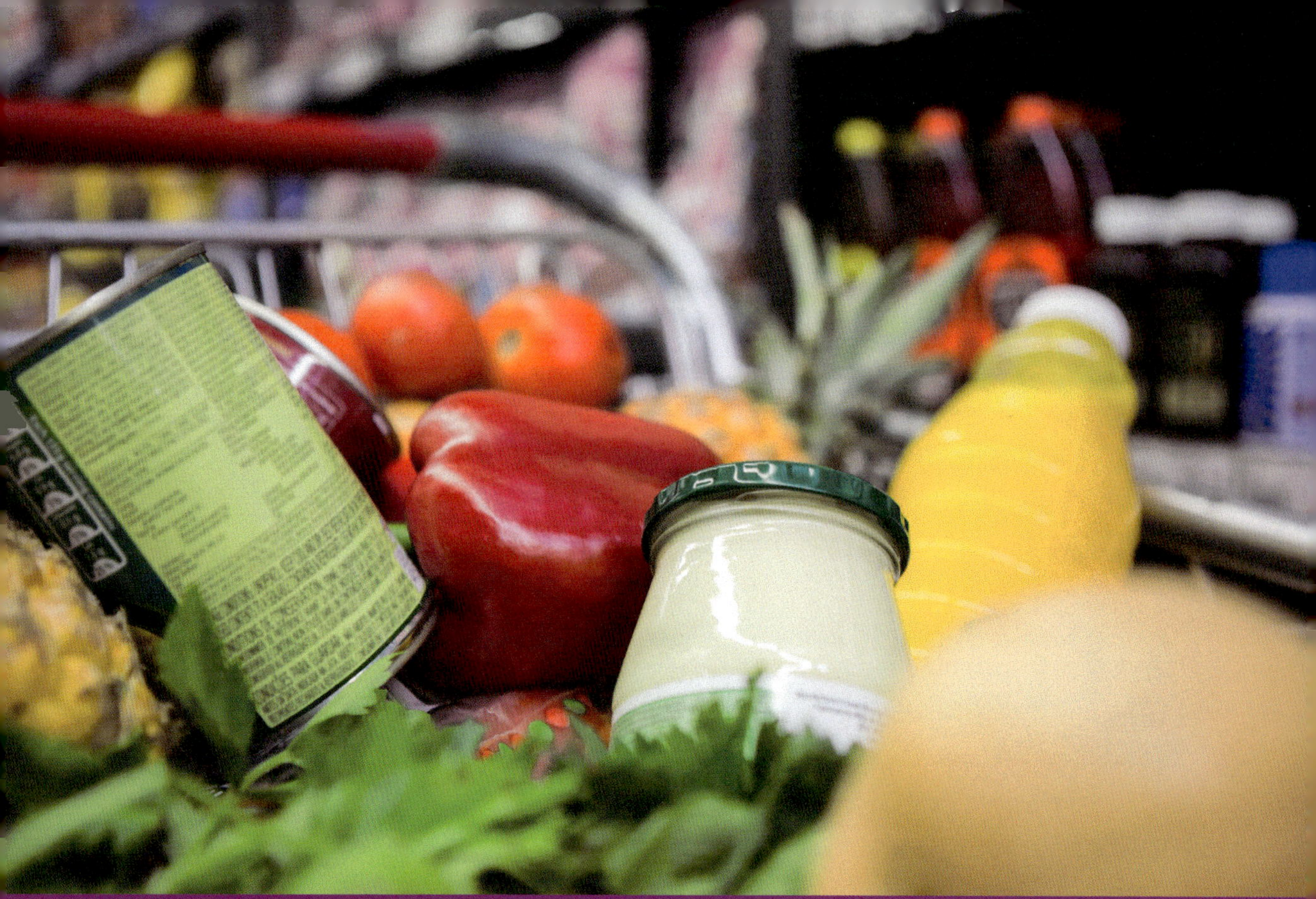

"Believe you can and you're halfway there."

CHAPTER 21

Traffic Light Food Labelling Explained

In the UK, repeating nutritional information on the front of pre-packaged foods and drinks is voluntary but most of the major supermarkets and many food manufacturers now provide this. The information has to be displayed as either:

- Energy (kJ and kcal) only

or

- Energy (kJ and kcal)
- Fat
- Saturated fat
- Sugars (total sugars)
- Salt

This information will be written per 100g/100ml, per portion or both. The government's recommended format is red, amber, green colour-coding and percentage 'reference intakes', or as you may better recognise it; traffic light labelling.

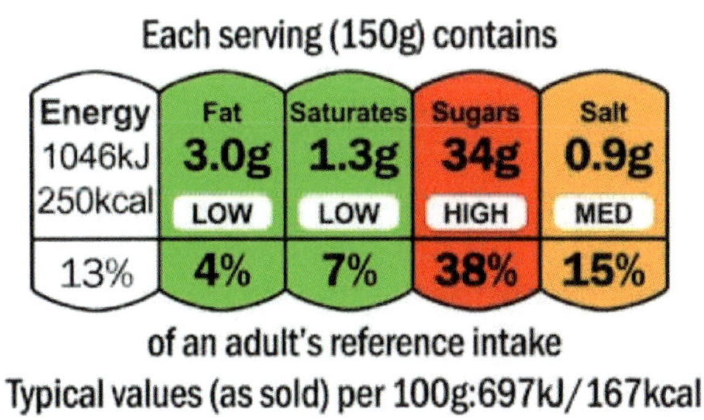

Using the front of pack labels is really useful when you want to quickly compare different food products while shopping. A simple combination of colour coding traffic lights and nutritional information is used to show, at a glance, whether a product is high (red), medium (amber) or low (green) in fat, saturated fat, salt and sugars, and how much energy (calories and kilojoules) it provides. This can help you make comparisons between foods to allow you to make a healthier choice; for example selecting a sandwich for lunch. Remember that 600 calories will take about two hours to exercise off.

Top tips about traffic light labelling

What does green mean?	What does amber mean?	What does red mean?
If there is mostly green on the label, then this is telling you straight away it is low in that nutrient and a healthier choice!	This means the product is neither high nor low in the specific nutrient. You can eat foods with all or mostly amber on the label most of the time.	Red doesn't mean you cannot eat the product but means the food is high in fat, saturated fat, salt or sugar. We should be cutting down on foods with lots of red on the label, or if they are eaten, to have less often and in small amounts.

When choosing between similar products, try to opt for more greens and ambers and fewer reds.

Alongside these traffic lights, the label generally shows the amount of these nutrients in a portion of the food or drink and the percentage of your reference intake (RI) a portion of the product provides, see the example below (the figures at the bottom of the label). In some cases, where there isn't much room on the label, just energy values will be displayed but the full nutrition information will be available on the back of the pack.

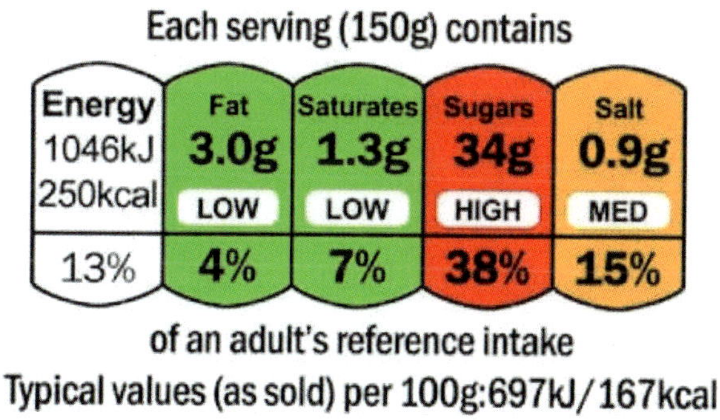

You may also see a label like this for the RI values:

Nutrition

Typical values	100g contains	Each slice (typically 44g) contains	% RI*	RI* for an average adult
Energy	985kJ 235kcal	435kJ 105kcal	 5%	8400kJ 2000kcal
Fat	1.5g	0.7g	1%	70g
of which saturates	0.3g	0.1g	1%	20g
Carbohydrate	45.5g	20.0g		
of which sugars	3.8g	1.7g	2%	90g
Fibre	2.8g	1.2g		
Protein	7.7g	3.4g		
Salt	1.0g	0.4g	7%	6g

This pack contains 16 servings

*Reference intake of an average adult (8400kJ / 2000kcal)

As part of a healthy balanced diet, an adult's RIs for a day are:

Energy or Nutrient	Reference Intake
Energy	8400kJ/2000kcal
Fat	70g
Saturates	20g
Carbohydrate	260g
Sugars	90g
Protein	60g
Salt	6g

What are the guidelines for high, medium and low on a front of pack label?

The table below shows how high, medium and low levels of fat, saturates, total sugars and salt in foods are classified for front of pack labels. These levels have been decided by the UK government. The 'per portion' in red is used where portions are 260g or more. Remember that 600 calories will take about two hours to exercise off.

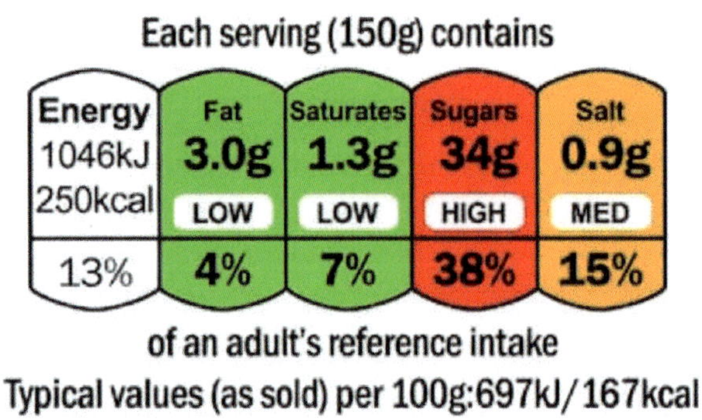

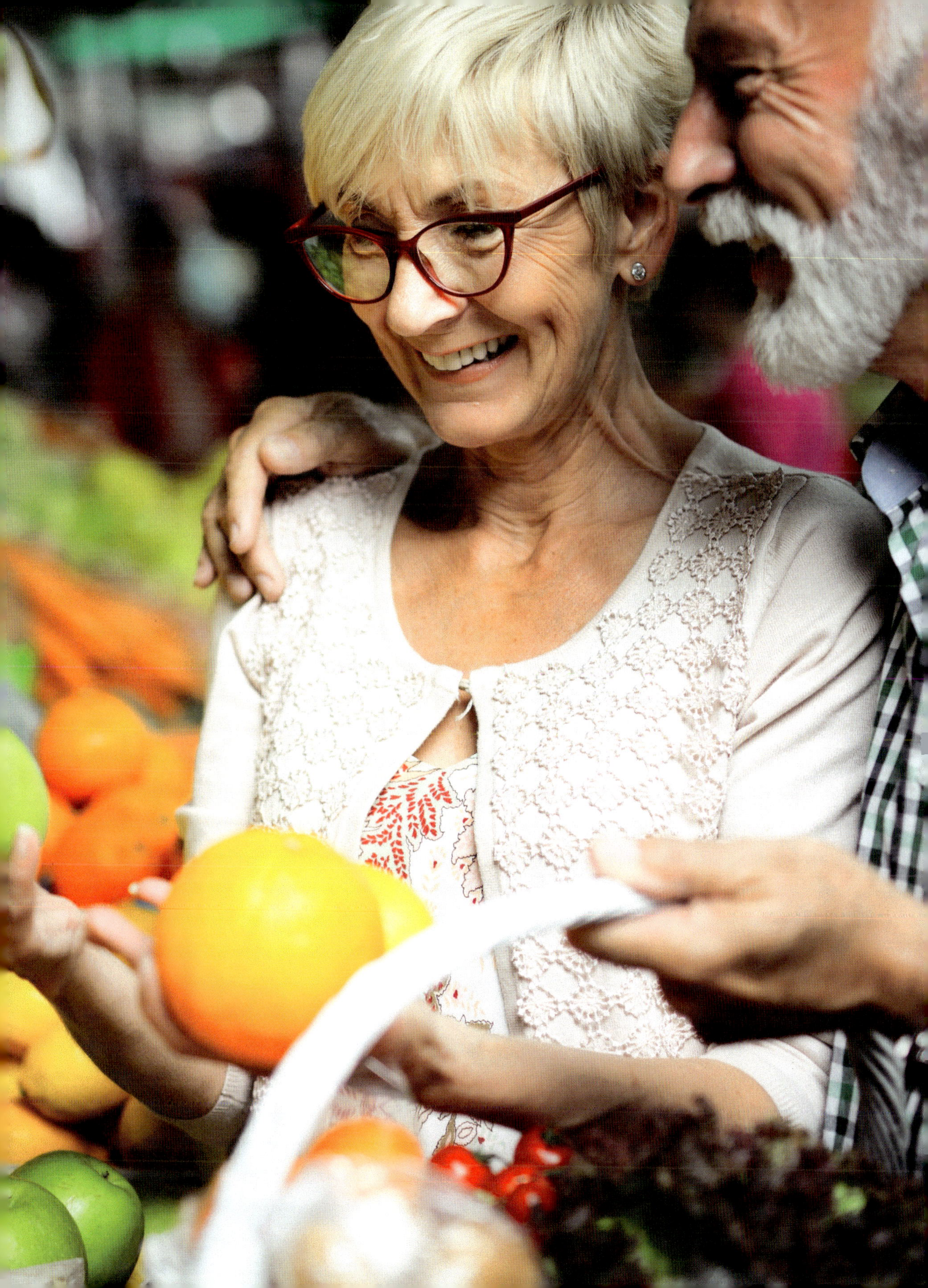

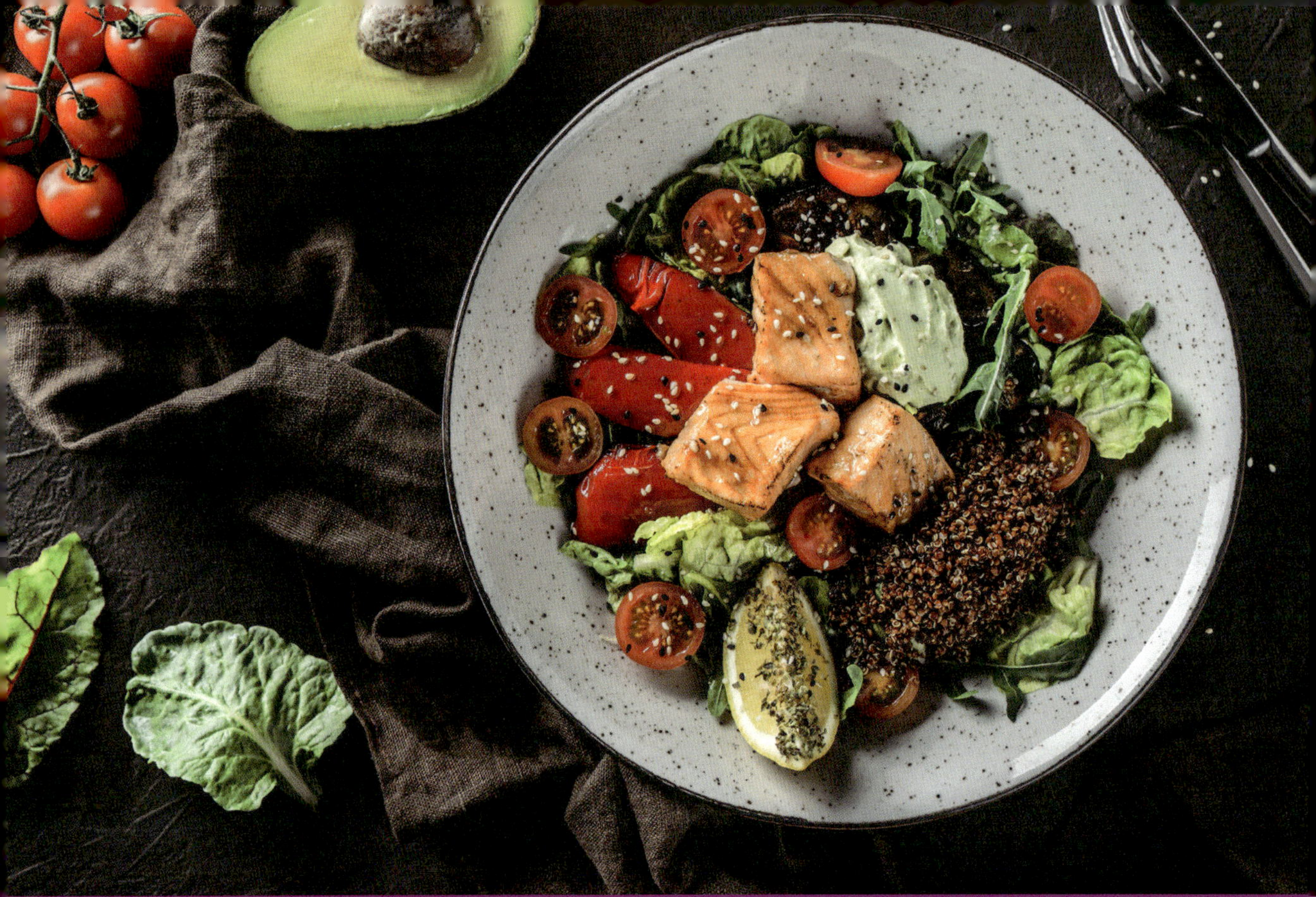

"You are what you eat."

CHAPTER 22

The Best Weight Loss Foods

Just as all people are not created equal, the same can be said of calories. Different foods travel through your body's different metabolic pathways. And this can cause dramatic differences in how hungry you feel and the number of calories you use up. Here for your delectation are twenty of the most weight loss-friendly foods that are scientifically proven to help you lose weight, and I've used many of them to help control mine. So, include these in your diet and remember that if you are trying to lose weight aim to lose 0.5 to 1 kilo (1 to 2 pounds) per week. Losing weight at this rate is far more likely to be sustained, particularly if you increase the amount of exercise you do.

1. Apple Cider Vinegar

Apple cider vinegar enjoys much popularity amongst the natural health community. It's regularly used in condiments such as dressings and vinaigrettes. Several studies suggest that apple cider vinegar can be useful for weight loss. Taking vinegar at the same time as a high-carb meal can increase feelings of fullness and make people eat fewer calories for the rest of the day. Vinegar has also been shown to reduce blood sugar spikes after meals, which may have various beneficial health effects over the long term.

2. Avocado

Avocados are unique amongst fruits as they are packed with healthy fats rather carbs. They are particularly high in monosaturated oleic acid, the same type of fat found in olive oil. Because of the high-water content, they are not as calorific as you might think and they contain loads of important nutrients, including potassium and vitamin K.

3. Boiled Potatoes

Seemingly no longer in vogue, boiled potatoes have several properties that make them great for weight loss and optimal health. This is down to the fact that they contain a wide range of nutrients with a bit of nearly everything you need. They are particularly high in potassium which plays an important role in blood pressure control. If you let boiled potatoes cool for a while, they form large amounts of resistant starch, a fibre-like substance which amongst other things has been shown to promote weight loss. For a bit of variety sweet potatoes, turnips, parsnips and other root vegetables are also good choices.

4. Chia Seeds

Chia seeds are among the most nutritious foods around. They contain 12 grams of carbohydrates per ounce or 28 grams, which is fairly high, but 11 of these grams are fibre! This combines to make chia seeds a low-carbohydrate friendly food and one of the best sources of fibre you can get and due to its high fibre content, chia seeds can absorb up to 12 times their weight in water, turning gel-like and expanding in your stomach which will help make you feel full.

5. Chili Pepper

This might be a surprise entry, but chilli pepper really can help with weight loss. They contain something called capsaicin, which studies have shown to reduce appetite and increase fat burning.

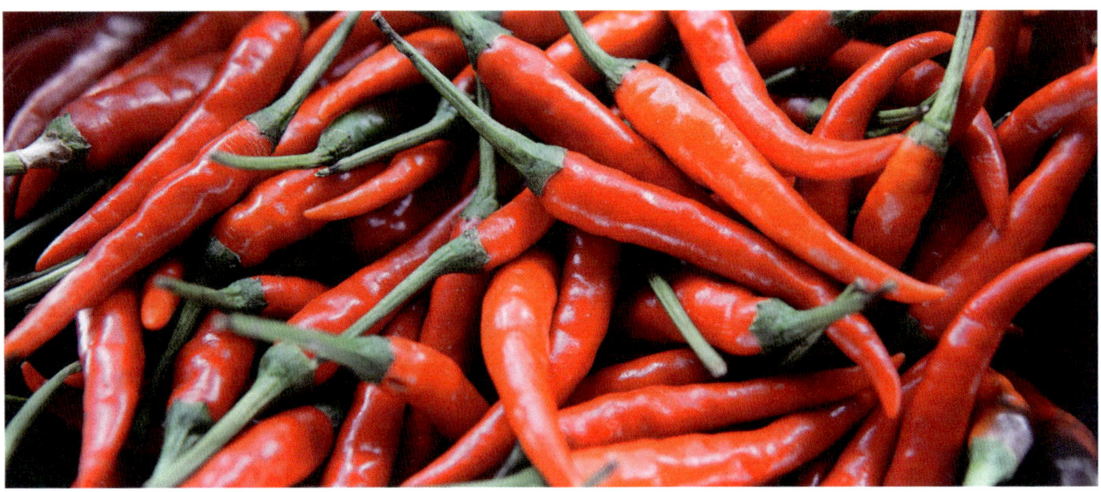

6. Coconut Oil

Just as not all calories are created equal the same principle applies to fats. Coconut oil is high in fatty acids of a medium length, called medium-chain triglycerides which have been shown to boost satiety better than other fats while increasing the number of calories burned. Of course, coconut oil still contains calories, so adding it on top of what you're already eating is not a good idea. However, a much better idea is to replace some of your other cooking fats with coconut oil. Extra virgin olive oil is also worth noting, as it's probably one of the healthiest fats around.

7. Cottage Cheese

Dairy products all tend to have a large amount of protein. One of the best options is cottage cheese because it is mostly protein with a relatively low amount of carbohydrates and only a little fat. It's also very satiating, meaning you feel fuller for longer on a relatively low number of calories, and like all other dairy products, it is high in calcium, which may help you with fat burning.

8. Cruciferous Vegetables

Think broccoli, cabbage, Brussels sprouts and cauliflower and much like other vegetables cruciferous vegetables are high in fibre and tend to be very filling. Better still these types of vegetables have decent amounts of protein. A simple combo of fibre, protein and low energy density makes them the perfect foods to include in your meals if weight loss is your primary goal. There's also the added bonus of being packed with nutrients with cancer fighting-substances.

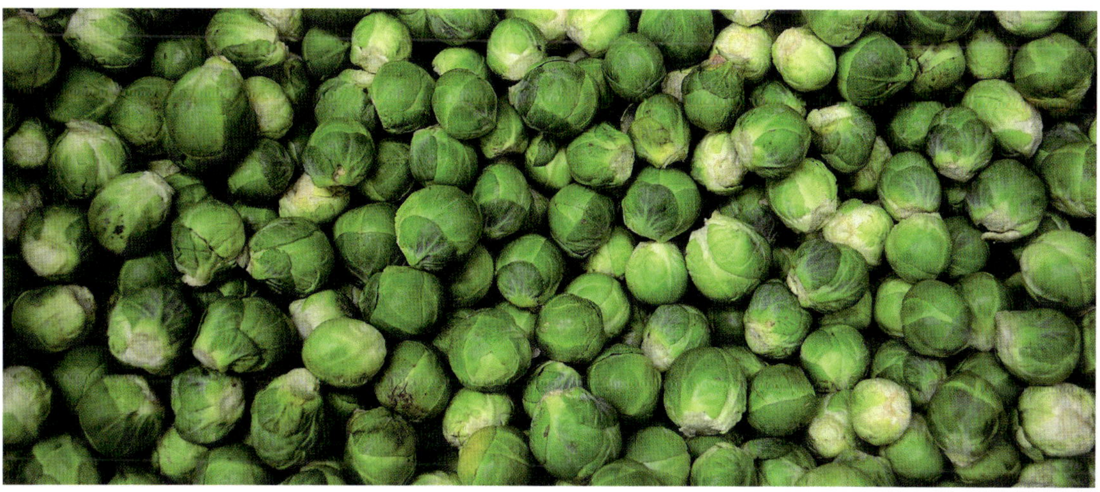

9. Eggs

Once avoided for being a 'cholesterol bombs' eggs are now firmly back in vogue. They are filling, dense with nutrients which are found mainly in the yolk. And eggs will help suppress your appetite until later in the day promoting weight loss.

10. Fruit

Most health and nutrition experts agree that fruit is good for you. Numerous studies have shown that people who eat the most fruit and vegetables tend to be healthier than people who don't manage their 5 a day fruit and vegetable quota. Of course, correlation does not equal causation, so these studies don't really prove anything. However, fruits have properties that make them weight loss-friendly as they have a low energy density and take a while to chew. Plus, the high amount of fibre found in fruit helps prevent sugar from being released too quickly into your bloodstream. Save for the few people that sadly can't tolerate them, fruit can be an effective and delicious addition to your weight loss diet.

11. Full Fat Yogurt

Yogurt is another fantastic dairy food. Some types of yogurt contain probiotic bacteria that can improve the function of your gut. There are two main benefits of a healthy gut; 1.) It may help protect you against inflammation 2.) It may also help with leptin resistance, which is one of the main hormonal drivers of obesity. It's important to note that some studies have shown that full-fat dairy rather than low-fat dairy is closely associated with a reduced risk of obesity and type 2 diabetes over time. It may be contrary to your thinking, but low-fat yogurt is often loaded with sugar, so it's best to avoid it, as it's really not good for you.

12. Grapefruit

One fruit that deserves to be singled out is grapefruit. Its effects on weight control have been studied specifically. In one 12-week study in 91 obese individuals, eating half a fresh grapefruit before meals led to a weight loss of 1.6 kg. The grapefruit group of fruits also had reduced insulin resistance, a metabolic abnormality that is implicated in various chronic diseases. Therefore, eating half a grapefruit about half an hour before some of your daily meals may help you feel fuller for longer while eating fewer calories.

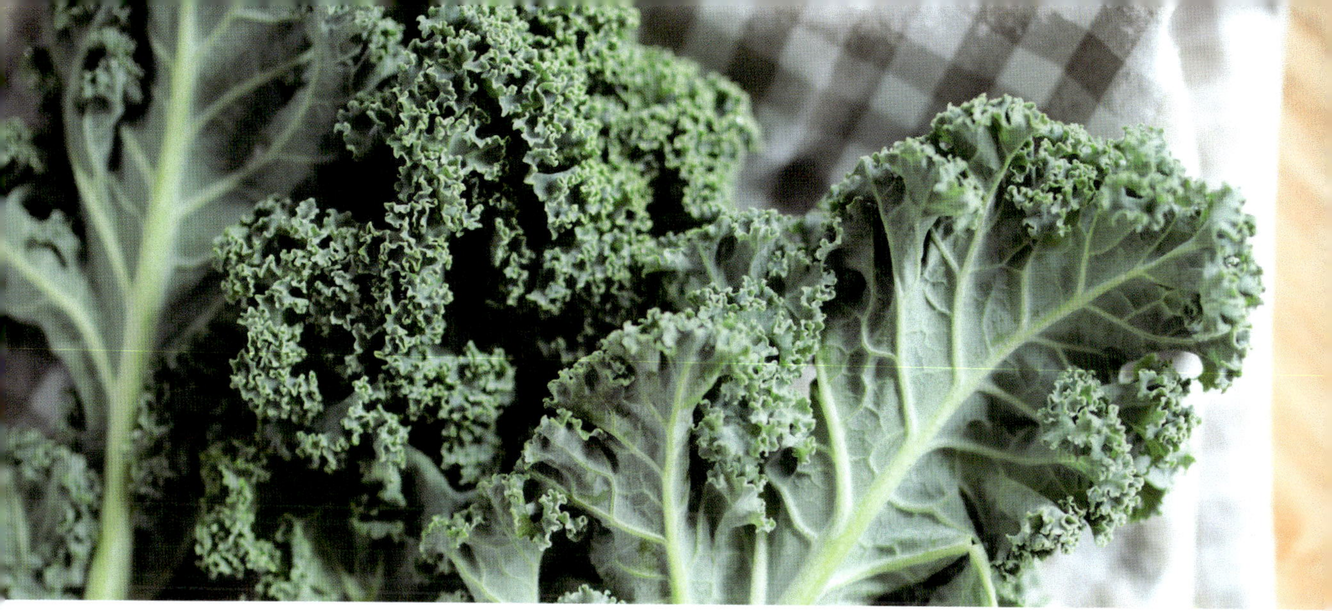

13. Leafy Greens

I bet as a kid your mum told you to 'eat your greens' which at the time you probably didn't appreciate! Turned out your mum was right! Kale, Swiss chards, collards, spinach and a few other leafy greens have numerous properties that make them suited for a weight loss diet, by increasing the volume of your plate of food without increasing calories. Studies have revealed that meals with a low energy density make you and me eat fewer calories overall. Leafy greens are also very nutritious and incredibly packed with vitamins, minerals and antioxidants including calcium. Leafy greens have also been found in some scientific studies to help fat burning.

14. Lean Red Meat

Meat has been unfairly blamed for various health problems despite a lack of evidence to back up these damning claims. Although processed meat is widely acknowledged to be unhealthy, studies show that unprocessed red meat does not raise the risk of heart disease or diabetes. According to two large studies, red meat has only a weak correlation with cancer in men and no correlation whatsoever in women. The simple truth is, meat is a weight loss-friendly food because it's high in protein not to mention packed with nutrients.

15. Legumes & Beans

Several legumes and beans can help in weight loss including kidney beans, lentils, black beans and a few others. They tend to be high in protein and fibre and help you feel fuller for longer while clocking up only a modest calorie count.

16. Nuts

While nuts are packed with fats, they are not quite as fattening as you might think. And they make the perfect snack with balanced amounts of protein, fibre and healthy fats. There have been some scientific studies that have shown them to improve metabolic health as well as promoting weight loss. Be careful not to eat too many though as they are fairly-high on the calorie count.

17. Salmon

Fatty fish should be in your diet twice a week and is very healthy and great at keeping you feeling full for hours on end with relatively few calories. This tasty fatty fish is packed with high-quality protein, numerous important nutrients and healthy fats.

18. Soups

As already mentioned above, diets with a low energy density, tend to make people eat fewer calories. The majority of foods with a low energy density are those that contain large amounts of water, for example, fruit and vegetables. But you can also just add water to your food, making a nutritious and healthy soup. Some scientific studies have shown that eating the exact same food turned into a soup rather than as solid food, makes people feel fuller for longer while eating significantly fewer calories. Be careful not to add too much fat to your soup, for example, cream or coconut milk, as this can significantly increase the calorie content.

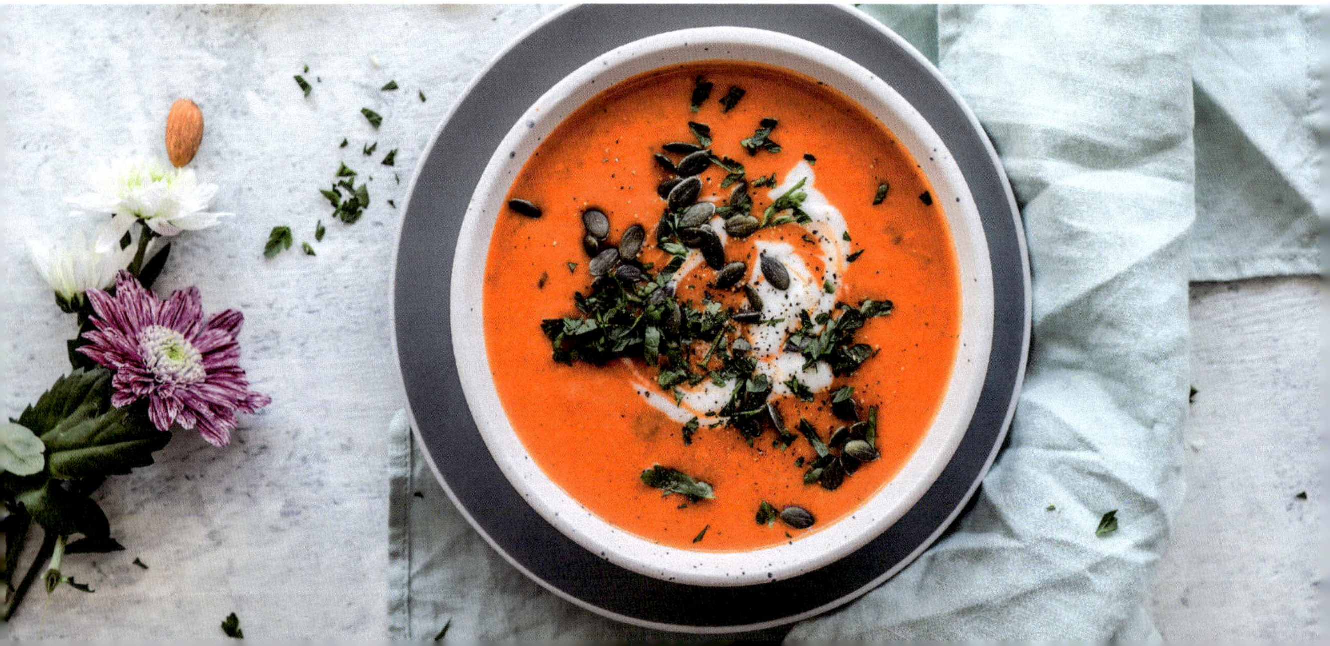

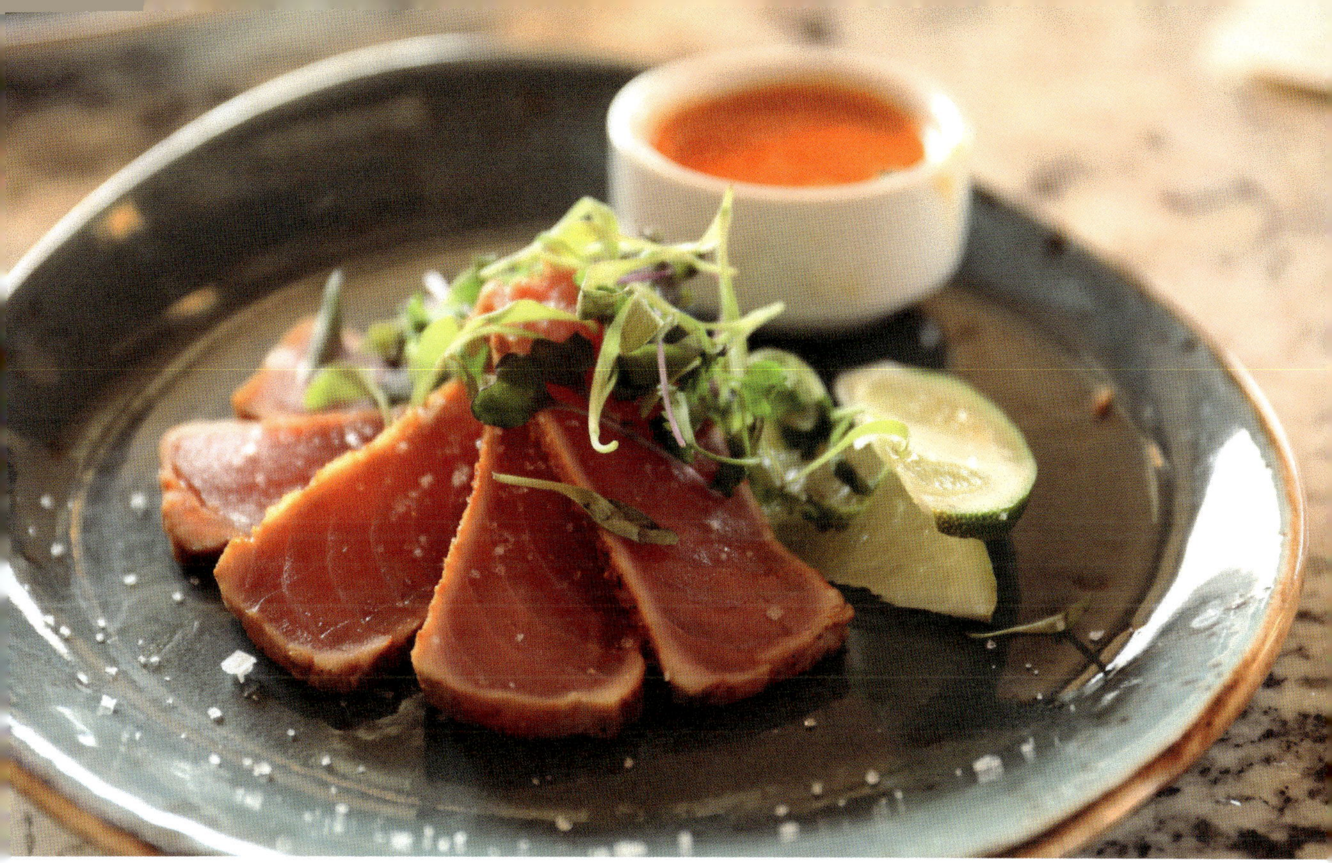

19. Tuna

This lovely fish is another low-calorie, high protein food. It's very lean (low in fat) and is popular amongst bodybuilders who are on a cutting cycle. If you're focused on protein intake, make sure to choose tuna canned in water rather than oil or go one better and buy tuna steaks from the fresh fish counter.

20. Whole Grain

Although some cereal grains have received a bad press in recent years, many types are definitely-healthy, filled with fibre while containing a fair amount of protein, for example, oats, brown rice and quinoa. Oats are loaded with beta-glucans, soluble fibres that have been shown to make you feel fuller for longer while improving your metabolic health. Brown and white rice can contain significant amounts of resistant starch, particularly if cooked and then allowed to cool down before consumption. Please be aware that refined grains are not a healthy choice, and sometimes foods that have 'whole grains' listed on the food label are highly processed sugar-laden junk foods that are harmful and very fattening. Of course, for some people, whole grains are a no go, but if you can tolerate them, then they're a great choice for weight loss.

So, there you have it, some of the very best foods around to help you with a weight loss goal, of course, diet is just one side of the coin, to get achieve sustainable-long term weight loss you'll need to add in regular exercise, and if you lack the motivation to start this, or simply do not know where to begin, then having a qualified personal trainer can help you achieve your weight loss goal.

In the UK, you can find a personal trainer near you by downloading the My Coach App. You can download this here: **www.fibodo.com** and if you live in or around Brighton & Hove, you'll find my details here too.

The next time you go shopping think about trying some of the foods listed here as part of a balanced and or calorie controlled diet.

Caution: Food Allergies I'm among one of the lucky ones, a personal trainer who can eat pretty much anything without suffering any unpleasant allergic reactions. Dairy products, cereals and nuts don't pose any problem to my health. While these are my top foods and drinks for weight loss, they may not be suitable for everyone. Always read the food label!

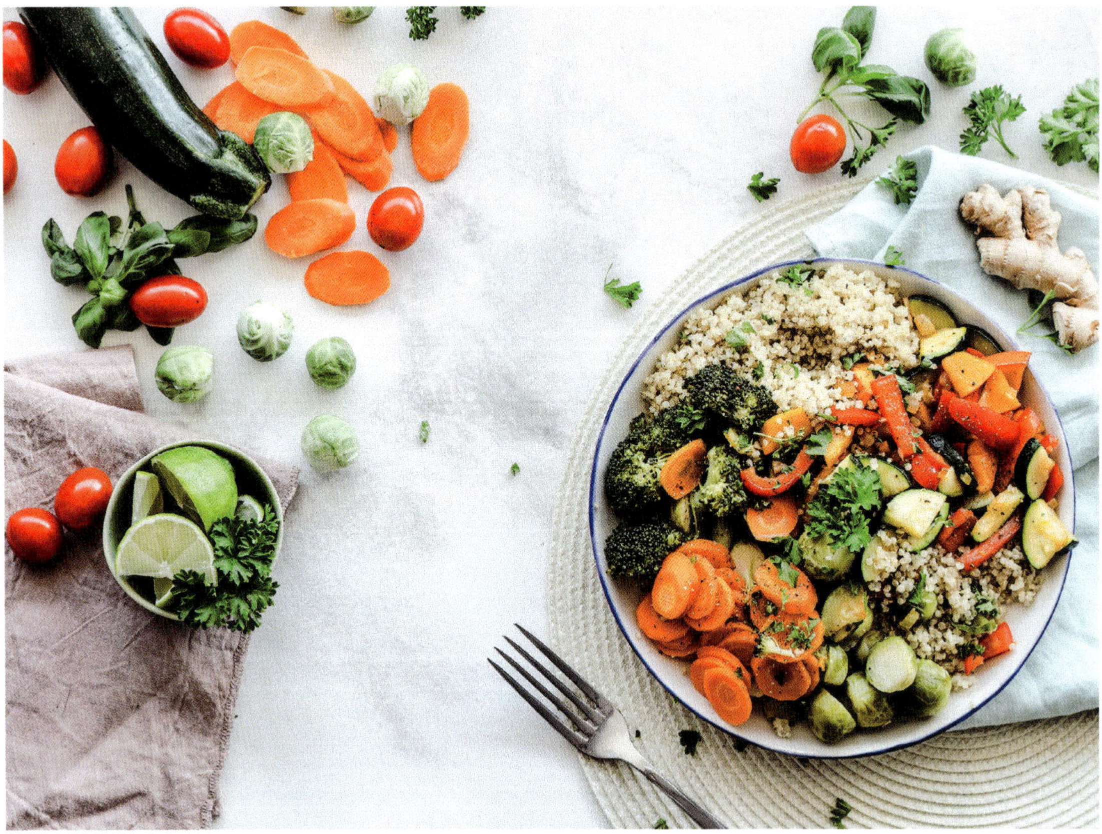

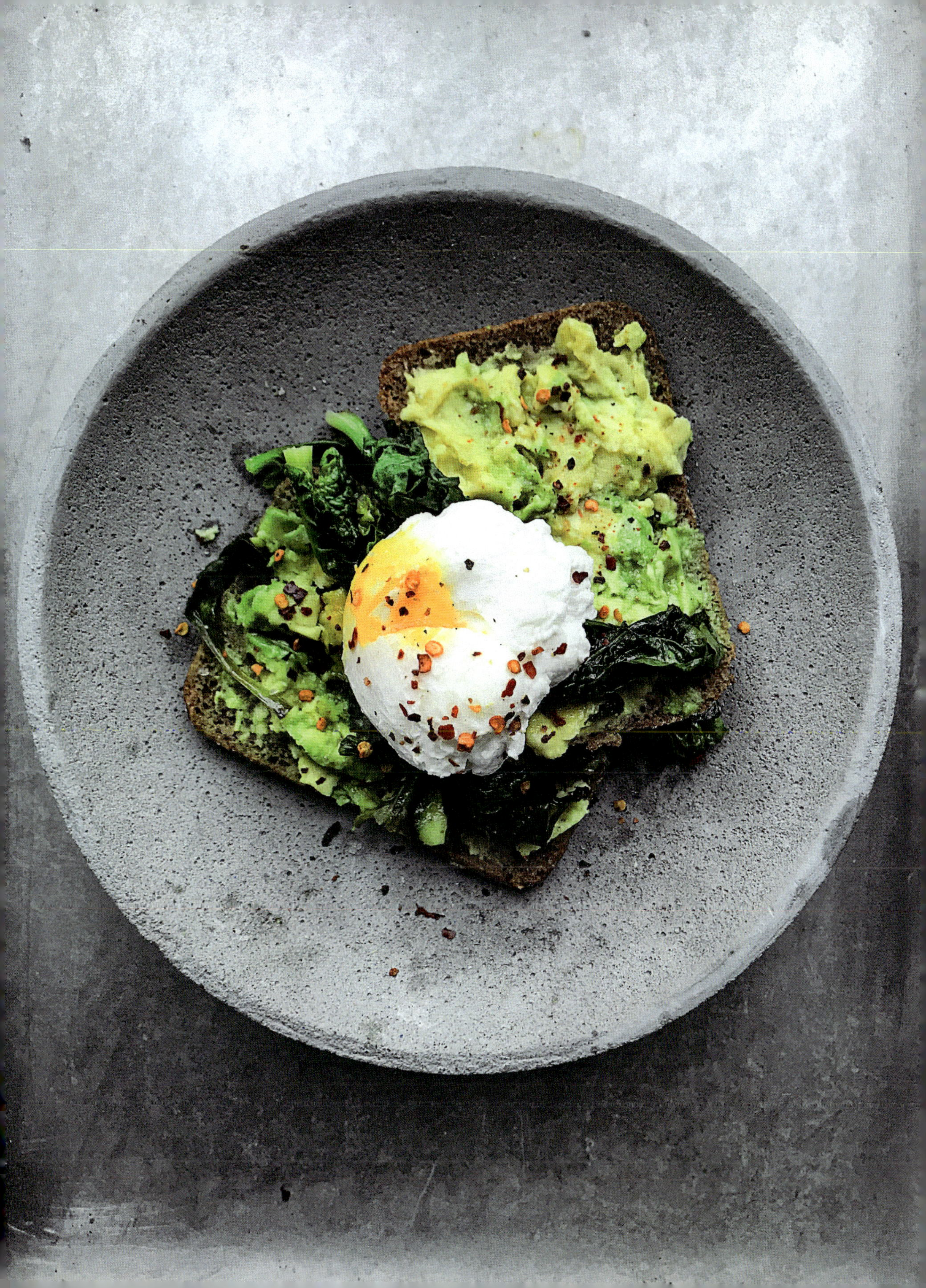

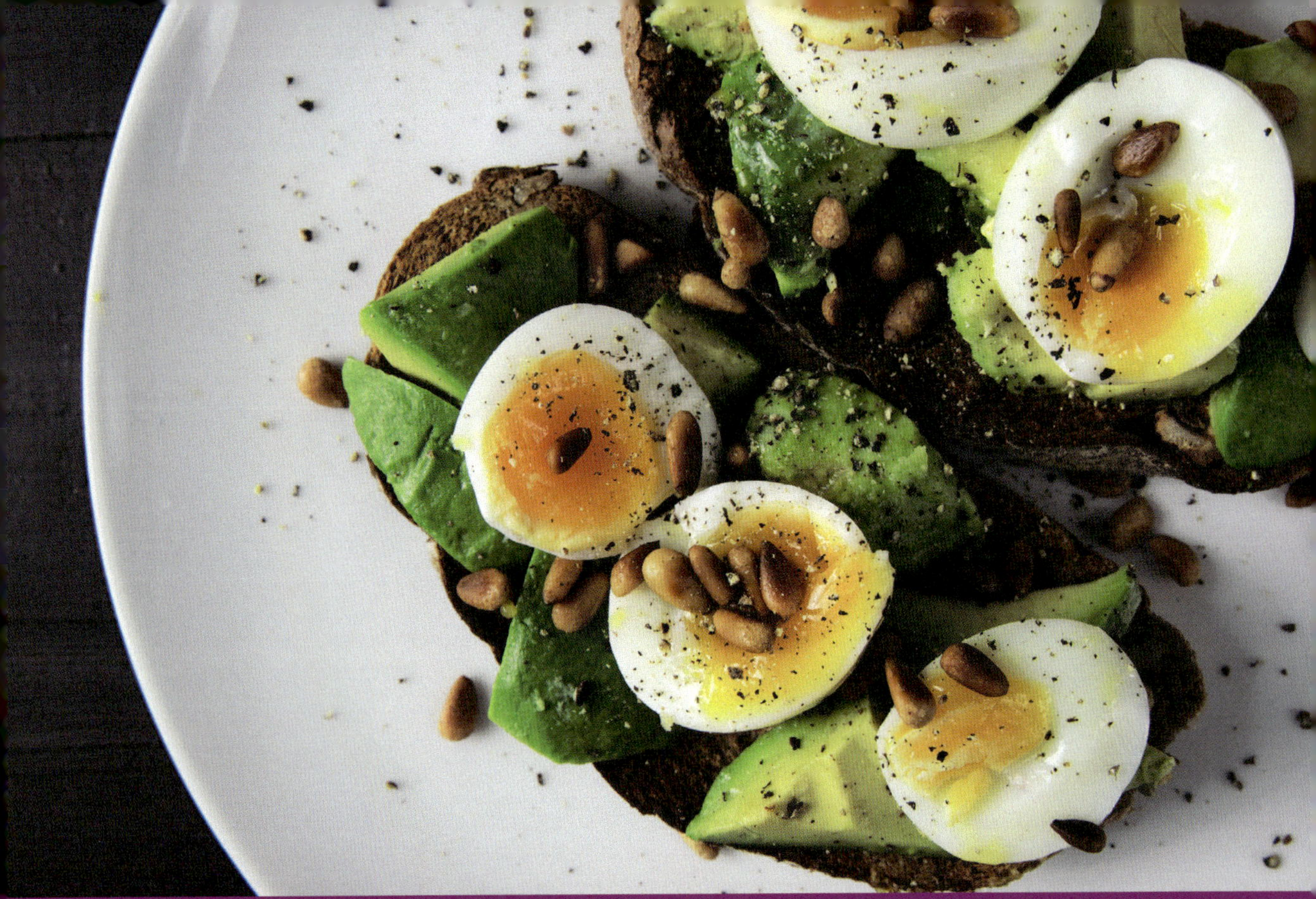

"It won't always be easy but it will always be worth it."

CHAPTER 23

The Best Foods & Drinks To Boost Energy Levels

Picture this; perhaps you had a rotten night's sleep or you're fast approaching that mid-afternoon energy slump, either way, you're in desperate need of an energy fix. Don't reach for your favourite sugar-laden energy drink. Instead, check out my top 20 go-to healthier options that are better for you in providing that much-needed energy boost.

All food, even junk food will give you energy, but there are some foods that are simply in a league of their own. As we grow older our energy levels decline. So on days when you really need your 'A-game' firing on all cylinders, try eating and in some cases drinking my top 20 go-to energy-boosting favourites.

1. Apples

With the high abundance of vitamins and minerals, an apple is basically the poster child for healthy food. It's made up of simple carbohydrates, which can offer a quick burst of fuel at any time of the day. I rarely leave my home without a few apples in my sports bag.

2. Bananas

We all know about eating your five-a-day fruit and veg. One of the easiest and cheapest foods for an instant pick-me-up at any point in your day is the banana. They contain glucose which provides a great energy boost to help you murder your High-Intensity interval training workout. This personal trainer has at least one of these a day!

3. Beans

Not only will beans keep you feeling full and satisfied, but they can also prevent you from feeling sluggish during the middle of your day. Protein helps keep blood sugar levels steady to keep you feeling energised, plus the complex carbohydrate provides energy for your body and brain.

4. Beetroot

Beetroot has gained popularity due to their ability to improve energy and stamina. Studies have shown that beetroot may be able to improve blood flow due to its antioxidant content and naturally occurring nitrates. As with leafy green vegetables, nitrates are compounds that help increase nitric oxide and improve blood flow throughout the body, allowing more oxygen delivery to tissues. This has the ability to increase energy levels.

5. Blueberries

Snacking on these powerful berries can help you beat that post-lunch slump. They're low in sugar, but high in fibre, a powerful combination to keep your body running with energy. The best part is that you can throw them into pretty much anything: salads, yogurt, smoothies, or just enjoy them on their own. They also possess powerful antioxidant properties. Try them with some fat-free Greek yogurt and a little honey.

6. Coffee

Early morning starts are part of my daily routine as a personal trainer. We all know that caffeine can provide a much-needed pick-me-up to get through a busy day and is a feature of how I start my day. But a study also found that drinking coffee before your workout can improve your ability to exercise. Men who drank about 2-3 cups of coffee found that they were able to complete more reps of bench presses and leg presses than workout days that were devoid of coffee.

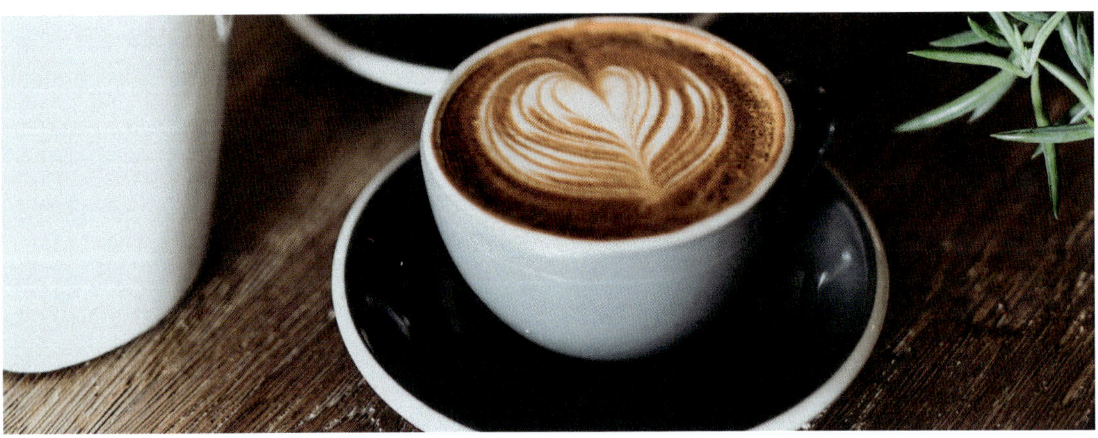

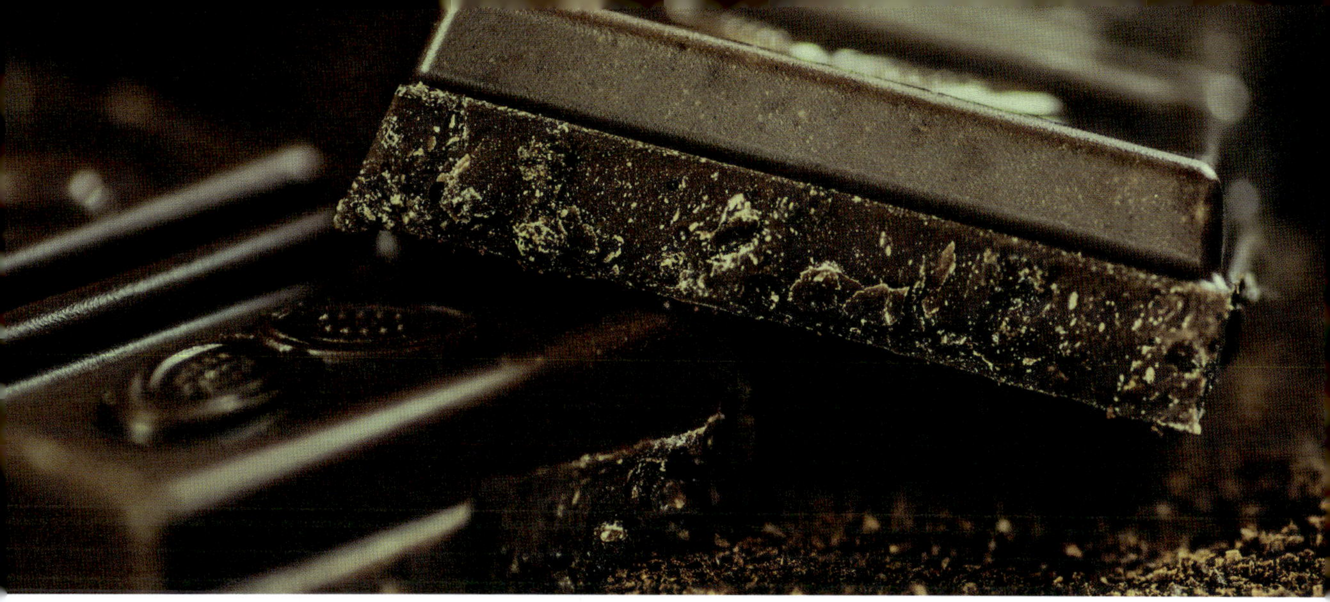

7. Dark Chocolate

Of course, I've read that researchers found that eating dark chocolate increases both alertness and attentiveness. Sadly, their findings don't give either you or me the green light to devour the entire large chocolate bar in one go (yeah, you got me banged to rights!). However, a small piece (do as I say and not as I do!) is just enough to get you going when you feel that you're flagging. Remember to choose a dark chocolate bar with at least 70 per cent cocoa.

8. Eggs

They're the nation's top breakfast food (as part of a full English) for a good reason! Eggs provide you with high-quality protein and heart-healthy monounsaturated and polyunsaturated fatty acids that combine to help you stay energised. And there are ways you can cook a healthier full English breakfast too, check this option out: **www.bbcgoodfood.com/recipes/5820/the-ultimate-makeover-full-english-breakfast**. Scrambled eggs on a slice of wholemeal bread toast are how I take this energy-boosting, personal trainer power meal for lunch.

9. Green Tea

Green tea is well known for its list of healthy attributes. It has a high concentration of powerful antioxidants that can help prevent oxidative stress and inflammation. Rather like coffee, green tea contains caffeine, which can increase energy levels. However, green tea also contains a compound called L-theanine, which can moderate the effects of caffeine, such as anxiety and the jitters, and it produces a smoother boost of energy.

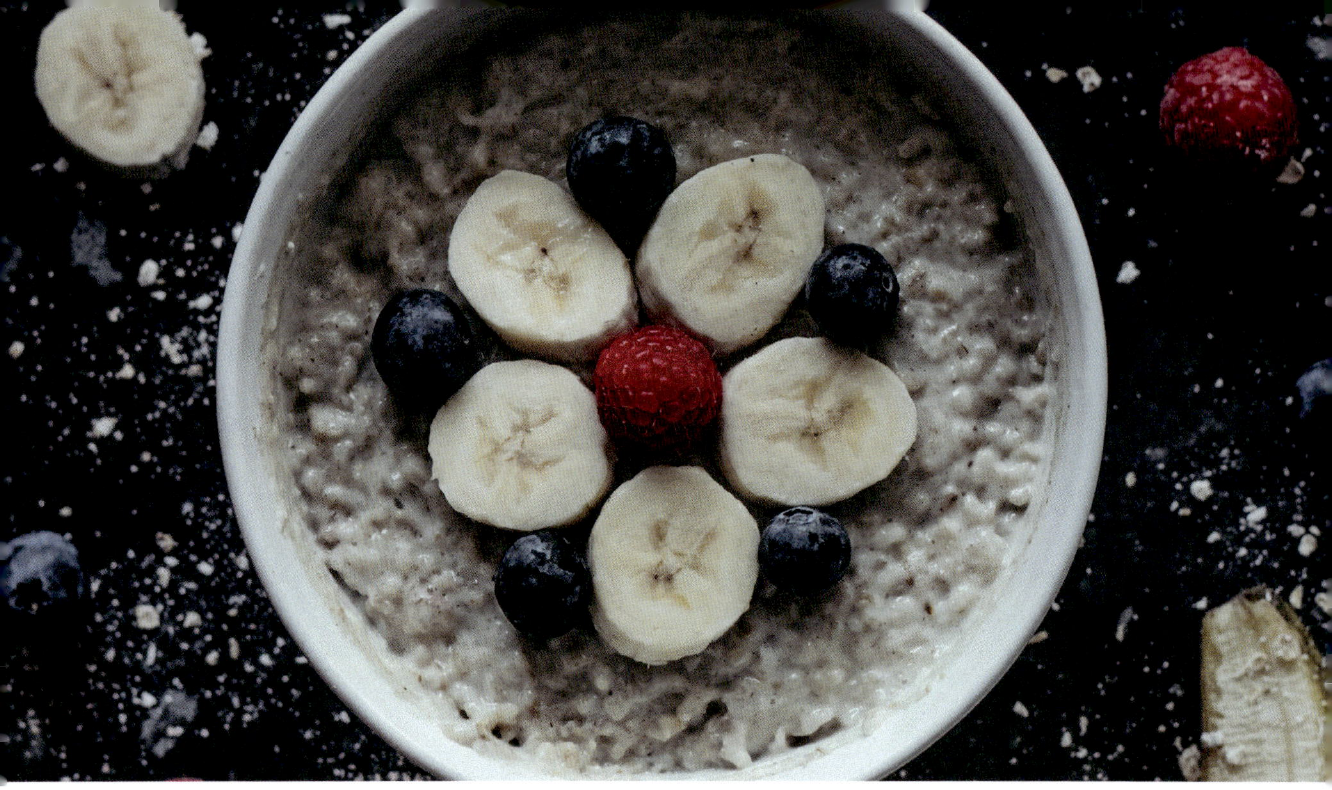

10. Oatmeal

Oatmeal contains beta-glucan, a soluble fibre that forms a thick gel when combined with water. The presence of this gel in the digestive system delays stomach emptying and the absorption of glucose into the blood. In addition, oats are rich in vitamins and minerals that help the energy production process. These include B vitamins, iron and manganese. The combined effect of all these nutrients makes oatmeal the optimal food for sustained energy release.

11. Oranges

Known the world over for their high levels of vitamin C, oranges can make you feel less tired just two hours after eating them. A small glass of orange juice will do exactly the same job. As a personal trainer, I couldn't get through my busy week without a few oranges to keep me energised.

12. Nuts

Most nuts like almonds, walnuts, Brazil and cashews are brimming with trace nutrients, healthy fats, as well as being an excellent source of protein. Past studies have found that their nutrition content can help sustain energy levels. Plus, they're easy to take wherever you go.

13. Quinoa

Packed with more protein than any other grain and rich in amino acids quinoa is the perfect food for your midday energy boost. It's high in folate, phosphorus, magnesium and manganese, making it a nutrient-packed source of carbohydrates for long-lasting energy levels.

14. Salmon

Honestly, there is nothing fishy about this entry in my top 20 list! Not only is salmon great for muscle development it's also a rich source for omega-3 fatty acids and protein, which can help you maintain high energy levels during even your most hectic days. I make sure this, along with tuna steaks or smoked haddock features in my evening meals during the week.

15. Strawberries

Strawberries are another good energy-boosting fruit. They can provide you with carbohydrates, fibre and sugars that can enhance energy levels. In addition to helping fight inflammation in the body, the antioxidants found in strawberries may help fight fatigue and give you energy. Try adding them to your breakfast cereal or fruit salad as part of your 5 a day.

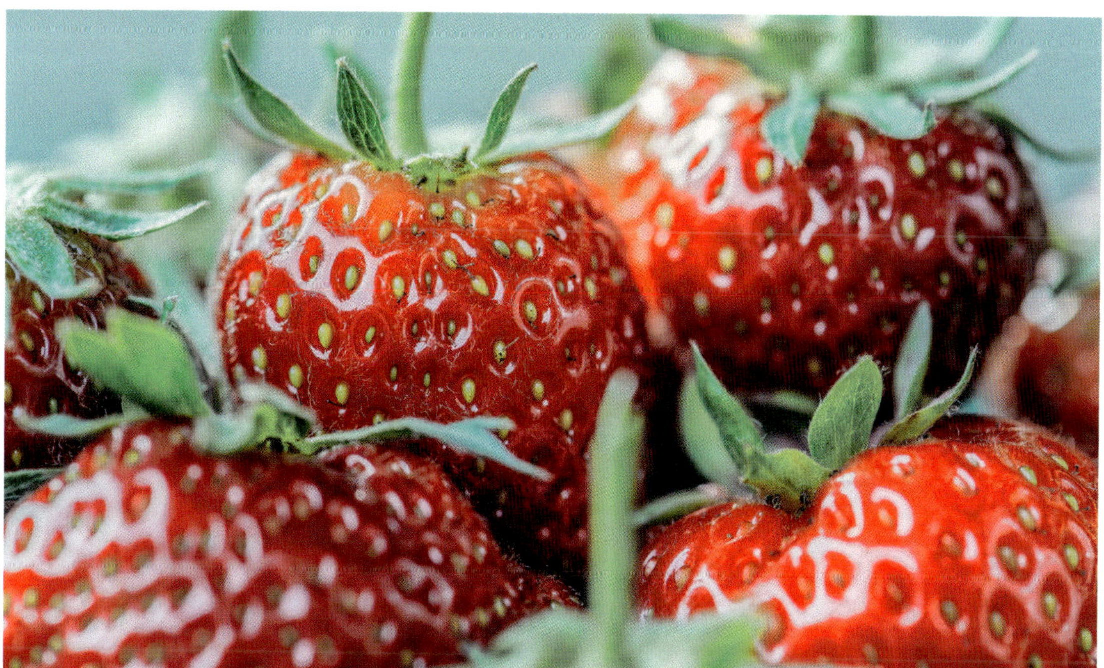

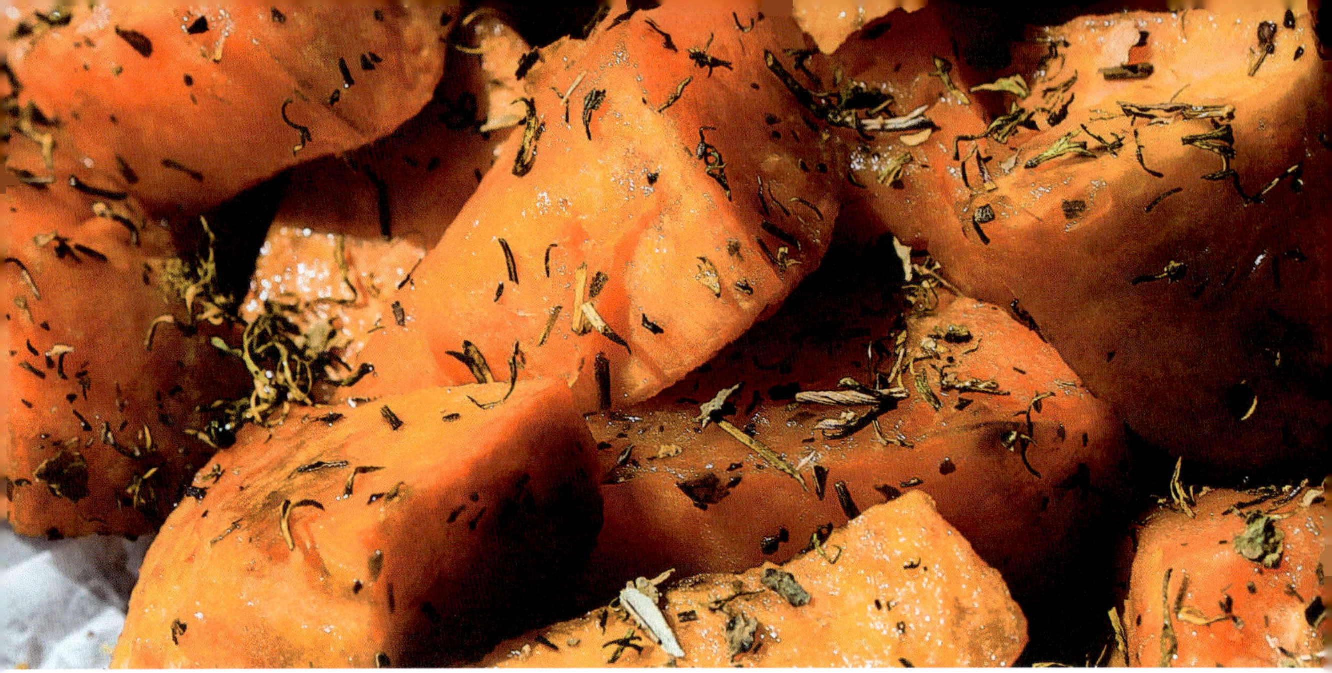

16. Sweet Potatoes

Sweet potatoes are a delicious nutritious source of energy for those looking for an extra boost. Due to sweet potatoes' fibre content and complex carbohydrates, the body digests them at a slow pace, which provides you with a steady supply of energy. Sweet potatoes are also a great source of manganese, which helps in the breakdown of nutrients to produce energy. I bake these and eat the skin.

17. Tuna

Loaded with protein and vitamin B, eating this type of fish can provide you with a great source of energy. I go for the canned in brine water variety which is a great option for weight loss too. Eating tuna for lunch can perk up your energy levels no end. Add a green salad and a hard-boiled egg for the perfect energy power lunch which is my personal trainer favourite dish!

18. Water

Past studies have found that dehydration is the main culprit as to why we feel so tired all of the time or the reason we think we're hungry enough to eat the entire contents of the fridge in a single sitting. So, the next time you're feeling particularly sluggish or ravenously hungry, guzzle down some cool tap water or even your favourite fancy mineral water for that much-needed energy boost. You can always add a little fruit squash for flavour if the thought of drinking only water bores you. Aim for 6-8 glasses each day.

19. Whole Grain Cereal

In my humble personal trainer opinion, there's nothing bland about whole grain cereal and I invariably start my day with a nice big bowl of the stuff, topped with some sliced banana. Eating this in the morning is a great way to pump up your energy levels. The high-fibre whole grain cereals slow the release of glucose into your bloodstream which translates to more consistent energy levels throughout your day.

20. Yogurt

Yogurt is a great source of high-quality protein to not only fill you up but provide basic energy for your brain. For me, the best part about yogurt is that it pairs well with pretty much everything. Add some granola, muesli, nuts, sliced banana or handful of blueberries to max up its flavour. My nearest and dearest often refers to me as 'the yogurt monster'. There's a good reason why this food features in this list.

So, there you have it, some of the very best foods around to boost your energy levels, of course, diet is just one side of the equation as you get fit for later life, you'll need to add in regular exercise, and if you lack the motivation to start this, or simply do not know where to begin, then having a qualified personal trainer can help you achieve your health and fitness goal.

In the UK, you can find a personal trainer near you by downloading the My Coach App. You can download this here: **www.fibodo.com** and if you live in or around Brighton & Hove, you'll find my details here too.

The next time you go shopping consider trying some of the foods listed here as part of a balanced and or calorie-controlled diet.

Caution: Food Allergies I'm among one of the lucky ones, a personal trainer who can eat pretty much anything without suffering any unpleasant allergic reactions. Dairy products, cereals and nuts don't pose any problem to my health. While these are my top foods and drinks for boosting energy levels, they may not be suitable for everyone. Always read the food label!

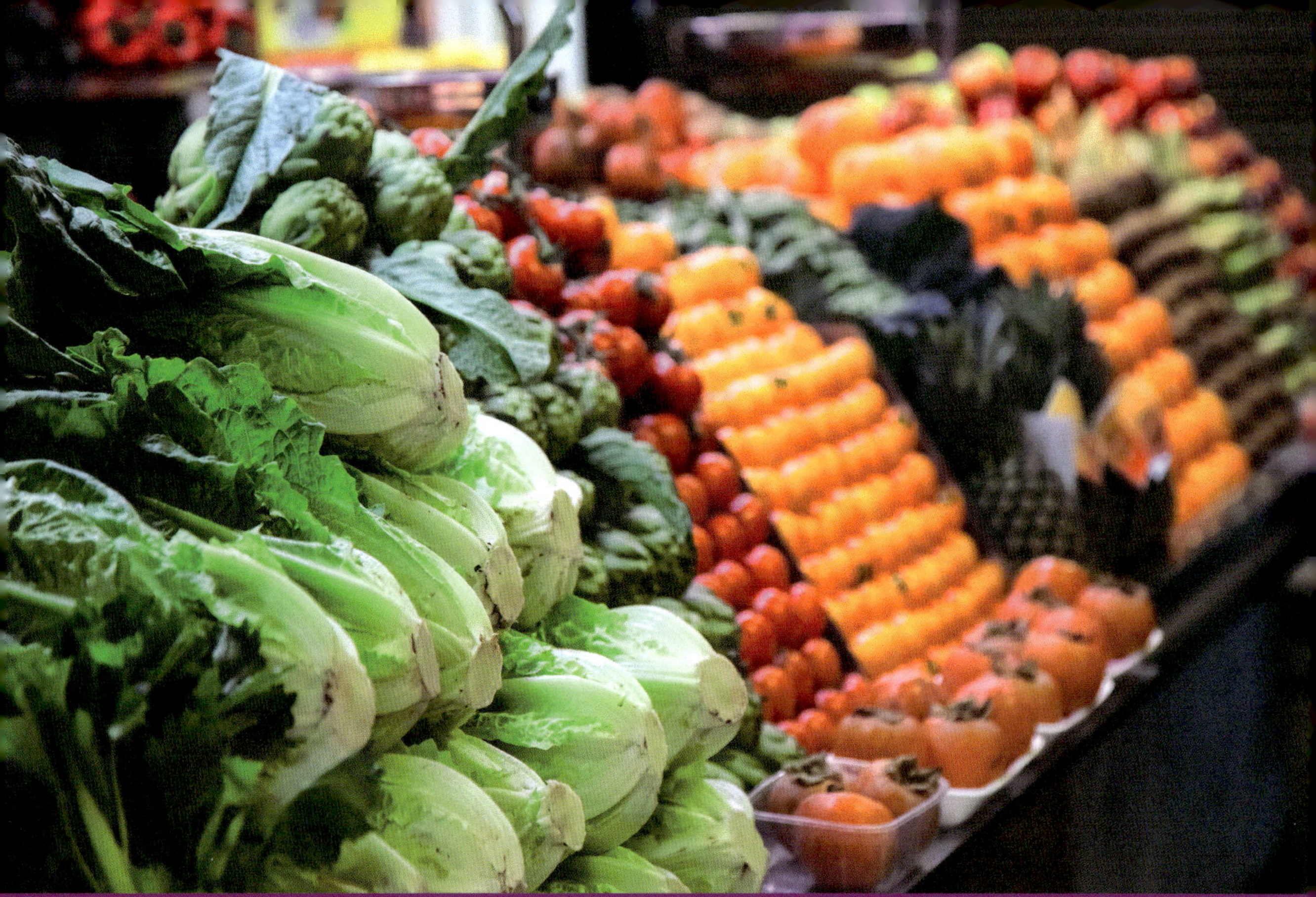

"The way to get started is to quit talking and start doing."

CHAPTER 24

The Best Foods To Boost Your Immune System

Having a healthy balanced diet filled with certain foods can help keep your immune system super-charged. I routinely include many of the foods listed below specifically for this purpose. If you're looking for ways to prevent colds, flu, and other infections then your first step should be a visit to your local supermarket and or farmer's market rather than the chemist. So, plan your meals to include these powerful immune system boosting foods.

1. Almonds

When it comes to preventing and fighting off colds, vitamin E tends to take a backseat to vitamin C. However, this powerful antioxidant is key to maintaining a healthy immune system. It's a fat-soluble vitamin, which means it requires the presence of fat to be absorbed properly. Nuts, such as almonds are packed with vitamin E and also have healthy fats. Adults only need about 15 mg of vitamin E each day. Almonds are a favourite and I take a small tubful while on the go.

2. Black Cumin Seed Oil

This oil has been extensively studied over the last fifty years. Used in traditional healing for thousands of years, it may be effective in supporting the immune and nervous systems. One such study tested how effective black cumin seed oil, as well as a number of antibiotics, is on superbugs. The study found that most bugs were indeed resistant to antibiotics, but that black cumin oil successfully stopped the growth of 97 out of 144.

3. Bone Broth

Chicken soup is the one of the oldest cold and flu remedies in the book, and, it's currently seeing a surge in popularity in the form of bone broth, which is the fashionable for what we all knew as chicken soup growing up. Bone Broth helps keep you hydrated which is useful when you're dehydrated from the dry winter air or seasonal colds and flu.

4. Broccoli

Broccoli is supercharged with vitamins and minerals. Packed with vitamins A, C, and E, as well as fibre and many other antioxidants, broccoli is one of the healthiest vegetables you can eat. The key to keeping its power intact is to cook it as little as possible, so steamed is ideal as research has shown it is the best way to keep more nutrients in.

5. Cinnamon

Many of us sprinkle cinnamon on our coffee or porridge. Cinnamon's power is in its antiviral, antibacterial and antifungal effect on the body. It can reduce bacteria's ability to multiply, and if you do end up suffering from a cold, it should help it clear up quicker. Adding this to porridge is a favourite of mine with a drizzle of honey.

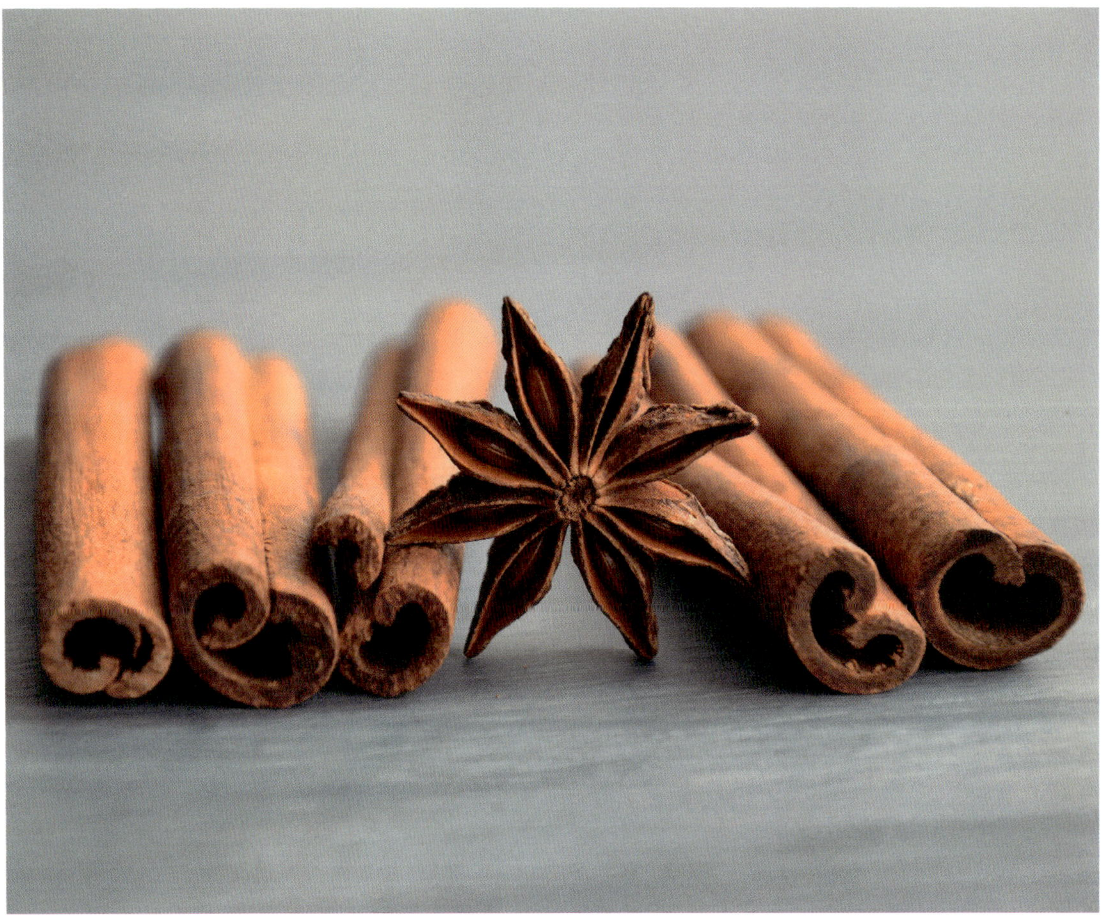

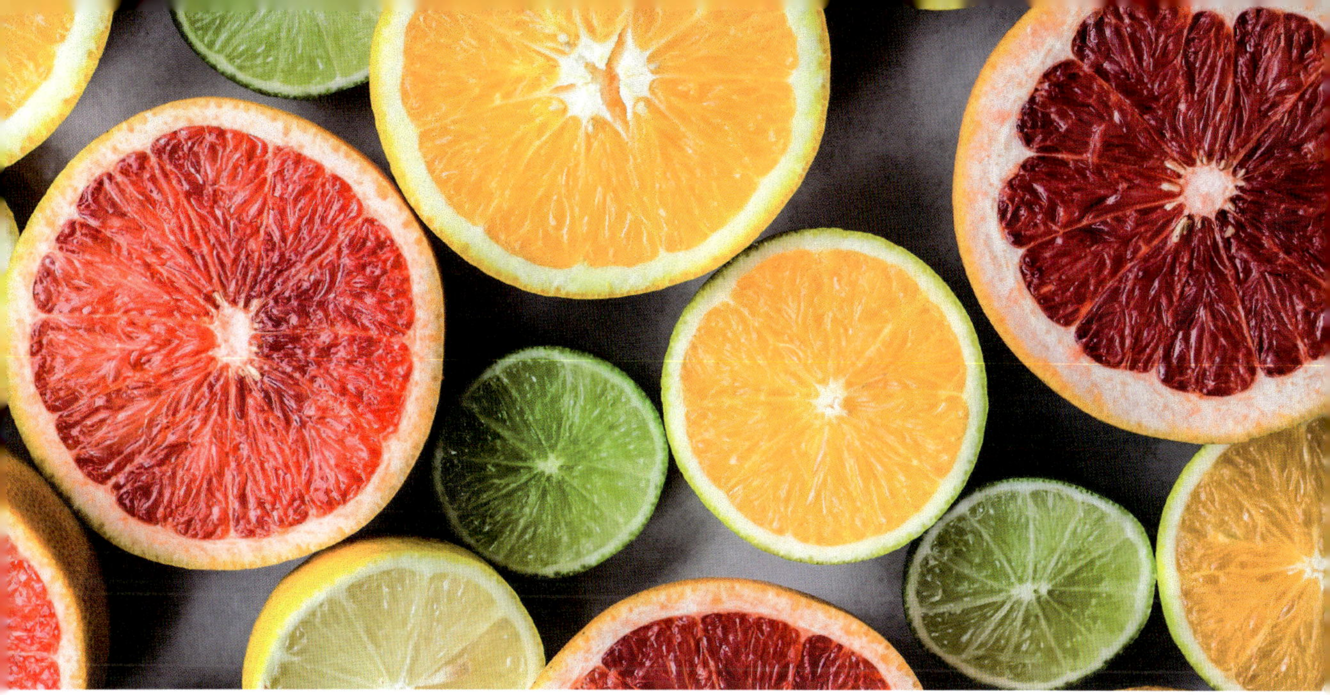

6. Citrus Fruits

Most people turn straight to vitamin C after they've caught a cold. That's because it helps build up your immune system. Vitamin C is thought to increase the production of white blood cells, which are key to fighting infections.

Almost all citrus fruits are high in vitamin C. With such a wide variety to choose from, it's easy to add a squeeze of this vitamin to any meal. Popular citrus fruits include grapefruit, oranges, clementines, mandarins, tangerines, kumquats, lemons and limes. As a personal trainer, I couldn't get through my busy week without a few oranges to keep me energised.

Because your body doesn't produce or store it, you need daily vitamin C for continued health. The recommended daily allowance for most adults is 75 mg for women and 90 mg for men. Keep in mind that while vitamin C might help you recover from a cold quicker. Sadly there's no evidence yet that it's effective against the new Covid-19.

7. Garlic

Garlic is found in almost every cuisine around the world. It adds a flavour and zest to food and it's a must-have for your health. Ancient civilisations recognised its value for fighting infections. Garlic may also slow down hardening of the arteries. Garlic's immune-boosting properties seem to come from a heavy concentration of sulphur-containing compounds, such as Allicin.

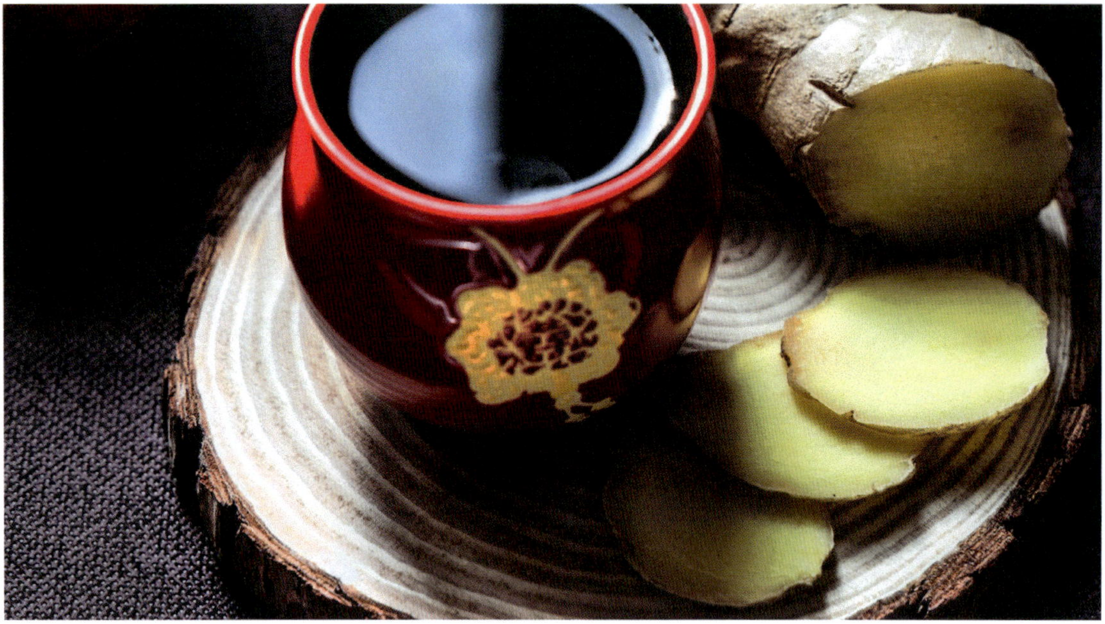

8. Ginger

Ginger is another ingredient many people turn to after falling unwell. Ginger may help to decrease inflammation, which can help reduce a sore throat and other inflammatory illnesses. While it's used in many sweet desserts, ginger packs some heat in the form of Gingerol, a relative of Capsaicin. Ginger may also possess cholesterol-lowering properties. This versatile spice tastes great in a stir fry.

9. Green Tea

Green tea is packed with flavonoids, a type of antioxidant. Where green tea really excels is in its levels of epigallocatechin gallate (EGCG), another powerful antioxidant. In scientific studies, EGCG has been shown to enhance immune function. Green tea is also a good source of the amino acid L-theanine. L-theanine may aid in the production of germ-fighting compounds in your T cells.

10. Kiwi Fruit

Like papayas, kiwis are naturally loaded full of essential nutrients, including folate, potassium, vitamin K, and vitamin C. Vitamin C boosts the white blood cells to fight infection, while kiwi's other nutrients keep the rest of your body functioning properly. These liven up any fruit salad or smoothie.

11. Mushrooms

There is a growing body of evidence that indicates people who eat mushrooms on a regular basis have increased immunity. One study found that people who ate a cooked shiitake mushroom every day for four weeks had stronger immune systems as a result. Mushrooms are rich in vitamin B6, vitamin D, potassium, copper and selenium.

12. Papaya

Papaya is another fruit loaded with vitamin C. You can find double the daily RDA of vitamin C in a single medium fruit. Papayas also have a digestive enzyme called papain that has anti-inflammatory effects. Papayas also have decent amounts of potassium, magnesium, and folate, all of which are beneficial to your overall general health.

13. Poultry

When you're sick and you reach for chicken soup, it's more than just the placebo effect that makes you feel better. The soup may help lower inflammation, which could improve symptoms of a cold. Poultry, such as chicken and turkey, is high in vitamin B-6. About 3 ounces of light turkey or chicken meat contains nearly one-third of your daily recommended amount of B-6. Vitamin B-6 is an important player in many of the chemical reactions that happen in the body. It's also vital to the formation of new and healthy red blood cells. Stock or broth made by boiling chicken bones contains gelatine, chondroitin, and other nutrients helpful for gut healing and immunity. I eat a lot of chicken, probably 3-days of each week.

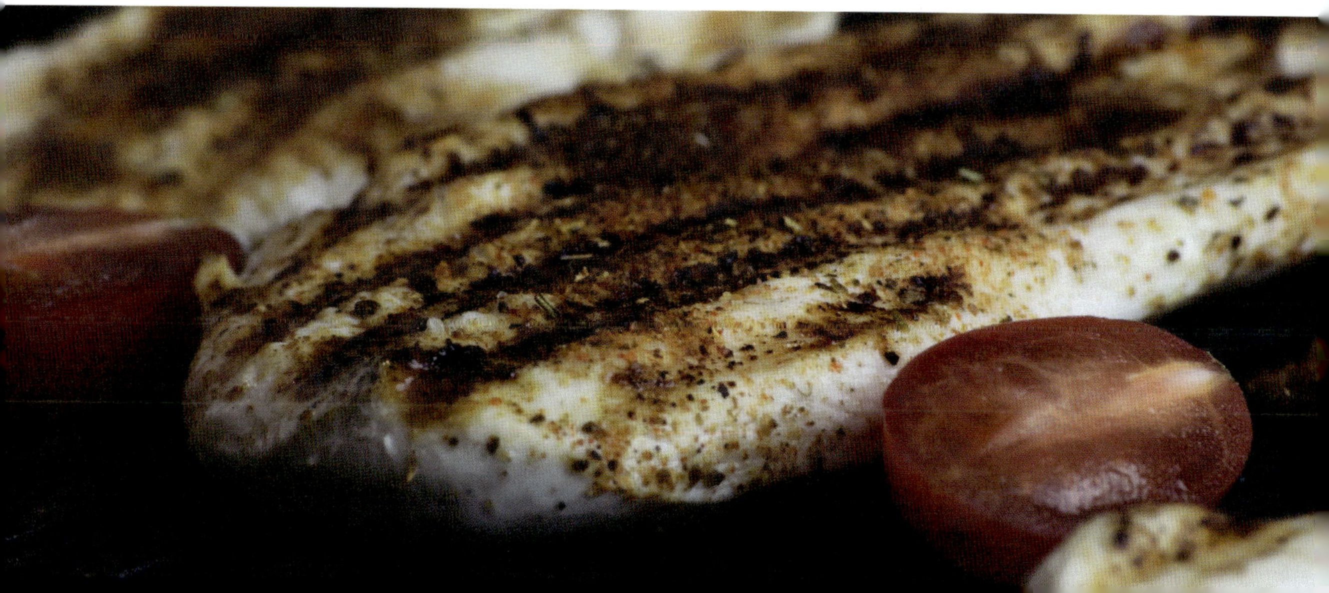

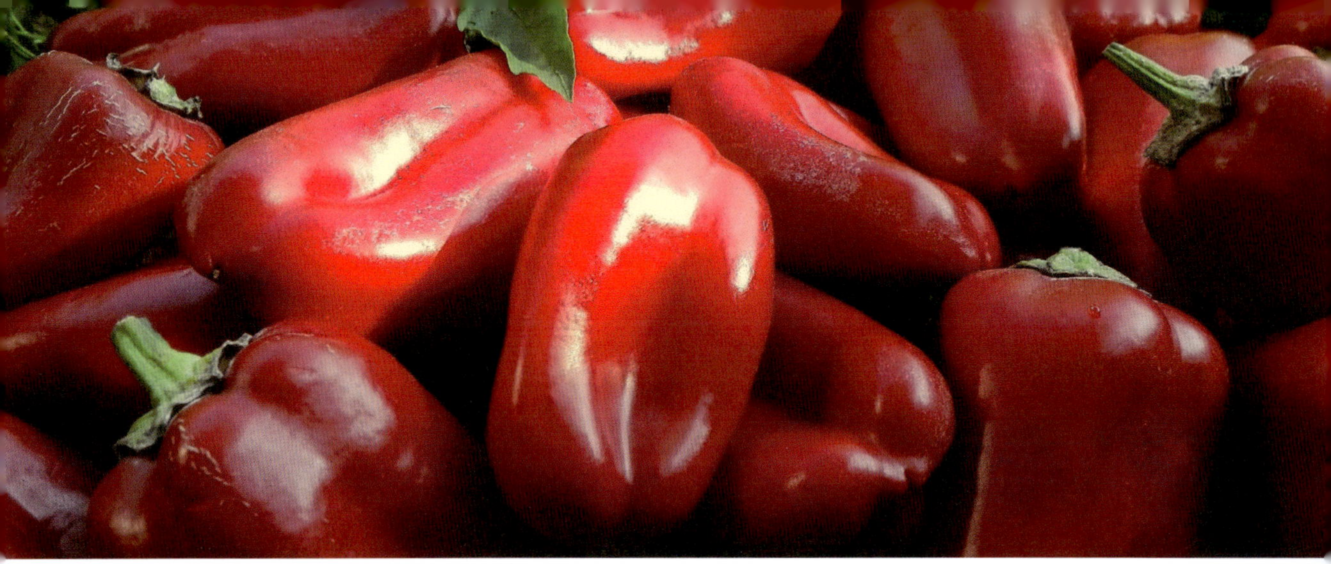

14. Red Bell Peppers

If you think citrus fruits have the most vitamin C of any fruit or vegetable, you're in for surprise. Gram for gram, red bell peppers-contain almost 3 times as much vitamin C when compared to a Florida orange. They're also a rich source of beta carotene. In addition to boosting your immune system, vitamin C may help you maintain healthy skin and complexion. Beta carotene, which your body converts into vitamin A, also helps keep your eyes and skin healthy.

15. Shellfish

Shellfish isn't the obvious choice when looking for a way to boost your immune system, but some types of shellfish are packed with zinc. Zinc doesn't get as much attention as many other vitamins and minerals, but our bodies need it so that our immune cells can function as intended. Popular varieties of shellfish that are high in zinc include oysters, crab, lobster and mussels. Keep in mind that you don't want to have more than the daily recommended amount of zinc in your diet 11 mg for adult men and 8 mg for most adult women. Too much zinc can actually inhibit immune system function.

16. Spinach

Spinach is crammed full with numerous antioxidants as well as Beta Carotene, which may both increase the infection-fighting ability of our immune systems. Similar to broccoli, spinach is healthiest when it's cooked as little as possible so that it retains its nutrients. However, light cooking makes it easier to absorb vitamin A and allows other nutrients to be released from oxalic acid, an antinutrient. I generally go down the light cooking route.

17. Sunflower Seeds

Sunflower seeds are full of nutrients, including phosphorous, magnesium, and vitamins B-6 and E. Vitamin E is important in regulating and maintaining immune system function. Other foods with high amounts of vitamin E include avocados and dark leafy greens. Sunflower seeds are also incredibly high in selenium. I snack on these, in place of crisps.

18. Turmeric

You may know turmeric as a key ingredient in many curries. This bright yellow, bitter spice has also been used for years as an anti-inflammatory in treating both osteoarthritis and rheumatoid arthritis. Research has shown that high concentrations of curcumin, which gives turmeric its distinctive colour, can help decrease exercise-induced muscle damage.

19. Water

Keeping hydrated is of paramount importance, whether you are trying to avoid getting sick or already fighting a cold. Downing fruit juices when you're under the weather will only lead to a blood sugar crash, making you feel worse. Since our body's fluid needs increase when we're fighting infection, drinking your daily minimum plus a few extra glasses can help flush bacteria through your system.

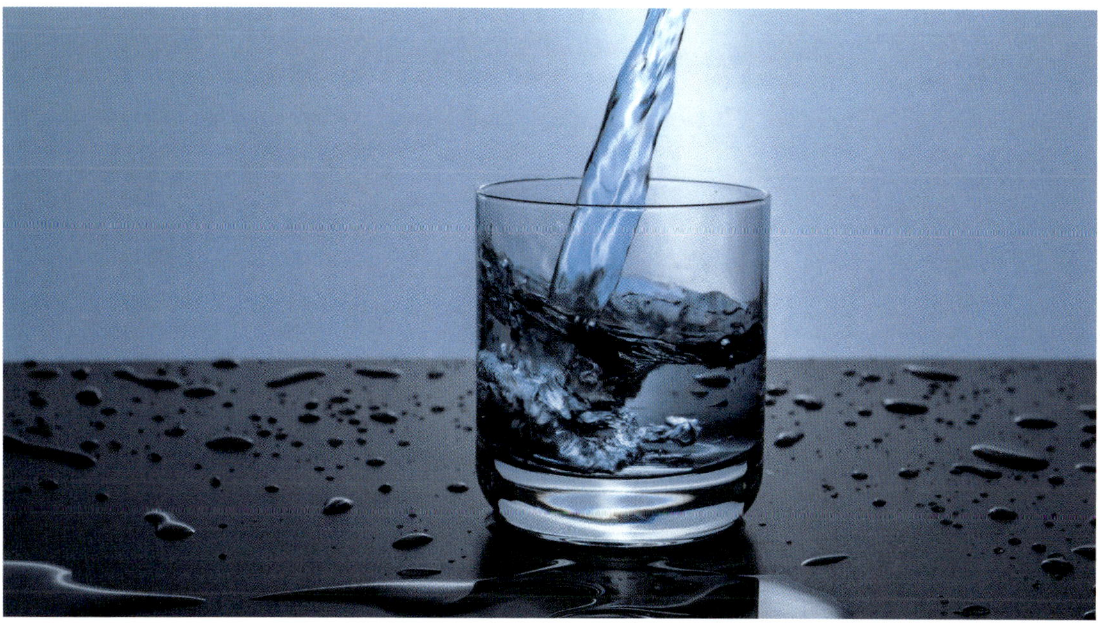

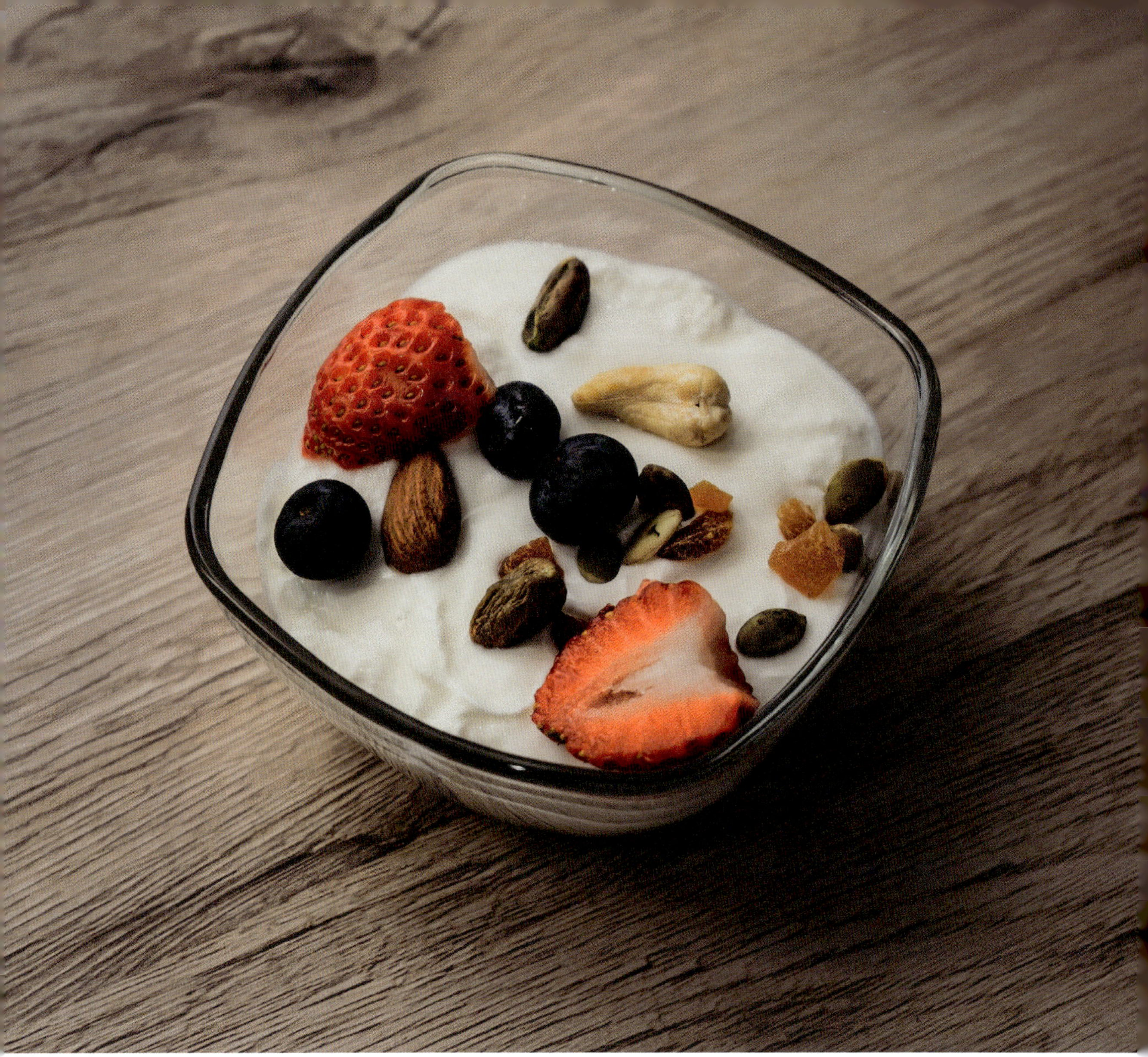

20. Yogurt

Look for yogurts that contain the phrase 'live and active cultures' on the label, like Greek yogurt. These cultures may stimulate your immune system to help fight diseases. Try to get plain yogurt rather than the kind that are flavoured as these are often loaded with sugar. You can easily sweeten plain yogurt yourself with healthy fruits and a drizzle of honey instead. Yogurt can also be a great source of vitamin D, so try to select brands fortified with this vitamin. Vitamin D helps regulate the immune system and is thought to boost our body's natural defences against diseases. It may also better protect you from Covid-19.

So, there you have it, some of the best foods to boost your immune system, of course, you'll need to add in regular exercise to improve your overall general health, and if you lack the motivation to start this or simply do not know where to begin, then having a qualified personal trainer can help you achieve your health and fitness goal.

In the UK, you can find a personal trainer near you by downloading the My Coach App. You can download this here: **www.fibodo.com** and if you live in or around Brighton & Hove, you'll find my details here too.

The next time you go shopping consider trying some of the foods listed here as part of a balanced and or calorie-controlled diet.

Caution: Food Allergies I'm among one of the lucky ones, a personal trainer who can eat pretty much anything without suffering any unpleasant allergic reactions. Dairy products, cereals and nuts don't pose any problem to my health. While these are my top foods for boosting the immune system, they may not be suitable for everyone. Always read the food label!

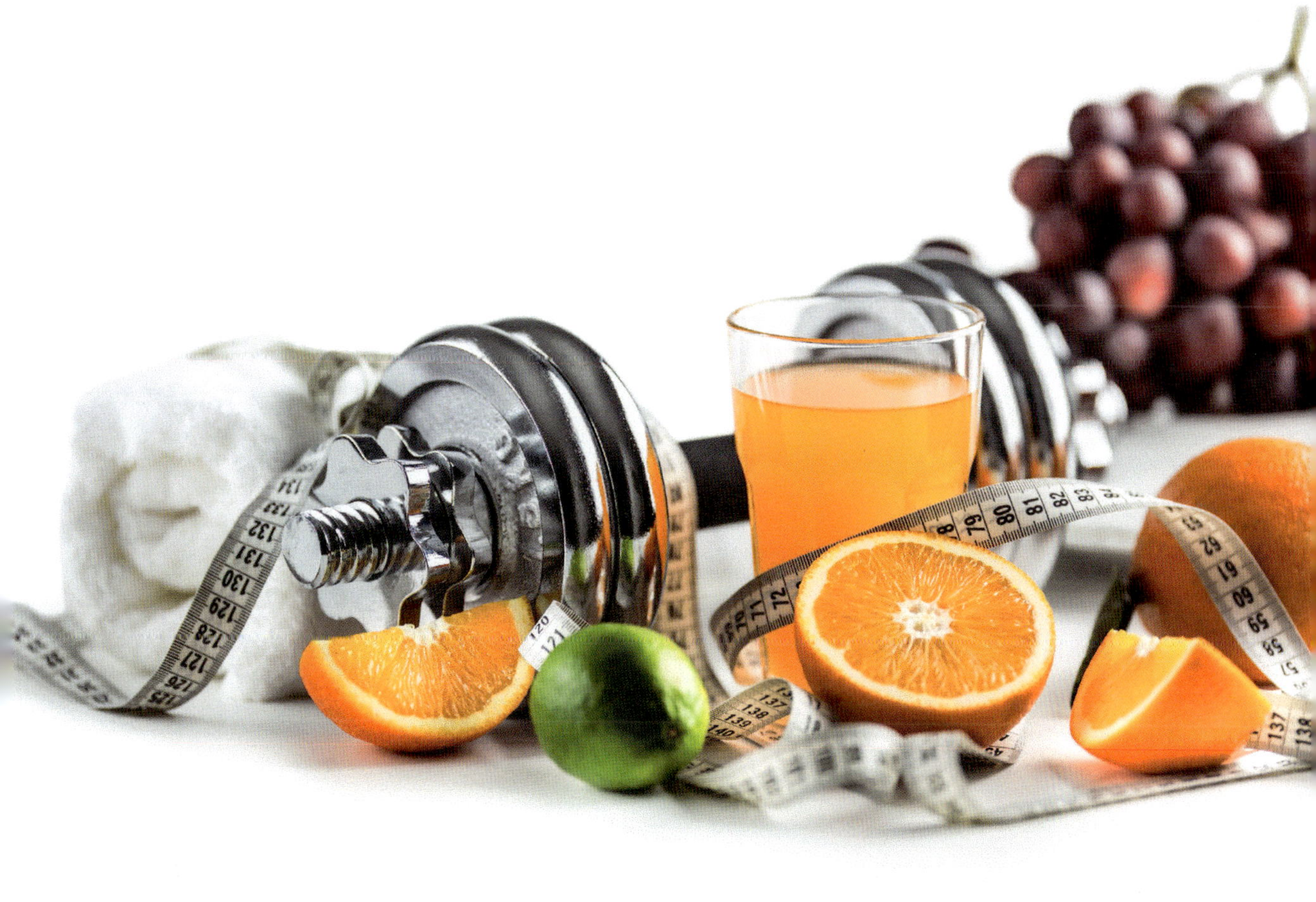

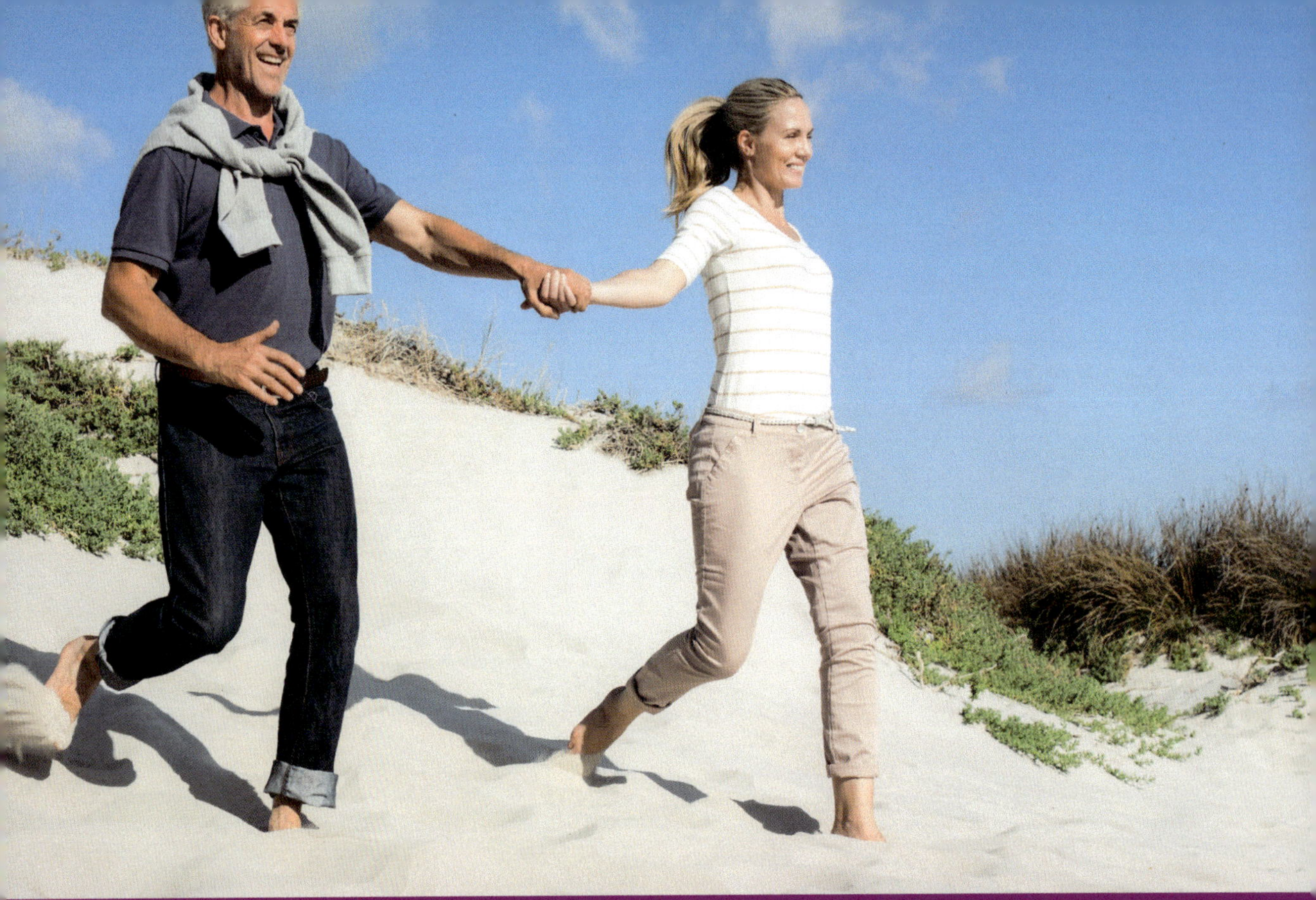

"A journey of a thousand miles begins with a single step. You've just taken your first step. Keep going!"

CHAPTER 25

Get Started On Your How To 2 Get Fit 4 Later Life Challenge

I said right at the start of this book that my wish for you is to take up my **HOW 2 GET FIT 4 LATER LIFE 12-WEEK CHALLENGE**, and discover for yourself, how great a healthier and fitter you feels. You should now have collated all your answers and already have downloaded your **GET FIT TOOL KIT**. Your answers will guide you as to whether your **12-WEEK CHALLENGE** is to start exercising or to start exercising combined with a calorie-controlled diet. Either-way, please discuss your intention with your doctor. It is important to know that it is safe for you to start exercising, and your doctor can also provide guidance on dieting.

Within the **GET FIT TOOL KIT**, you'll find everything you need to start the 12-week challenge. Download the **GET FIT TOOL KIT** at **www.3fspt.co.uk/toolkit**.

Your Answers Sheet

If you haven't already answered the questions you'll need to revisit the ends of chapter 2, 3, 4, 5, 6, 7, 8 and 16.

Blank 3-Day Food Diary

Use this to record a typical 3-days worth of what you eat and drink. You'll get the most from it by not altering your current dietary habits. You'll be able to work out how many calories you typically eat each day using the A-Z CALORIE COUNTS FOR POPULAR FOOD LIST and to see how healthy or otherwise your current diet is. Remember that not eating enough calories is as much a threat to your physical health as eating too much. If you find that you are underweight and are not eating enough calories, please go and see your doctor.

If you decide to go on a diet, then I typically recommend my personal training clients to use the NHS WEIGHT LOSS PLAN which has been developed in conjunction with THE BRITISH DIETIC ASSOCIATION. Please exercise caution using celebrity diets and 'fad' and or extreme weight loss diets. These can be potentially harmful, and while you may get dramatic results fairly quickly, the weight loss is unlikely to be sustainable. The NHS knows best! Learn more here: **www.nhs.uk/live-well/healthy-weight/start-the-nhs-weight-loss-plan**

Blank 12-Week Exercise Planner

If you've read through my **12-WEEK EXERCISE PLANNER** and feel that the exercises aren't all appropriate, for example, you may prefer more or indeed only chair-based options, then use this template to design your own **12-WEEK EXERCISE PLAN**. If you have limited mobility in your legs but are more able with your arms and hands, then you might want to consider buying a portable pedal exerciser. You can use this sitting at a table, using your arms and hands on the pedals, and this will provide you with a good aerobic workout in place of taking regular walks. Prices vary, but you can get a decent one from between £20 to £35. Drive DeVilbiss Healthcare has one at £24.99.

Exercise Planner As Per The Book

This is my recommendation on how to go from doing little or no exercise to the recommended weekly minimum of 150-minutes of moderate-intensity exercise. There are small time and number of repetition increments each week to steadily take you to your goal.

A-Z Calorie Counts For Popular Food List

Use this helpful calorie counter to help you keep to a calorie-controlled diet.

The Individual Step-By-Step Exercise Sections:

- Warm-Up Exercises
- Aerobic Exercises
- Balance Exercises
- Chair-Based Exercises
- Strength Exercises
- Core Exercises
- Stretching Exercises

These are repeated from earlier in the book for your convenience. Keep these in handy reach as you try the exercises for the first few times, going step-by-step.

How 2 Get Fit 4 Later Life 12-Week Challenge App

If you really get stuck and you use a Smartphone you can have an App version of the 12-week programme, with instructional videos of me to show you good form for each of the exercises, daily prompts and the opportunity through the Facebook Group to contact me each week to report your progress, and to get some all important encouragement and support! The App version for the 12-week course costs £89. For more information please email **gav@3fspt.co.uk**.

How 2 Get Fit 4 Later Life Facebook Group

Whether you decide to use the App version of the 12-week programme or not, I highly recommend you join the **HOW 2 GET FIT 4 LATER LIFE FACEBOOK GROUP**. I've set this up for everyone who takes up the 12-week challenge to provide peer support, motivation and to share progress. The group already has over 100 members to help encourage and support you through the 12-week programme. I also want to encourage your friends and family members to join, so that they can lend their support in your quest for a healthier and fitter you. To join the Facebook Group use this link: **www.tiny.cc/H2GF4LL**

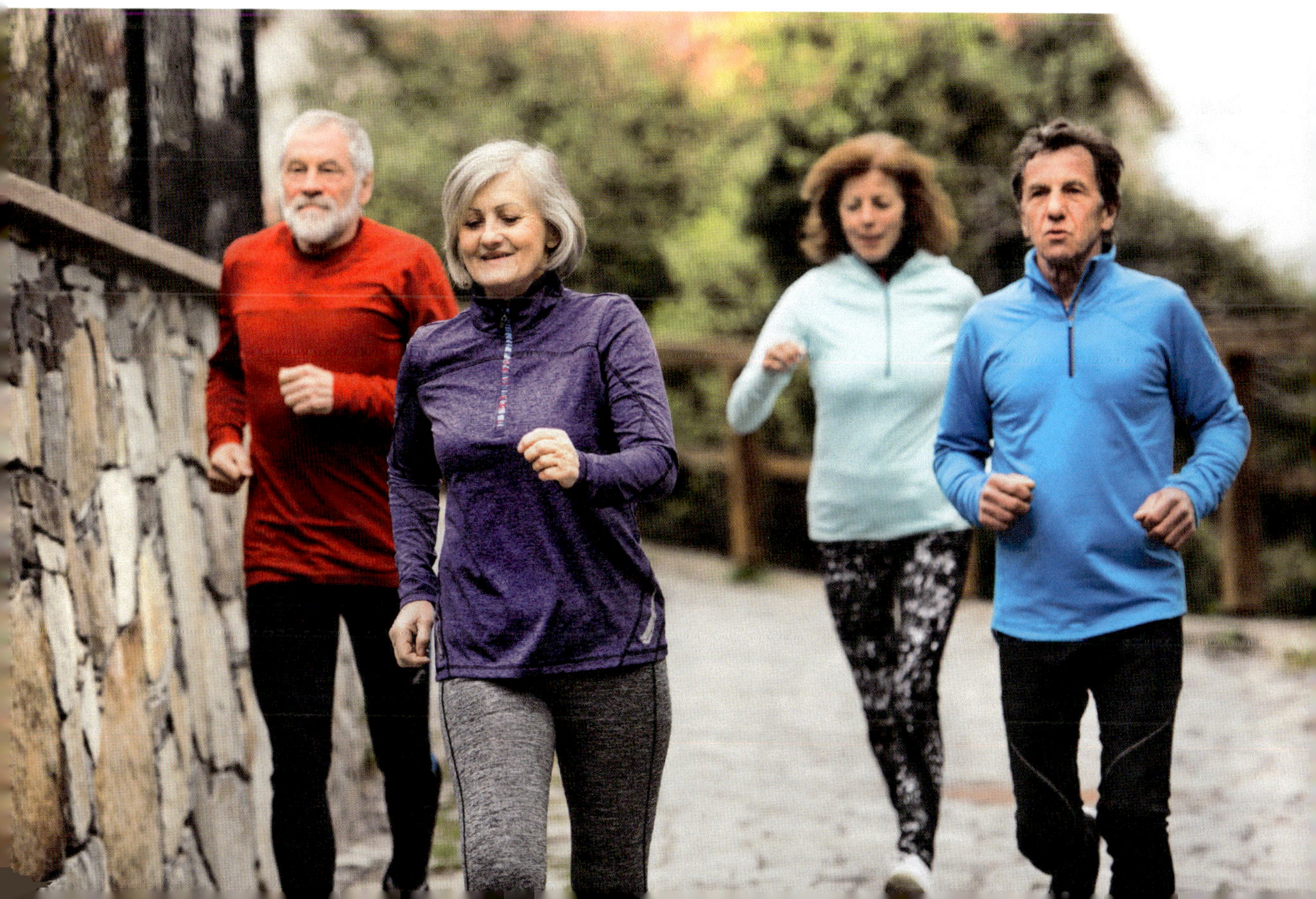

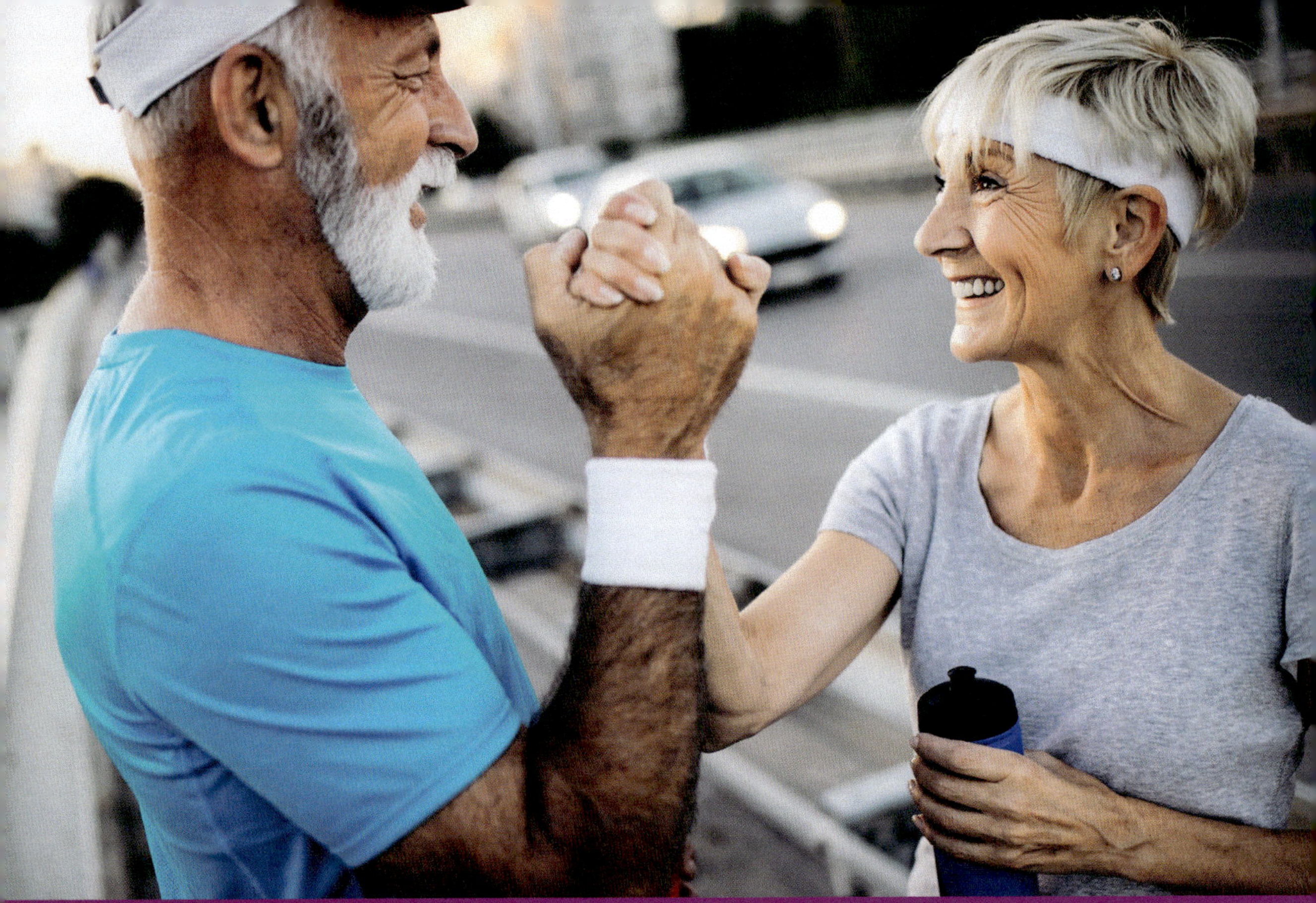

"Good luck in your
HOW 2 GET FIT 4 LATER
LIFE CHALLENGE!"

Contact

Questions

Thank you for reading **HOW 2 GET FIT 4 LATER LIFE - EXERCISE & NUTRITION FOR PEOPLE AGED 60+**. I hope you found it useful and motivational to get you regularly exercising and to change your diet for a healthier active lifestyle. If you have any questions about the exercises featured or the food and nutritional advice, please feel free to email **gav@3fspt.co.uk**.

Personal Training

If you are new to exercise and live in and around Brighton and Hove, I offer one-on-one personal training sessions, email **gav@3fspt.co.uk** for more information. I also do remote video linked personal training sessions, so if you live some distance away, I could still help you. In the UK, you can find a personal trainer near you by downloading the My Coach App. You can download this here: **www.fibodo.com** and you'll find my details here too, search for Gavin O'Brien.

Downloads

The **HOW 2 GET FIT 4 LATER LIFE TOOL KIT** is available as a digital download, visit **www.3fspt.co.uk/toolkit**.

Facebook Group

Join the **HOW 2 GET FIT 4 LATER LIFE FACEBOOK GROUP**. I've set this up for everyone who takes up the 12-week challenge to provide peer support, motivation and to share progress. I also want to encourage your friends and family members to join, so that they can lend their support in your quest for a healthier and fitter you. To join the Facebook Group use this link: **www.tiny.cc/H2GF4LL**

Glossary of terms

ATP - ATP transports chemical energy within cells for metabolism. Every cell in your body uses ATP for energy. It consists of a base (adenine) and three phosphate groups.

BMI - BMI (Body Mass Index) is a measurement that is a ratio of your weight and height. Knowing your BMI can help you and your doctor determine any health risks you may face if it's outside of the healthy range of 18.5 to 24.9.

BMR - BMR (Basal Metabolic Rate) is the amount of energy your body burns at rest daily. In other words, it is the number of calories required to keep your body functioning while you are not doing any physical activities.

COPD - Chronic obstructive pulmonary disease (COPD) is a common lung disease. Having COPD makes it hard to breathe. There are two main forms of COPD: Chronic bronchitis, which involves a long-term cough with mucus and Emphysema which involves damage to the lungs.

Hypermobility - Hypermobility means your joints are more flexible than in other people. You may think of yourself as being double-jointed. When this causes pain it might be joint hypermobility syndrome.

Osteoblasts - Large cell responsible for the synthesis and mineralisation of bone during both initial bone formation and later bone remodelling.

PARmed-X - The PARmed-X is a physical activity-specific checklist to be used by a doctor and or personal trainer with people who have had positive responses to the Physical Activity Readiness Questionnaire (PAR-Q).

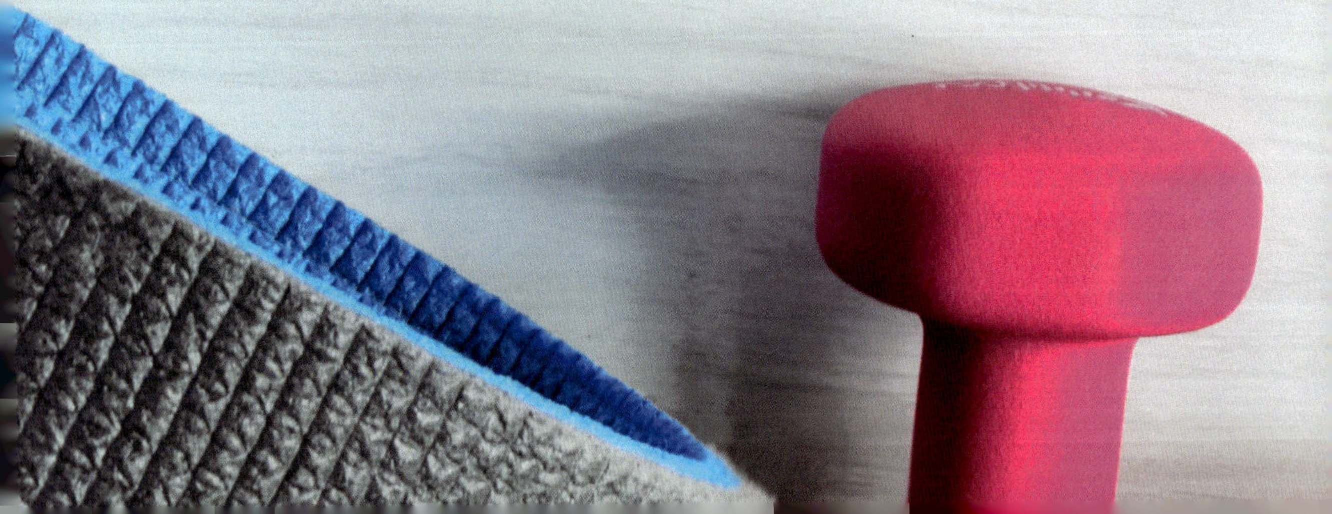

PAR-Q - The Physical Activity Readiness Questionnaire (PAR-Q) is a common method of uncovering health and lifestyle issues prior to an exercise programme starting. The questionnaire is short and easy to administer and reveals any family history of illness.

PNF - PNF stretching is an advanced form of flexibility training. It involves the contraction and stretching of muscles. The technique was first used in clinical rehabilitation. It spread into mainstream gyms because of its perceived effectiveness.

RDA - Stands for recommended dietary allowance and is the basis for the per cent daily values you see on nutrition and supplement labels. A group that became the Food and Nutrition Board established the values during World War II. They represent what the vast majority of healthy people need to stay well.

RI - Stands for 'Reference Intake', and refers to amounts of nutrients, as set out in law. They are there to provide a guideline of the contribution nutrients can make to a balanced diet. Reference Intakes are the same across Europe and are based on a healthy adult eating a 2000kcal diet.

SMART goals - SMART is an acronym that stands for Specific, Measurable, Achievable, Realistic, and Timely. Therefore, a SMART goal incorporates all of these criteria to help focus your efforts and increase the chances of achieving that goal.

Synovial fluid - Synovial fluid is the thick liquid that lubricates your joints and keeps them moving smoothly. It's on all of your joints, including in your knees, shoulders, hips, hands, and feet.

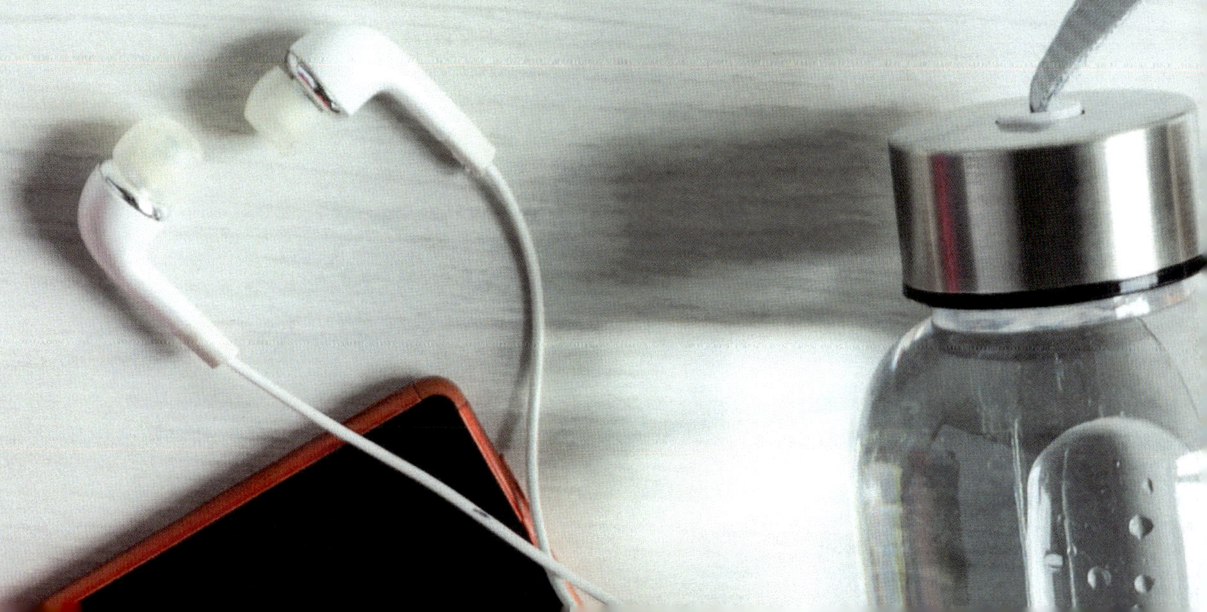

How 2 Get Fit 4 Later Life!

TOOL KIT

Welcome to the How 2 Get Fit 4 Life Tool Kit!

In this **HOW 2 GET FIT 4 LATER LIFE TOOL KIT** you have everything you need to go from doing little or no exercise step-by-step, week-by-week over 12-weeks to doing 150-minutes of exercise. You'll be working towards this with a mix of regular brisk walks, and at home exercise routines that focus on:

- **Flexibility**
- **Balance**
- **Strength**

My hope for you is that you have the motivation and determination to complete the 12-weeks, and then from there to keep on going with regular exercise and plenty of brisk walking, keeping you active, mobile and most importantly independent so that you live life to the full!

If you feel that you'd like the helping hand of a personal trainer, then there is a way we can work together over the **HOW 2 GET FIT 4 LATER LIFE 12-WEEK CHALLENGE**. You can have an App version of the programme, with instructional videos of me to show you good form, daily prompts and the opportunity through the Facebook Group to contact me each week to report your progress, and to get some all important encouragement and support!

For a one off fee of £89, you'll receive the App to download on your Smartphone or Tablet with weekly contact. Your goal of a new fitter, healthier and happier you, is my goal too. I understand that sometimes making changes is easier said than done. So, if you have any doubts about your ability to succeed, then give this option of additional support some serious thought.

How do I get the How 2 Get Fit 4 Later Life App?

For more information on the App and the additional help available, simply email **gav@3fspt.co.uk**. Please let me know a contact number, and the best time to call. However you decide to approach this **HOW 2 GET FIT 4 LATER LIFE 12-WEEK CHALLENGE**, I wish you the very best of luck, grit and determination to succeed! I know **YOU** can do it!

Tool Kit Contents

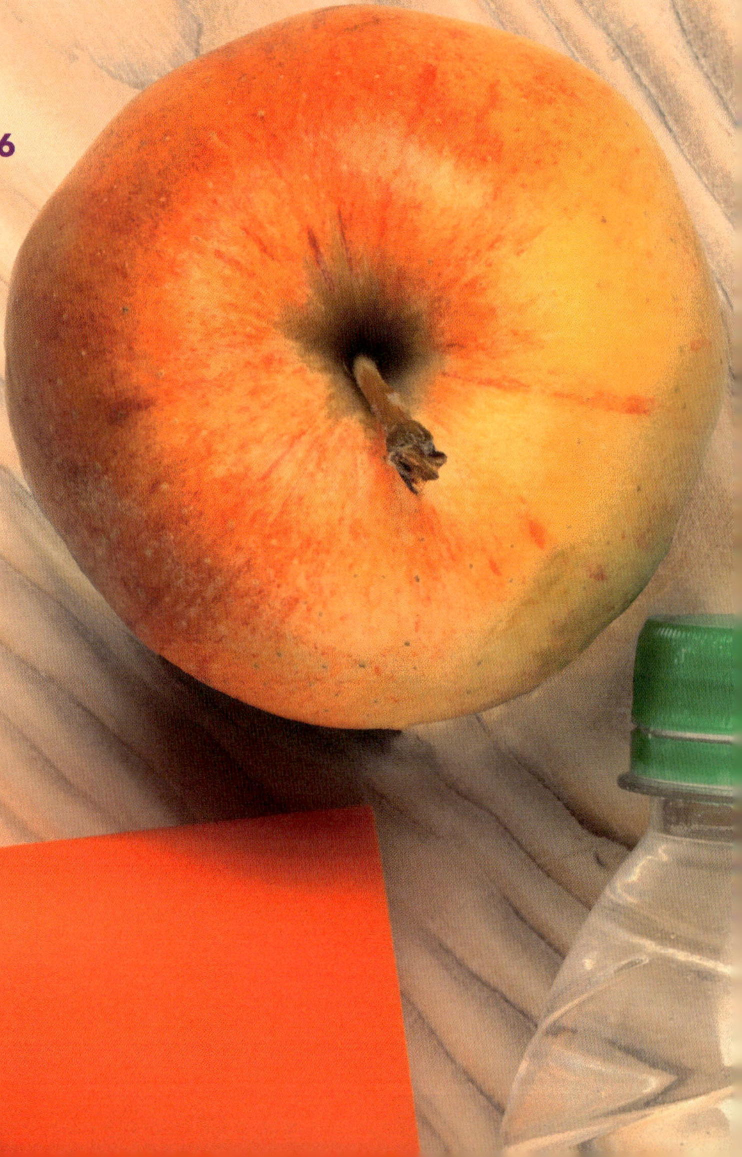

Get Fit 4 Later Life Exercise Answers

TYPE of EXERCISE	TIME SPENT	NUMBER of DAYS
AEROBIC Page 29		
BALANCE Page 38		
CHAIR-BASED Page 49		
STRENGTH Page 61		
CORE Page 71		
STRETCHING Page 78		

Guidance

- Aim to be physically active every day. Any activity is better than none. The more you do the better, even if it's just light activity.
- Aim to do activities that improve strength, balance and flexibility on at least 2 days a week.
- Aim to do at least 150 minutes of moderate intensity activity a week or 75 minutes of vigorous intensity activity if you are already active, or a combination of both.
- Aim to reduce time spent sitting or lying down and break up long periods of not moving with some activity.
- Use the **GET FITTER IN 12-WEEKS CHALLENGE** to go from zero to 150 minutes of activity. Speak to your doctor if you have any concerns about exercising. **Exercises are covered on pages 254 to 287**.

Get Fit 4 Later Life BMI & BMR Answers

Body Mass Index (Tick Box)

UNDERWEIGHT 18.5 or less	HEALTHY WEIGHT 18.5 - 24.9	OVERWEIGHT 25 - 29.9	OBESE 30 or above

Page 167

Basal Metabolic Rate (BMR)

MAINTAIN WEIGHT	GAIN WEIGHT ADD 500 CALS	LOSE WEIGHT MINUS 500 CALS

Page 168

Activity Level Adjustment for BMR	Calories
Sedentary: little or no exercise	
Exercise 1-3 times per week	
Exercise 4-5 times per week	
Daily exercise or intense exercise 3-4 times per week	
Intense exercise 6-7 times per week	
Very intense exercise daily, or physical job	

How 2 Get Fit 4 Later Life Facebook Group

Join the **HOW 2 GET FIT 4 LATER LIFE FACEBOOK GROUP**. I've set this up for everyone who takes up the 12-week challenge to provide peer support, motivation and to share progress. I also want to encourage your friends and family members to join, so that they can lend their support in your quest for a healthier and fitter you. To join the Facebook Group use this link: **www.tiny.cc/H2GF4LL**

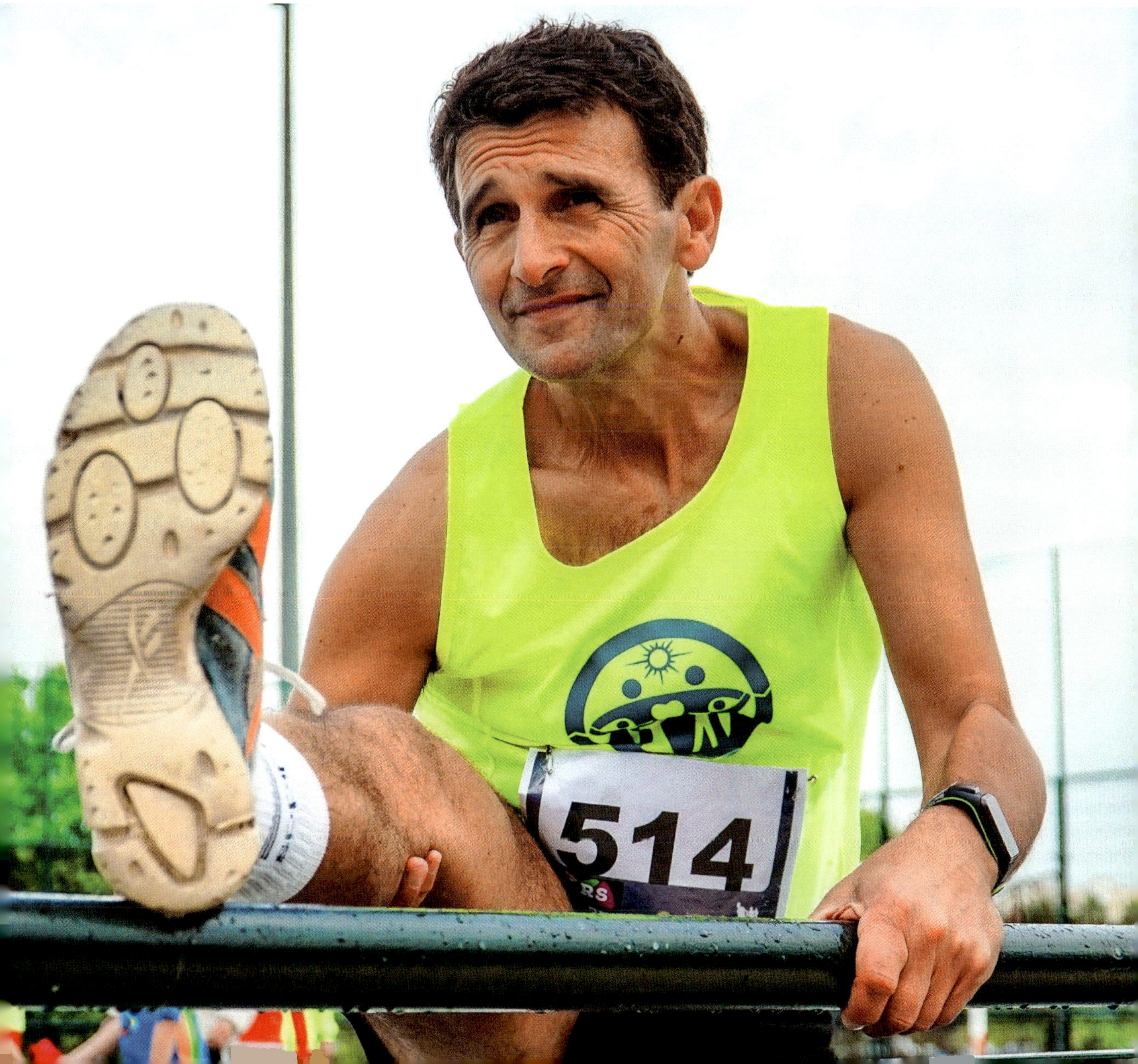

How 2 Get Fit 4 Later Life
3 Day Food Diary

	DAY 1	DAY 2	DAY 3
BREAKFAST			
SNACK			
LUNCH			
SNACK			
DINNER			
SNACK			

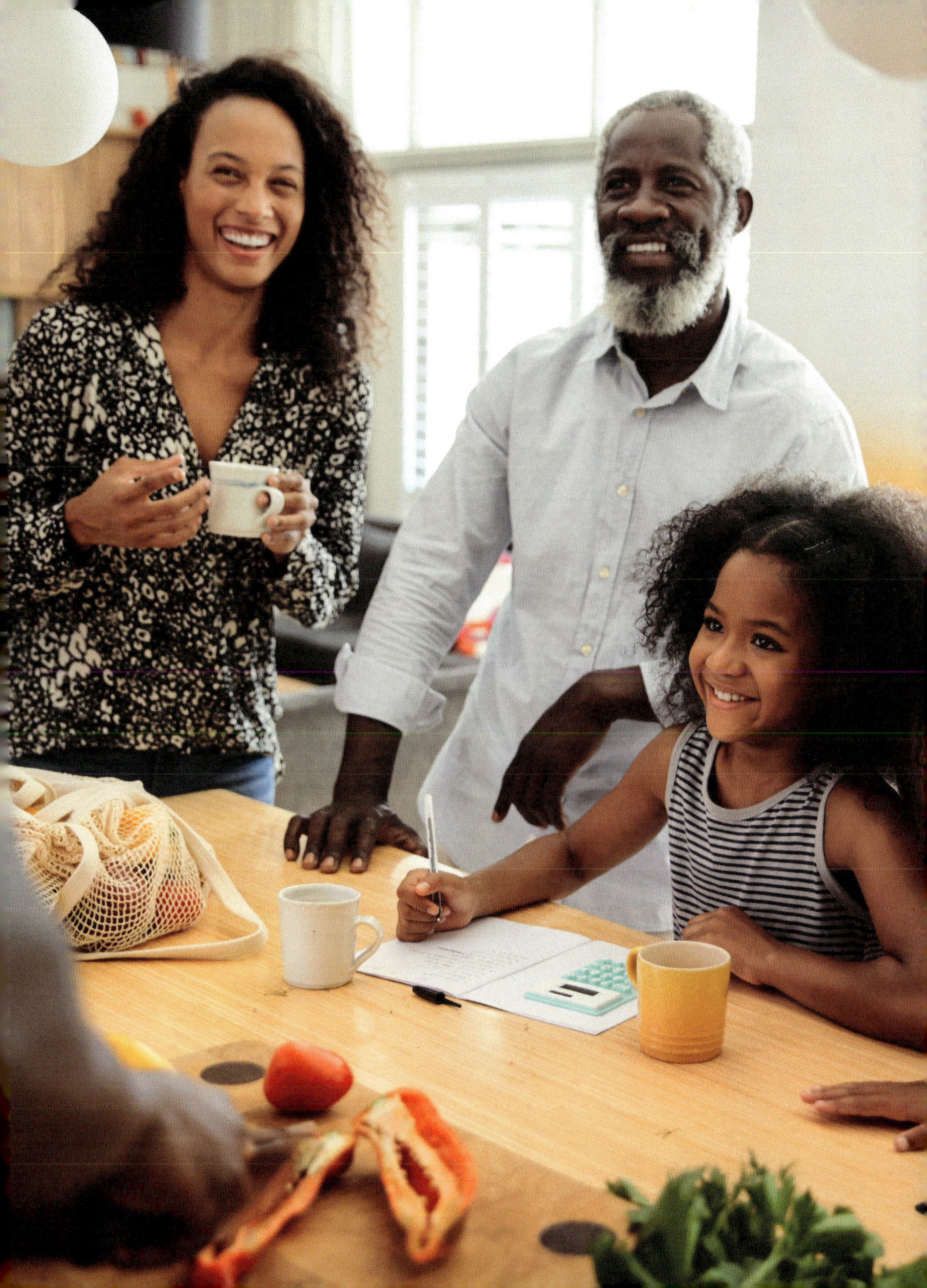

12-Week Workout Planner – Get Fit 4 Later Life

WEEK	MON	TUES	WEDS	THURS	FRI	SAT	SUN
1							
2							
3							

"Every workout counts even if it's just for 10 minutes."

ADD: WALK DAYS / WORKOUT DAYS / REST DAYS / REWARD DAYS

12-Week Workout Planner – Get Fit 4 Later Life

WEEK	MON	TUES	WEDS	THURS	FRI	SAT	SUN
4							
5							
6							

"It won't always be easy, but it will always be worth it."

ADD: WALK DAYS / WORKOUT DAYS / REST DAYS / REWARD DAYS

12-Week Workout Planner – Get Fit 4 Later Life

WEEK	MON	TUES	WEDS	THURS	FRI	SAT	SUN
7							
8							
9							

"A bad workout is the one that didn't happen."

ADD: WALK DAYS / WORKOUT DAYS / REST DAYS / REWARD DAYS

12-Week Workout Planner – Get Fit 4 Later Life

WEEK	MON	TUES	WEDS	THURS	FRI	SAT	SUN
10							
11							
12							

"If it doesn't challenge you, it won't change you!"

ADD: WALK DAYS / WORKOUT DAYS / REST DAYS / REWARD DAYS

Week 1

Day 1: Walk 10 minutes

Day 2: Rest day

Day 3: Walk 10 minutes

Day 4: Rest day

Day 5: Flexibility, Balance & Strength Exercise Routine 10 minutes

Day 6: Rest day

Day 7: Rest day

TOTAL ACTIVITY: 30 Minutes, Target 150 Minutes plus

REWARD: Well done, you're making progress so don't forget to do or have something nice.

Week 2

Day 1: Walk 10 minutes

Day 2: Rest day

Day 3: Walk 10 minutes

Day 4: Flexibility, Balance & Strength Exercise Routine 10 minutes

Day 5: Rest day

Day 6: Rest day

Day 7: Flexibility, Balance & Strength Exercise Routine 10 minutes

TOTAL ACTIVITY: 40 Minutes, Target 150 Minutes plus

REWARD: Well done, you're making progress so don't forget to do or have something nice.

Week 3

Day 1: Walk 10 minutes

Day 2: Rest day

Day 3: Walk 10 minutes

Day 4: Flexibility, Balance & Strength Exercise Routine 15 minutes

Day 5: Rest day

Day 6: Rest day

Day 7: Flexibility, Balance & Strength Exercise Routine 15 minutes

TOTAL ACTIVITY: 50 Minutes, Target 150 Minutes plus

REWARD: Well done, you're making progress so don't forget to do or have something nice.

Week 4

Day 1: Walk 15 minutes

Day 2: Rest day

Day 3: Walk 15 minutes

Day 4: Flexibility, Balance & Strength Exercise Routine 15 minutes

Day 5: Rest day

Day 6: Rest day

Day 7: Flexibility, Balance & Strength Exercise Routine 15 minutes

TOTAL ACTIVITY: 60 Minutes, Target 150 Minutes plus

REWARD: Well done, you're making progress so don't forget to do or have something nice.

Week 5

Day 1: Walk 15 minutes
Day 2: Rest day
Day 3: Walk 15 minutes
Day 4: Flexibility, Balance & Strength Exercise Routine 20 minutes
Day 5: Rest day
Day 6: Rest day
Day 7: Flexibility, Balance & Strength Exercise Routine 20 minutes

TOTAL ACTIVITY: 70 Minutes, Target 150 Minutes plus

REWARD: Well done, you're making progress so don't forget to do or have something nice.

Week 6

Day 1: Walk 15 minutes
Day 2: Rest day
Day 3: Walk 15 minutes
Day 4: Flexibility, Balance & Strength Exercise Routine 20 minutes
Day 5: Rest day
Day 6: Walk 15 minutes
Day 7: Flexibility, Balance & Strength Exercise Routine 20 minutes

TOTAL ACTIVITY: 85 Minutes, Target 150 Minutes plus

REWARD: Well done, you're making progress so don't forget to do or have something nice.

Week 7

Day 1: Walk 15 minutes

Day 2: Rest day

Day 3: Walk 15 minutes

Day 4: Flexibility, Balance & Strength Exercise Routine 25 minutes

Day 5: Rest day

Day 6: Walk 15 minutes

Day 7: Flexibility, Balance & Strength Exercise Routine 25 minutes

TOTAL ACTIVITY: 95 Minutes, Target 150 Minutes plus

REWARD: Well done, you're making progress so don't forget to do or have something nice.

Week 8

Day 1: Walk 15 minutes

Day 2: Rest day

Day 3: Walk 15 minutes

Day 4: Flexibility, Balance & Strength Exercise Routine 30 minutes

Day 5: Rest day

Day 6: Walk 15 minutes

Day 7: Flexibility, Balance & Strength Exercise Routine 30 minutes

TOTAL ACTIVITY: 105 Minutes, Target 150 Minutes plus

REWARD: Well done, you're making progress so don't forget to do or have something nice.

Week 9

Day 1: Walk 20 minutes
Day 2: Rest day
Day 3: Walk 20 minutes
Day 4: Flexibility, Balance & Strength Exercise Routine 30 minutes
Day 5: Rest day
Day 6: Walk 20 minutes
Day 7: Flexibility, Balance & Strength Exercise Routine 30 minutes

TOTAL ACTIVITY: 120 Minutes, Target 150 Minutes plus

REWARD: Well done, you're making progress so don't forget to do or have something nice.

Week 10

Day 1: Walk 20 minutes
Day 2: Rest day
Day 3: Walk 20 minutes
Day 4: Flexibility, Balance & Strength Exercise Routine 35 minutes
Day 5: Rest day
Day 6: Walk 20 minutes
Day 7: Flexibility, Balance & Strength Exercise Routine 35 minutes

TOTAL ACTIVITY: 130 Minutes, Target 150 Minutes plus

REWARD: Well done, you're making progress so don't forget to do or have something nice.

Week 11

Day 1: Walk 20 minutes
Day 2: Rest day
Day 3: Walk 20 minutes
Day 4: Flexibility, Balance & Strength Exercise Routine 40 minutes
Day 5: Rest day
Day 6: Walk 20 minutes
Day 7: Flexibility, Balance & Strength Exercise Routine 40 minutes

TOTAL ACTIVITY: 140 Minutes, Target 150 Minutes plus

REWARD: Well done, you're making progress so don't forget to do or have something nice.

Week 12

Day 1: Walk 20 minutes
Day 2: Rest day
Day 3: Walk 20 minutes
Day 4: Flexibility, Balance & Strength Exercise Routine 45 minutes
Day 5: Rest day
Day 6: Walk 20 minutes
Day 7: Flexibility, Balance & Strength Exercise Routine 45 minutes

TOTAL ACTIVITY: 150 Minutes, Target 150 Minutes plus

REWARD: Success! You're now doing the recommended weekly exercise, don't forget to do or have something nice. KEEP THIS UP!

Flexibility, Balance & Strength Workout Weeks 1 to 3
TIME: 10 to 15 MINUTES
WARM-UP Neck, Shoulders, Back, Wrists, Hips, Knees & Ankles Pulse Raiser Knees into Elbows
ARMS Bicep Curls Seated - 6 to 8 reps
SHOULDERS Upright Rows Seated - 6 to 8 reps Lateral Raises Seated - 6 to 8 reps
LEGS Sit Down Stand Ups - 6 to 8 reps Leg Extensions - 6 to 8 reps
BALANCE Single Limb Stance - Aim for a minimum 20 seconds Side Leg Raises - 6 to 8 reps each leg
END STRETCH Hamstring Seated Lower Back Seated Arms Across Seated Obliques Reach in Air Stand Chest Stretch Seated Shoulders Arms Out Triceps Seated or Standing Quads Hold on Chair

Flexibility, Balance & Strength Workout Weeks 4 to 6

TIME: 15 to 20 MINUTES

WARM-UP
Neck, Shoulders, Back, Wrists, Hips, Knees & Ankles
Pulse Raiser Knees into Elbows

ARMS
Bicep Curls Seated – 8 to 10 reps

SHOULDERS
Upright Rows Seated – 8 to 10 reps
Lateral Raises Seated – 8 to 10 reps

LEGS
Sit Down Stand Ups – 8 to 10 reps
Leg Extensions – 8 to 10 reps

NEW: WEIGHTS/ DUMBBELLS
Goblet Squats – 6 to 8 reps
Triceps Extensions – 6 to 8 reps
Figure of Eights – 6 to 8 reps
Lateral Side Bends – 6 to 8 reps

BALANCE
Single Limb Stance – Aim for a minimum 30 seconds
Side Leg Raises – 8 to 10 reps each leg

END STRETCH
Hamstring Seated
Lower Back Seated
Arms Across Seated
Obliques Reach in Air Stand
Chest Stretch Seated
Shoulders Arms Out
Triceps Seated or Standing
Quads Hold on Chair

Flexibility, Balance & Strength Workout Weeks 7 to 9

TIME: 25 to 30 MINUTES

WARM-UP
Neck, Shoulders, Back, Wrists, Hips, Knees & Ankles
Pulse Raiser Knees into Elbows

ARMS
Bicep Curls Seated - 8 to 10 reps

SHOULDERS
Upright Rows Seated - 8 to 10 reps
Lateral Raises Seated - 8 to 10 reps
NEW: Shoulder Press - 8 to 10 reps

LEGS
Sit Down Stand Ups - 8 to 10 reps
Leg Extensions - 8 to 10 reps

WEIGHTS/ DUMBBELLS
Goblet Squats - 8 to 10 reps
Triceps Extensions - 8 to 10 reps
Figure of Eights - 8 to 10 reps
Lateral Side Bends - 8 to 10 reps
NEW: Calf Raises - 10 to 15 reps

BALANCE
Single Limb Stance - Aim for a minimum 40 seconds
Side Leg Raises - 8 to 10 reps each leg
NEW: Walking Heel To Toe - 20 steps each way
NEW: Tiptoe Lifts - 20 reps

END STRETCH
Hamstring Seated
Lower Back Seated
Arms Across Seated
Obliques Reach in Air Stand
Chest Stretch Seated
Shoulders Arms Out
Triceps Seated or Standing
Quads Hold on Chair

Flexibility, Balance & Strength Workout Weeks 10 to 12

TIME: 35 to 45 MINUTES

WARM-UP
Neck, Shoulders, Back, Wrists, Hips, Knees & Ankles
Pulse Raiser Knees into Elbows

ARMS
Bicep Curls Seated - 2 sets of 10 to 12 reps

SHOULDERS
Upright Rows Seated - 2 sets of 10 to 12 reps
Lateral Raises Seated - 2 sets of 10 to 12 reps
Shoulder Press - 2 sets of 10 to 12 reps

LEGS
Sit Down Stand Ups - 2 sets of 10 to 12 reps
Leg Extensions - 2 sets of 10 to 12 reps

WEIGHTS/ DUMBBELLS
Goblet Squats - 2 sets of 10 to 12 reps
Triceps Extensions - 2 sets of 10 to 12 reps
Figure of Eights - 2 sets of 10 to 12 reps
Lateral Side Bends - 2 sets of 10 to 12 reps
Calf Raises - 2 sets of 15 to 20 reps

BALANCE
Single Limb Stance - Aim for a minimum 60 seconds
Side Leg Raises - 10 to 12 reps each leg
Walking Heel To Toe - 20 steps each way x 2 sets
Tiptoe Lifts - 20 reps x 2 sets

END STRETCH
Hamstring Seated
Lower Back Seated
Arms Across Seated
Obliques Reach in Air Stand
Chest Stretch Seated
Shoulders Arms Out
Triceps Seated or Standing
Quads Hold on Chair

A-Z Calorie Counts For Popular Food List

Portion sizes will vary and can be subjective depending on the bowl, cup or plate used.

BREADS & CEREALS	CALORIES PER PORTION SIZE	CALORIES PER 100g
Bagel (1 average)	140 (45g)	310
Biscuit digestives	86 (per biscuit)	480
Jaffa cake	48 (per biscuit)	370
Bread white (thick slice)	96 (1 slice 40g)	240
Bread wholemeal (thick)	88 (1 slice 40g)	220
Chapatis	250	300
Cornflakes	130 (35g)	370
Crackerbread	17 per slice	325
Cream crackers	35 (per cracker)	440
Crumpets	93 (per crumpet)	198
Flapjacks basic fruit mix	320	500
Macaroni (boiled)	238 (250g)	95
Muesli	195 (50g)	390
Naan bread (normal)	300 (small plate size)	320
Noodles (boiled)	175 (250g)	70

Pasta (normal boiled)	330	110
Pasta (wholemeal boiled)	315	105
Porridge oats (water)	193	55
Rice (white boiled)	420	140
Rice (egg-fried)	500	200
Rice (Brown)	405	135
Rice cakes	28	373
Ryvita Multi grain	37	331
Ryvita + seed & Oats	180	362
Spaghetti (boiled)	303 (300g)	101

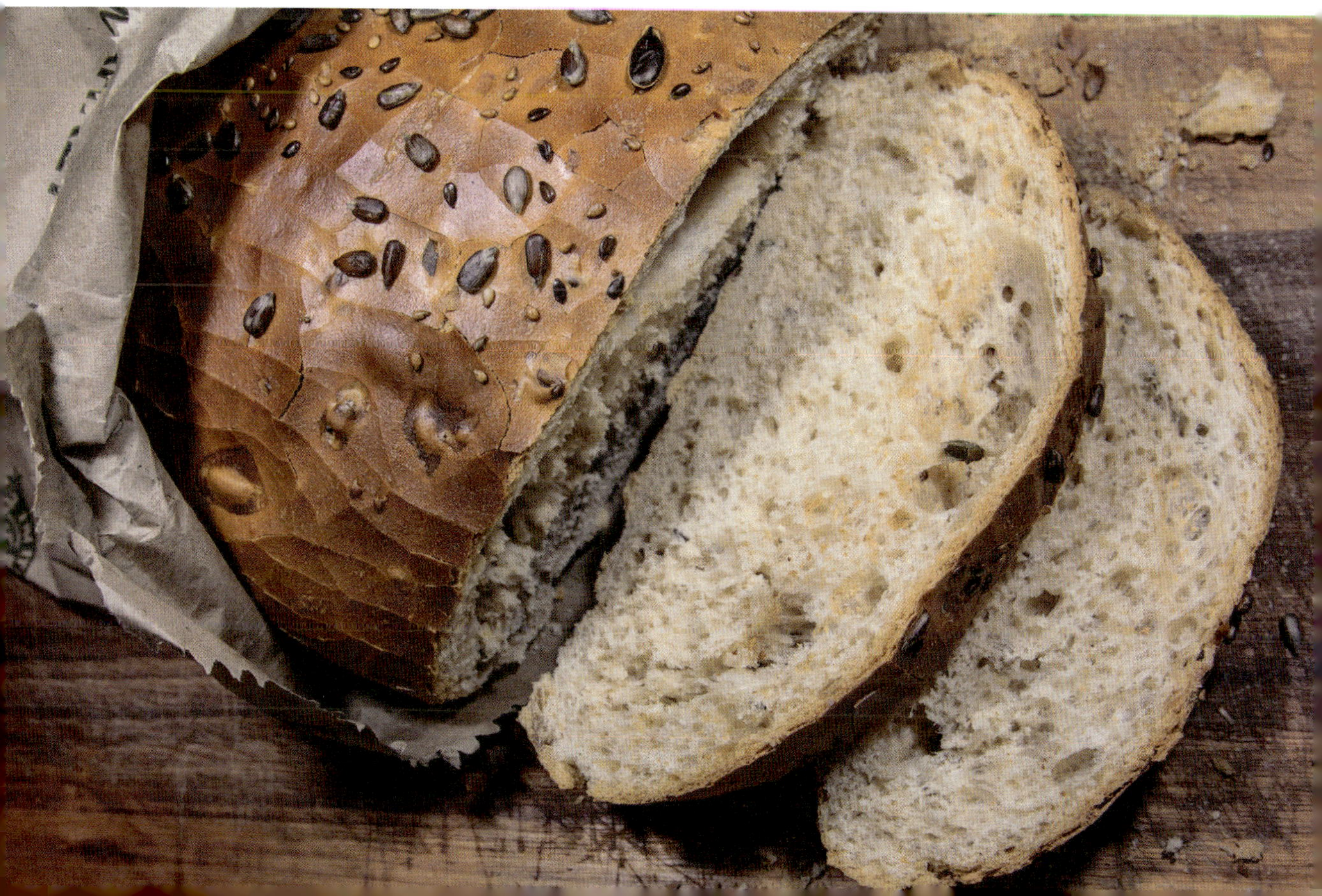

MEAT & FISH	CALORIES PER PORTION SIZE	CALORIES PER 100g
Anchovies tinned	300	300
Bacon average fried	250 (2 rashers)	500
Bacon average grilled	150	380
Beef (roast)	300	280
Beef burgers frozen	320	280
Chicken	220	200
Cockles	50	50
Cod fresh	150	100
Cod chip shop food	400	200
Crab fresh	200	110
Duck roast	400	430
Fish cake	90 (per cake)	200
Fish fingers	50 (per piece)	220
Gammon	320	280
Haddock fresh	200	110
Halibut fresh	220	125
Ham	6	240
Herring fresh grilled	300	200
Kidney	200	160
Kipper	200	120
Liver	200	150

Liver pate	150	300
Lamb (roast)	300	300
Lobster boiled	200	100
Luncheon meat	300	400
Mackerel	320	300
Mussels	90	90
Pheasant roast	200	200
Pilchards (tinned)	140	140
Prawns	180	100
Pork	320	290
Pork pie	320	450
Rabbit	200	180
Salmon fresh	220	180
Sardines tinned in oil	220	220
Sardines in tomato sauce	180	180
Sausages pork fried	250	320
Sausages pork grilled	220	280
Sausages roll	290	480
Scampi fried in oil	400	340
Steak & kidney pie	400	350
Taramasalata	130	490
Trout fresh	200	120

Tuna tinned water	100	100
Tuna tinned oil	180	180
Turkey	200	160
Veal	300	240

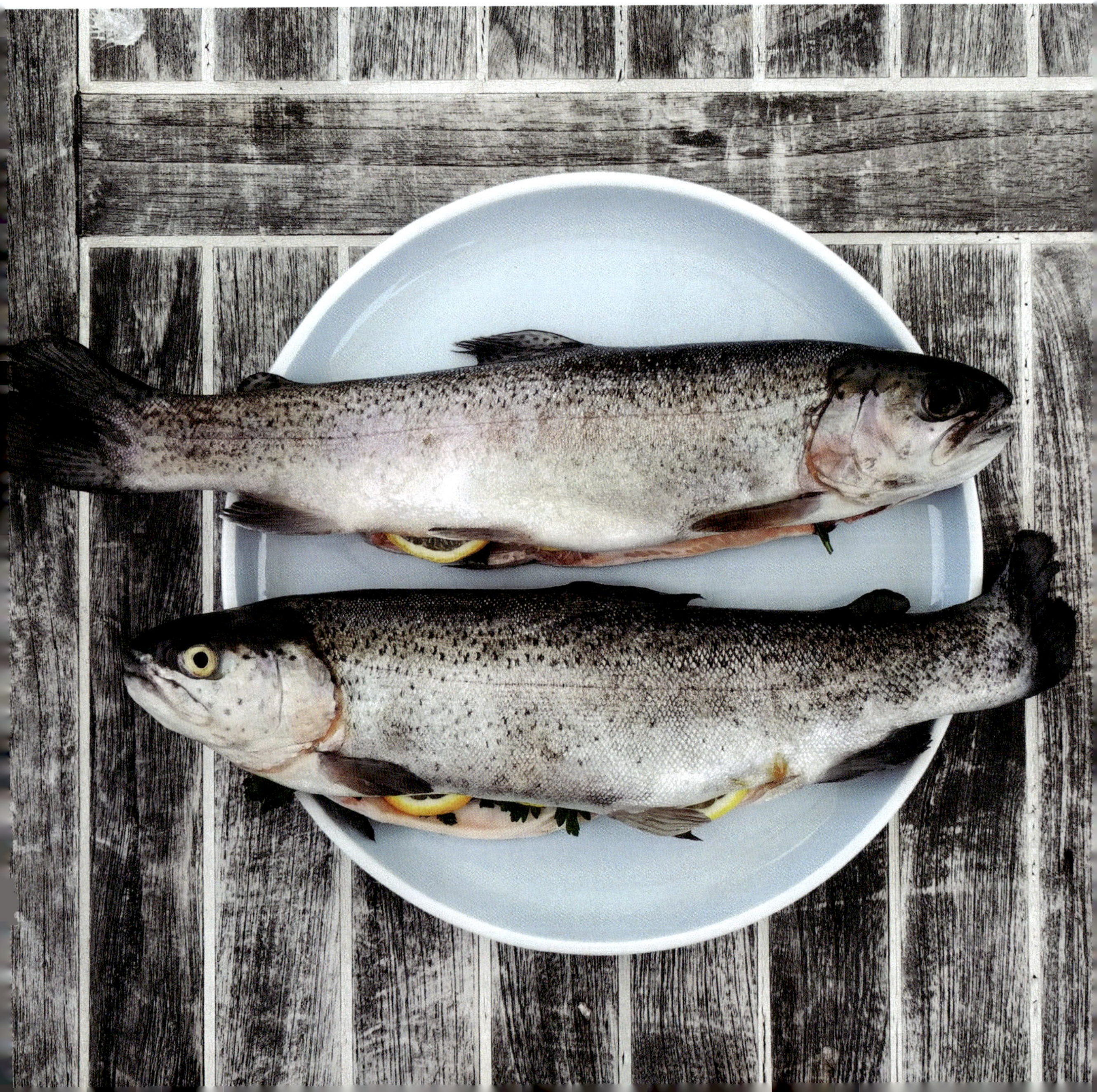

MILK & DAIRY	CALORIES PER PORTION SIZE	CALORIES PER 100g
Cheese average	110 (25g)	440
Cheese spreads	90	270
Cottage cheese low fat	40	80
Cottage cheese	49	98
Cream cheese	200	428
Cream fresh half	128	160
Cream fresh single	160	200
Cream fresh double	340	430
Cream fresh clotted	480	600
Custard	210	100
Eggs (1 average size)	90	150
Eggs fried	120	180
Fromage frais	125	125
Ice cream	200	180
Milk whole	175 (250ml/half pint)	70
Milk semi-skimmed	125 (250ml/half pint)	50
Milk skimmed	95 (250ml/half pint)	38
Milk Soya	90	36
Mousse flavoured	120	140
Omelet with cheese	300	266
Trifle with cream	290	190
Yogurt natural	90	60
Yogurt reduced fat	70	45

FATS & SUGARS	CALORIES PER PORTION SIZE	CALORIES PER 100g
Pure fat	9 (1 gram)	900
Bombay mix	250	500
Butter	112	750
Chewing gum	8 per piece	-
Chocolate	200	500
Cod liver oil	135 (1 tablespoon)	900
Corn snack	125	500
Crisps (average)	100	500
Honey	42	280
Jam	38	250
Lard	225	890
Low fat spread	50	400
Margarine	50	750
Mars bar	240	480
Mint sweets	10 per piece	-
Oils: corn, sunflower, olive	135 (1 tablespoon)	900
Popcorn (average)	150	460
Sugar (white)	20 (1 teaspoon)	400
Sweets (boiled)	100	300
Syrup	15	300

FRUIT & VEGETABLES	CALORIES PER PORTION SIZE	CALORIES PER 100g
Apple	44	44
Banana	107	65
Beans baked beans	170	80
Beans dried (boiled)	180	130
Blackberries	25	25
Blackcurrant	30	30
Broccoli	27	32
Cabbage (boiled)	15	20
Carrot (boiled)	16	25
Cauliflower (boiled)	20	30
Celery (boiled)	5	10
Cherry	35	50
Courgette	8	20
Cucumber	3	10
Dates	100	235
Grapes	55	62
Grapefruit	32	32
Kiwi	40	50
Leek (boiled)	10	20
Lentils (boiled)	150	100
Lettuce	4	15
Melon	14 c	28
Mushrooms (raw)	3	15

Mushrooms (boiled)	12	12
Mushrooms (fried)	100	145
Olives	50	80
Onion (boiled)	14	18
One red Onion	49	33
Onions spring	3	25
Onion (fried)	86	155
Orange	40	30
Peas	210	148
Peas dried & boiled	200	120
Peach	35	30
Pear	45	38
Pepper yellow	6	16
Pineapple	40	40
Plum	30	39
Spinach	8	8
Strawberries (1 average)	10	30
Sweetcorn	95	130
Sweetcorn on the cob	70	70
Tomato	30	20
Tomato cherry	6	17
Watercress	5 calories	20

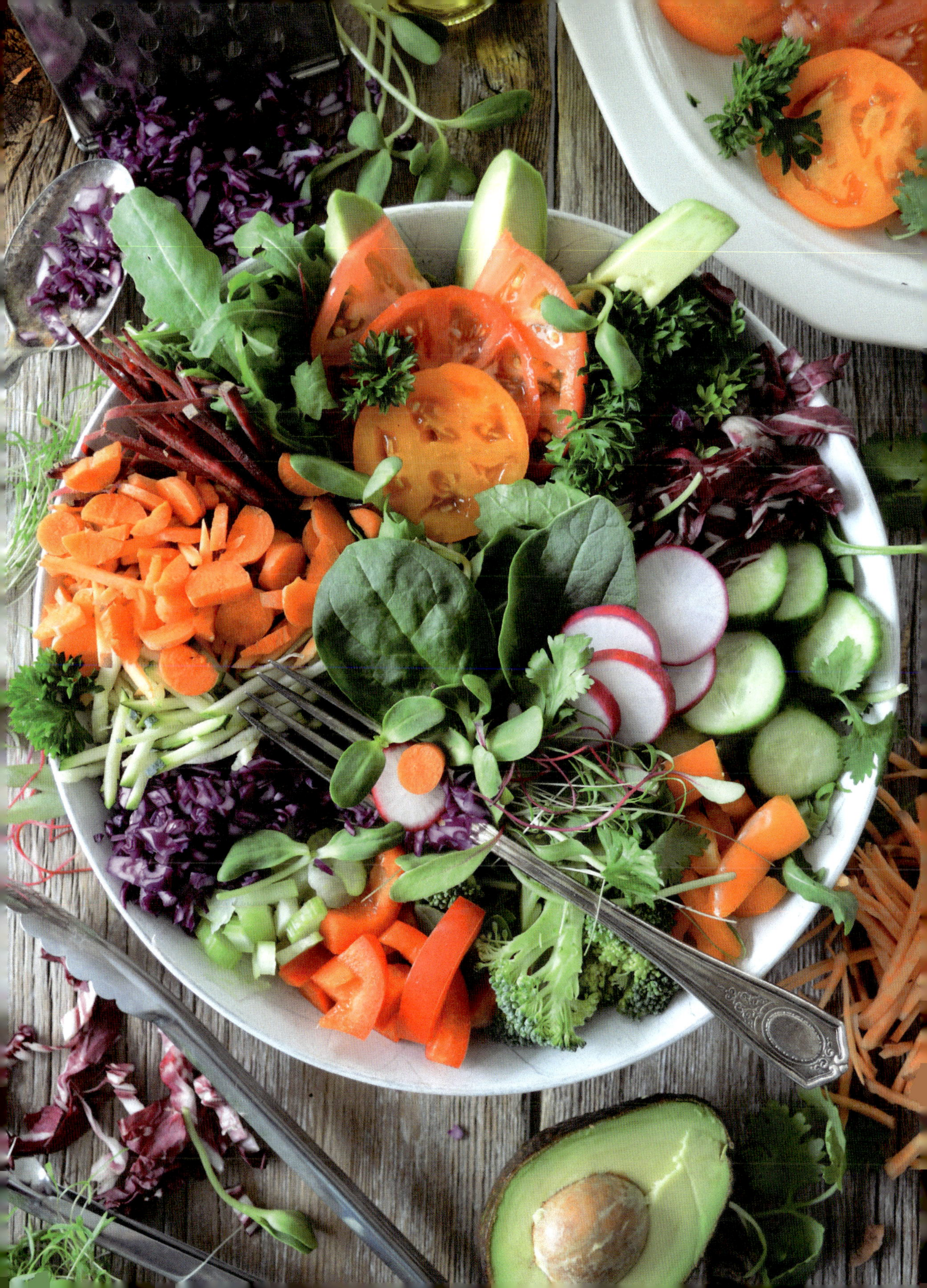

Step-By-Step Warm-Up Exercises

Neck

- **EQUIPMENT:** N/A
- Head side to side, for this warm-up exercise, start by moving your left ear towards the top of your left shoulder, same on the right side, repeat several times
- Head left to right, to start, look over to your left and then to the right, repeat several times
- Head forwards and backwards, to start, look up towards the ceiling, then look down towards the floor, repeat several times
- Breathe normally

Shoulders

- **EQUIPMENT:** N/A
- Backward circles of both arms, for this warm-up exercise first make vertical circles with your arms going up right above your head and then down by your sides, and then horizontally to the same height as your shoulder starting with big circles and then getting smaller and smaller, repeat several times, and then do all over again but this time forwards
- Move your arms forwards across the chest as though giving yourself a big hug, alternate the crossing of hands, hands high, then hands lower clapping behind your back, clapping in front, repeat several times
- Shoulder rolls, hands down by your side, rolling shoulders forwards, upwards then down
- Breathe normally

Back

- **EQUIPMENT:** N/A
- For this warm-up exercise stand with feet about shoulders width apart. Rotating, swing your arms and wrap around waist tapping your bum, take your head around, repeat several times
- Side to side reach out as though you're trying to touch something, keep your hips still, repeat several times
- Forwards and backwards, back of hands facing forwards your arms are down by your side, as you-breathe in pull your shoulders back, opening up your chest. As you-breathe out fold your shoulders back to the starting position, repeat several times
- Breathe normally

Wrists

- **EQUIPMENT:** N/A
- For this warm-up exercise, start with your hands together, fingers interlaced, rotate hands in a circle, then forwards and backwards, repeat several times
- Single hand, circles, side-to-side, forwards and backwards, repeat several times
- Breathe normally

Hips - Upper

- **EQUIPMENT:** N/A
- For this warm-up exercise start with your hands on hips rotate round in a circle, go in both directions, repeat several times
- Hands-on hip move side to side, repeat several times
- Breathe normally

Hips - Lower

- **EQUIPMENT:** Chair (optional for support)
- For this exercise start by standing on one leg, hold on to the back of a chair for balance, make circles with the other leg, repeat several times
- Standing on one leg, hold on to the back of a chair for balance, move the other leg forwards and backwards, repeat several times
- Breathe normally

Knees

- **EQUIPMENT:** Chair (optional for support)
- For this warm-up exercise start standing on one leg, hold on to the back of a chair for balance, kick heel back behind the other, repeat several times
- Shallow squats, stand behind a chair in case you need help with balance, bend knees and squat down, straighten legs, repeat several times
- Breathe normally

Ankles

- **EQUIPMENT:** Chair
- Heel to toe taps, for this warm-up exercise, hold on to a chair and shift weight onto one foot. Bring the heel of your other foot off the ground so only your toes are touching. Then move the heel to touch the ground as you lift your toes up. Repeat several times, then change legs
- Breathe normally

Dynamic Stretching - Walking around arms open stretch chest

- **EQUIPMENT:** N/A
- For this warm-up exercise start walking a brisk pace
- Walking open arms taking one hand higher shoulder height, while the other lower, waist height, then alternate, repeat several times
- Breathe normally

Dynamic Stretching - Walking around 3 steps then 2 shallow squats

- **EQUIPMENT:** N/A
- For this warm-up exercise start walking a brisk pace walking 3 strides then squat twice, keep back flat, bottom out, repeat several times
- Breathe normally

Dynamic Stretching - Walking around 3 steps then oblique stretch each side

- **EQUIPMENT:** N/A
- For this warm-up exercise start walking a brisk pace walking 3 strides
- Stop and stand with feet shoulder-width apart reach up with the left arm, then change sides and reach up with the right arm, repeat several times
- Breathe normally

Heart Rate Pulse Raiser

- **EQUIPMENT:** Chair (optional)
- For this warm-up exercise start marching on the spot, can do this seated, march as briskly as you can for two minutes
- Knees into elbows, bring left knee up and right elbow down towards knee, change sides, bring right knee up and left elbow down, continue alternating at a brisk pace, can do this seated
- Breathe normally

WARM-UP TIME GUIDELINES: You should spend at least 5 to 10 minutes warming up, longer if you feel you need to before you start your exercise routine.

Step-By-Step Aerobic Exercises

Knees into Elbows

- **EQUIPMENT:** N/A
- For this aerobic exercise, start by bringing your left knee up and right elbow down towards your knee
- Change sides, bring right knee up and left elbow down
- Continue alternating at a brisk pace
- You can do a variation of this seated
- Breathe normally

High Knees Marching on the Spot

- **EQUIPMENT:** N/A
- For this aerobic exercise, stand with your back straight and your head up looking forward
- Begin with your feet together and hands straight down by the side of your body
- Lift one foot at a time bringing your knee up to the height of your waist
- Move alternate hands forwards and backwards as though you are jogging
- You can do a variation of this seated
- Breathe normally

Step-Ups

- **EQUIPMENT:** Steps
- For this aerobic exercise, start on the bottom step of a set of steps or on your staircase. Step up onto the first step with your left foot, and then step up with your right foot, pause briefly

- Next, step back down with your right leg and then with your left leg
- Repeat on the other side
- You can make this a little more challenging by using weights; tins of food or dumbbells in each hand
- Breathe normally

Dancing

- A simple dance step of a brisk side to side, tap inside with your foot for a few minutes will do the job nicely
- You can of course, use any dance step; a Jive or Cha Cha etc as dancing is a great and indeed fun way to do aerobic exercise
- Put on your favourite music and let your feet loose and fancy-free for a nifty aerobic workout
- If dancing appeals, why not see if there's a local dance class to sharpen your moves as you get fit and have fun while doing it

Every day activities

- Any activity that leaves you slightly out of breath counts as aerobic exercise as you work towards your 150-minute weekly target
- Digging the vegetable garden, mowing and raking up the lawn, hand washing the car, brisk walk to the shops and carrying your shopping home, brisk walk with the dog, sports, for example, tennis and swimming

ACTIVITY TIME GUIDELINES: Older adults should aim to be active daily. Over a week, your activity should add up to at least 150-minutes of moderate-intensity activity in bouts of 10 minutes or more. One way to achieve this would be to do 30 minutes on at least 5 days of the week.

Step-By-Step Balance Exercises

Single Limb Stance

- **EQUIPMENT:** Chair
- For this balance exercise, start by standing behind a sturdy dining room chair and hold firmly on to the back initially using both hands, raise your right foot off of the floor and then balance on your left foot
- Hold the Single Limb Stance position for as long as you can, then change feet and repeat
- Your aim should be to stand in the Single Limb Stance position without holding onto the chair and hold it steady for up to one minute
- Breathe normally

Rock the Boat

- **EQUIPMENT:** N/A
- For this balance exercise, start by standing with your feet about hip-width apart, with both feet pressed firmly on the floor
- Next stand up straight with your head level looking out forward, then transfer your weight onto your right foot and slowly lift your left leg off of the ground. Hold that position for as long as possible aiming for up to 30 seconds
- To finish the Rock the Boat exercise carefully place your foot back onto the floor, transferring your weight to this foot, then slowly lift your other leg
- Begin by doing the Rock the Boat exercise five times each side, then gradually work your way up to more repetitions
- Breathe normally

Walking Heel to Toe

- **EQUIPMENT:** N/A
- For this balance exercise, start by placing your right foot in front of left foot so that the heel of the right foot touches the top of the toes of the left foot
- Next, move your left foot in front of your right foot, putting your full weight on the heel, shift weight to your toes
- Repeat the step with the left foot, walk this way for 20 steps, turn around and walk back
- Tip; doing this balance exercise in a hallway with walls either side can make this feel safer, or have someone with you to watch you to keep you safe and support you as you Walk Heel to Toe
- Breathe normally

Back Leg Raises

- **EQUIPMENT:** Chair
- For this balance exercise, start by standing behind the dining chair
- Next start lifting your right leg straight backwards, avoid bending at the knees and remain in this balanced position for a couple of seconds before returning the leg back down
- Repeat for the other leg to complete your Back Leg Raises exercises, aim for 8 to 12 reps for each leg
- Breathe normally

Side Leg Raises

- **EQUIPMENT:** Chair
- For this balance exercise, start by standing behind a sturdy dining room chair or kitchen countertop with one or both hands resting on it for support
- Lift your right leg out to the side and then bring it back to the standing position, repeat 10 times for each leg to complete the exercise
- Breathe normally

Balancing Wand

- **EQUIPMENT:** Chair and Broom Handle (without the broom head)
- For this balance exercise, start seated holding the bottom of the broom handle so that it is flat on the palm of your hand, the aim of this exercise is to keep the broom handle upright for as long as possible
- Alternate between hands so that you practice your balance skills on both sides
- Breathe normally

Clock Reach

- **EQUIPMENT:** Chair
- For this balance exercise, pretend that you're standing in the middle of a large clock with 12 o'clock directly in front of you and with 6 o'clock directly behind you
- Start by holding onto the dining room chair with your left hand, lift up your right leg and extend your right arm so it points to 12 o'clock
- Next, point your arm towards 3 o'clock and then finally point your arm behind you towards 6 o'clock
- Bring your arm back to 3 o'clock and then back to 12 o'clock, looking straight out ahead throughout the exercise
- Repeat the Clock Reach exercise three times each side
- Breathe normally

Tip Toe Lifts

- **EQUIPMENT:** Chair or Counter (optional)
- For this balance exercise, start by standing up with your back straight extend your arms right out directly in front of you
- Lift yourself up on your toes as high as you can and then gently lower yourself down again
- Try not to lean too far forward
- Repeat lifting yourself up on your toes and lowering yourself down 20 times, repeat this for 2 to 3 sets
- Breathe normally

Marching on the Spot

- **EQUIPMENT:** Chair
- For this balance exercise, start by standing straight, lift your right knee as high as you can. Lower it then lift the left leg, lift and lower your legs 20 times
- Breathe normally

3-Way Hip Kick

- **EQUIPMENT:** Chair or Counter
- For this balance exercise, stand with your feet shoulder-width apart, firmly hold onto a chair or counter and extend your leg forward and return to your starting position
- Next repeat this movement to the side this time returning to the starting position
- Finally end the 3-way hip kick by extending your leg back before returning it to the starting position
- Perform the 3-way hip kick 8 to 12 times on each leg. Repeat for 2 to 3 sets
- Breathe normally

Mini Lunges

- **EQUIPMENT:** Chair or Counter
- For this balance exercise, stand with your feet shoulder-width apart. Firmly hold onto a chair or counter and step forward with your front knee slightly bent. Return your leg back to the starting position. Repeat with your other leg
- Please note that these lunges do not need to be that deep. If you feel any knee or hip pain use the chair or counter for more support and or take smaller lunge steps.
- Aim for 8 to 12 mini lunges on each leg. Repeat for 2 to 3 times sets
- Breathe normally

Grapevine

- **EQUIPMENT:** N/A
- For this balance exercise, begin by standing with your arms by your sides with your feet together
- Next step across in front of your right foot with your left leg, continue sideways across the floor uncrossing and crossing your leg
- To finish reverse directions only this time crossing your left leg behind your right leg back to your starting position
- Aim to do the Grapevine 3 times in each direction
- Breathe normally

ACTIVITY TIME GUIDELINES: Older people should aim to do balance exercises at least twice a week, there is no set amount of time given but a sensible target would be at least 15 minutes each time.

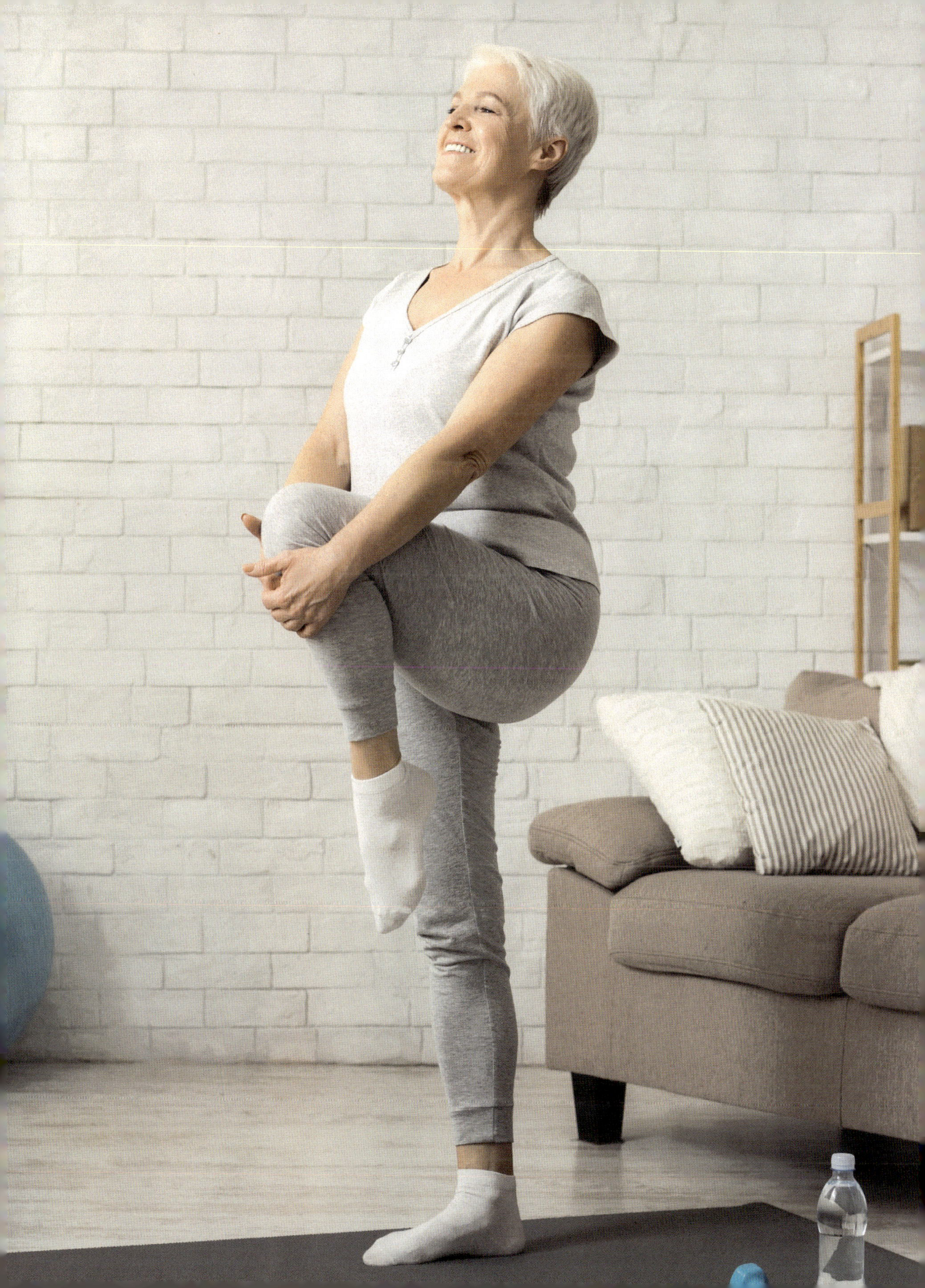

Step-By-Step Chair Based Exercises

Knees into Elbows

- **EQUIPMENT:** Chair
- For this aerobic exercise, start seated by bringing your left knee up and right elbow down towards the knee
- Change sides, bring right knee up and left elbow down
- Continue alternating at a brisk pace
- Breathe normally
- **TARGET**: As warm-up - 5 to 10 minutes, as aerobic exercise, 10 minutes and above

High Knees Marching on the Spot

- **EQUIPMENT:** Chair
- For this aerobic exercise, start seated sitting upright with your head up looking forward
- Begin with your feet together and hands straight down by the sides of the chair
- Lift one foot at a time bringing your knee up as high as you can
- Move alternate hands forwards and backwards as though you are jogging
- Breathe normally
- **TARGET:** As warm-up - 5 to 10 minutes, as aerobic exercise, 10 minutes and above

Bicep Curls

- **EQUIPMENT:** Chair, 2 Tins or 2 Dumbbells or Resistance Band
- For this strength exercise, sit towards the front of dining chair
- Holding a weight in each hand curl slowly upwards to your chest, keep your elbows fixed by your sides
- Lower the tins slowly, this is one complete rep
- Breathe in while lowering weights, breathe out while curling arms up
- **TARGET:** 2 to 3 sets of 8 to 12 repetitions

Triceps Extensions

- **EQUIPMENT:** Chair, Bottle of Water, Squash or a Dumbbell
- For this strength exercise, sit on a chair and hold the bottle in both hands extending it up overhead
- Keep your biceps close to your ears with your elbows pointing forward as you then lower the bottle behind your head until your elbows are at an angle of about 90-degrees
- Next straighten out your arms to the starting position, this is one rep
- Keep your abs engaged throughout the exercise, avoid arching your back
- Breathe in while lowering weight, breathe out while pushing arms up
- **TARGET:** 2 to 3 sets of 8 to 12 repetitions

Shoulder Rolls

- **EQUIPMENT:** Chair
- For this flexibility exercise, start seated and rotate your shoulders gently up towards the ceiling and then backwards and finally downwards
- Next, do the same movement but this time roll your shoulders upwards, forwards and then downwards
- Breathe normally
- **TARGET:** 2 to 3 sets of 8 to 12 repetitions

Upright Rows

- **EQUIPMENT:** Chair, 2 Tins or 2 Dumbbells or Resistance Band
- For this strength exercise, sit with a weight in each hand with your palms facing in towards your body
- Lift the weights by raising your elbows out to the sides until they line up with the height of your shoulders. Your hands should finish up just beneath your chin
- Next, slowly slide the weights down to your lap, this is one complete rep
- Breathe in while lowering weights, breathe out while moving arms up
- **TARGET:** 2 to 3 sets of 8 to 12 repetitions

Lateral Raises

- **EQUIPMENT:** Chair, 2 Tins or 2 Dumbbells or Resistance Band
- For this strength exercise, sit with a weight in each hand keep your arms down by your sides with your palms facing in
- Ensure that your shoulders are relaxed with your stomach muscles engaged
- Retaining this position, lift the weights out to the sides up to the height of your shoulders
- Pause and then slowly lower the weights back to your starting position, this is one complete rep
- Breathe in while lowering weights, breathe out while moving arms up
- **TARGET:** 2 to 3 sets of 8 to 12 repetitions

Front Raises

- **EQUIPMENT:** Chair, 2 Tins or 2 Dumbbells or Resistance Band
- For this strength exercise, sit with a weight in each hand with your arms down by your sides, palms facing your body
- Without bending your elbows, raise alternate arms straight up in front of the body until at shoulder-level height

- Lower the weights back down to starting position and then repeat with the other arm, this is one complete rep
- Breathe in while lowering weight, breathe out while moving arms up
- **TARGET:** 2 to 3 sets of 8 to 12 repetitions

Stomach Twists

- **EQUIPMENT:** Chair
- For this strength exercise, start seated, holding the top and bottom of the bottle of water or squash in both hands close to your stomach and elbows bent slightly
- Slowly rotate your body to the right as far as you can comfortably go while keeping the rest of your body stable and the move back across your body to finish on your left side, return to the centre, this is one complete rep
- Breathe normally
- **TARGET:** 2 to 3 sets of 8 to 12 repetitions each side

Leg Extensions

- **EQUIPMENT:** Chair
- For this strength exercise, sit towards the front of the chair while keeping your left foot on the floor and with your upper body quite still
- Next, extend your right leg until its parallel with the floor and hold it up for the count of two
- Bend knee to lower your right leg back to the starting position, repeat with left leg, this is a complete rep
- Breathe in while lowering legs, breathe out while moving legs up
- **TARGET:** 2 to 3 sets of 8 to 12 repetitions each leg

Shin Extensions

- **EQUIPMENT:** Chair
- For this strength exercise, start by sitting on the edge of a dining chair with both your legs extended and your heels firmly planted on the floor, keep your knees slightly bent
- Next point your toes downwards and then flex them back upwards
- Breathe normally
- **TARGET:** 2 to 3 sets of 12 to 15 repetitions

Seated Calf Raises

- **EQUIPMENT:** Chair
- For this strength exercise, start seated with your hips back as far back as possible
- Place both your hands down by the sides of the dining chair holding the seat to keep yourself stable
- Keep both legs at an angle of about 90-degrees with the chair, with both feet flat on the floor
- Slowly, raise the heels of your feet upwards while pushing your toes on the ground and lifting your heels in the air
- Place both feet back to the starting position, this is one complete rep
- Breathe in while lowering down, breathe out while moving up
- **TARGET:** 2 to 3 sets of 15 to 20 repetitions

ACTIVITY TIME GUIDELINES: Older adults should aim to be active daily. Over a week, your activity should add up to at least 150 minutes of moderate-intensity activity in bouts of 10 minutes or more. One way to achieve this would be to do 30 minutes on at least 5 days of the week. Ideally, you should aim to build up a routine of 8 to 12 exercises that strength train the major muscle groups 2 to 3 times a week on non-consecutive days to allow for recovery.

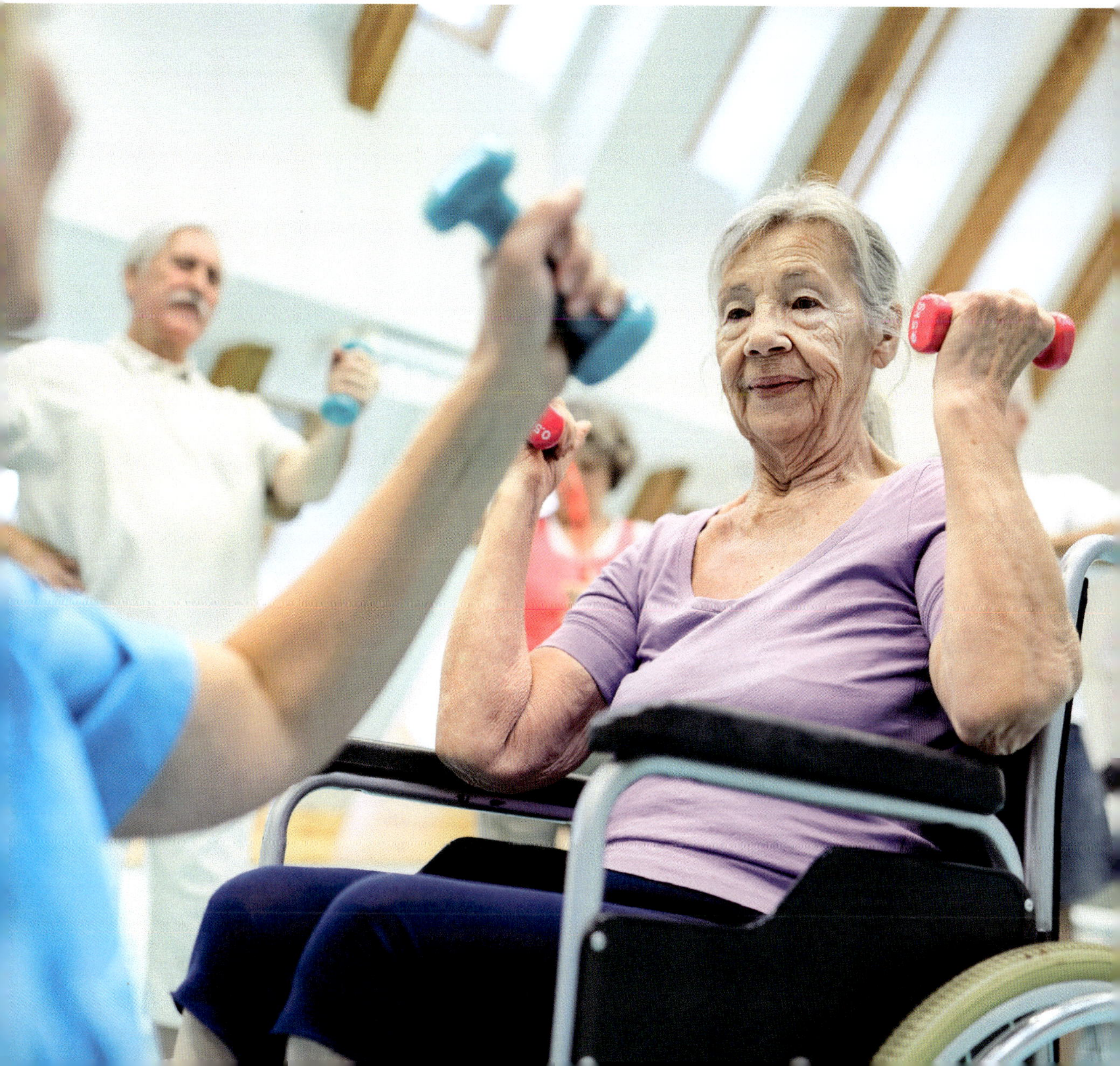

Step-By-Step Strength Exercises

Wall Push-ups

- **EQUIPMENT:** N/A
- For this strength exercise, stand about an arm's length in front of the wall (for your safety make sure the wall does not have any paintings, decorations, windows or doors)
- Lean forward slightly and put your palms flat on the wall at the same height and slightly wider than your shoulders, keep your feet firmly on the floor as you slowly move your body towards the wall
- Gently push yourself back so that your arms are straight to your starting position, this is one rep
- Take a deep breath while lowering yourself to the wall, breathe out as you push back
- **TARGET**: 2 to 3 sets of 8 to 12 repetitions

Bicep Curls

- **EQUIPMENT:** 2 Tins or 2 Dumbbells or Resistance Band
- For this strength exercise, stand upright with your feet hip-width apart
- Holding a weight in each hand curl slowly upwards to your chest, keep your elbows fixed by your sides
- Lower the tins slowly, this is one complete rep
- Breathe in while lowering weight, breathe out while curling arms up
- **TARGET:** 2 to 3 sets of 8 to 12 repetitions

Triceps Extensions

- **EQUIPMENT:** Bottle of Water, Squash or a Dumbbell
- For this strength exercise, stand upright with your feet hip-width apart
- Keep your biceps close to your ears with your elbows pointing forward as you then lower the bottle behind your head until your elbows are at an angle of about 90-degrees
- Next straighten out your arms to the starting position, this is one rep
- Keep your abs engaged throughout the exercise, avoid arching your back
- Breathe in while lowering weight, breathe out while pushing arms up
- **TARGET:** 2 to 3 sets of 8 to 12 repetitions

Upright Rows

- **EQUIPMENT:** 2 Tins or 2 Dumbbells or Resistance Band
- For this strength exercise, stand upright with your feet hip-width apart
- Lift the weights by raising your elbows out to the sides until they line up with the height of your shoulders. Your hands should finish up just beneath your chin
- Next, slowly slide the weights down to the starting position, this is one complete rep
- Breathe in while lowering weight, breathe out while moving arms up
- **TARGET:** 2 to 3 sets of 8 to 12 repetitions

Lateral Raises

- **EQUIPMENT:** 2 Tins or 2 Dumbbells or Resistance Band
- For this strength exercise, stand upright with your feet hip-width apart
- Ensure that your shoulders are relaxed with your stomach muscles engaged
- Retaining this position, lift the weights out to the sides up to the height of your shoulders
- Pause and then slowly lower the weights back to your starting position, this is one complete rep
- Breathe in while lowering weight, breathe out while moving arms up
- **TARGET:** 2 to 3 sets of 8 to 12 repetitions

Front Raises

- **EQUIPMENT:** 2 Tins or 2 Dumbbells or Resistance Band
- For this strength exercise, stand upright with your feet hip-width apart
- Start with a tin in each hand with arms by sides and palms facing your body
- Raise alternate arms without bending at your elbows straight up in front of your body up to the height of your shoulders
- Lower the weights back down to the starting position and then repeat with your other arm, this is one complete rep
- Breathe in while lowering the weights and back out while moving your arms up
- **TARGET:** 2 to 3 sets of 8 to 12 repetitions

Shoulder Press

- **EQUIPMENT:** 2 Tins or 2 Dumbbells or Resistance Band
- For this strength exercise, start your Shoulder Press exercise with your feet shoulder-width apart, weights (either tins or dumbbells) in hand at chest level, palms forward.
- Extend your arms straight up over your head, then lower back down to the starting position, this is one rep

- Breathe in while lowering the weights and back out while moving your arms up
- **TARGET:** 2 to 3 sets of 8 to 12 repetitions

Sit Down Stand-Ups

- **EQUIPMENT:** N/A
- For this strength exercise, sit towards the front of the chair with your knees bent and both your feet flat on the floor about shoulder-width apart
- Next, lean back slightly with both your hands crossed over your chest, keep your back and your shoulders straight
- Breathe in slowly
- Bring your upper body forward until sitting upright as you breathe out, extend your arms so they are parallel to the floor and slowly stand up pushing up through your heel
- Breathe in as you sit back down slowly under control, this is one rep
- **TARGET:** 2 to 3 sets of 8 to 12 repetitions

Goblet Squats

- **EQUIPMENT:** Bottle of Water, Squash or a Dumbbell
- For this strength exercise, start by standing with your feet about shoulder-width apart
- Hold the weight with both hands in front of your chest
- Remember to keep your chest up with your heels down throughout
- Perform a standard squat and when on the upward move raise the weight up above your head, then lower back down to finish in front of your chest, this is one rep
- Breathe in as you slowly squat down under control, breathe out as you stand back up
- **TARGET:** 2 to 3 sets of 8 to 12 repetitions

Squats

- **EQUIPMENT:** Chair for support (optional)
- For this strength exercise, start by standing up and using the dining chair as support
- Next, bend your knees as much as you can without your knees passing over your toes, then return to the starting position
- Breathe in as you slowly squat down, breathe out as you stand up
- **TARGET:** 2 to 3 sets of 8 to 12 repetitions

Standing Calf-Raises

- **EQUIPMENT:** Bottle of Water or Squash or a Dumbbell
- For this strength exercise, start by standing with your feet quite close together
- Hold the weight in front of you with both hands
- Push upwards through the balls of your feet and raise your heels until you are standing on your toes
- Next, lower slowly back to the start under control, this is one rep
- **TARGET:** 2 to 3 sets of 15 to 20 repetitions

Wrist Curls

- **EQUIPMENT:** Tin or Dumbbell, Chair with Arms
- For this strength exercise, start by placing your forearm on a chair's armrest with your hand hanging over the edge.
- Hold a tin with your palm facing upwards
- Slowly bend your wrist up and down and then repeat
- Change sides and perform with your other hand
- Breathe normally
- **TARGET:** 2 to 3 sets of 8 to 12 repetitions

Glute Bridges

- **EQUIPMENT:** Mat
- For this strength exercise, start by lying down on bed or floor with both your knees bent, your hips are in a neutral position
- Next, lift your bottom as high as you comfortably can off of the floor, pause briefly and then return the body to the starting position and repeat
- Breathe out completely and engage core before upward movement, breathe in during the downward movement
- **TARGET:** 2 to 3 sets of 8 to 12 repetitions

ACTIVITY TIME GUIDELINES: Older adults should aim to be active daily. Over a week, your activity should add up to at least 150 minutes of moderate-intensity activity in bouts of 10 minutes or more. One way to achieve this would be to do 30 minutes on at least 5 days of the week. Ideally, you should aim to build up a routine of 8 to 12 exercises that strength train the major muscle groups 2 to 3 times a week on non-consecutive days to allow for recovery.

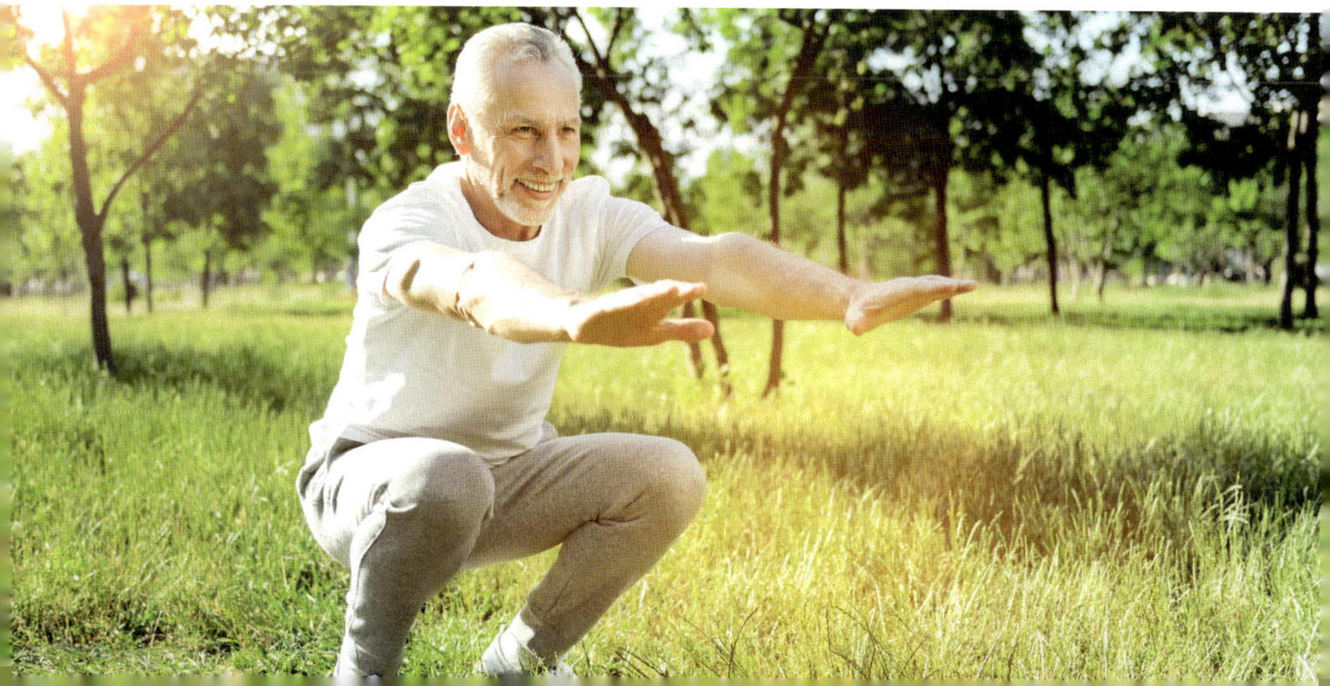

Step-By-Step Core Exercises

Lateral Side Bends

- **EQUIPMENT:** Chair, Tin or Dumbbell
- For this core exercise, start by holding a weight in your right hand
- Sit on the chair keeping your back straight and head held up, bend only at your waist
- Breathe in and bend down to your right side. Hold this position briefly and come back up to the starting position, keeping the rest of the body still, this is one rep
- Repeat the movement but bending towards your left side
- Breathe in while reaching down, breathe out while straightening up
- **TARGET:** 2 to 3 sets of 8 to 12 repetitions each side

Figure of Eights

- **EQUIPMENT:** Bottle of Water, Squash or Dumbbell
- For this core exercise, start seated on the chair with your feet about shoulder-width apart, bracing your stomach muscles, sitting up, holding the weight in both your hands, arms fully extended out
- With your arms fully extended draw big figures of eights, this is one complete rep
- Breathe normally
- **TARGET:** 2 to 3 sets of 8 to 12 repetitions

Leg Lifts

- **EQUIPMENT:** Mat
- For this core exercise, lie on your back with legs flat against the ground and feet relaxed
- Contract your abdominal muscles while raising one leg about 10 to 15 cm off the floor and hold for a few seconds
- Lower and repeat on your other leg
- Breathe in on the downward movement, breathe out while raising your leg back up
- **TARGET:** 2 to 3 sets of 8 to 12 repetitions

Seated Knee Lifts

- **EQUIPMENT:** Mat
- For this core exercise, begin seated on the floor
- Start by bringing both of your knees up towards your chest slowly under control, and continue by slowly extending your legs back out to the starting position, this is one complete rep
- Breathe in on the downward movement, breathe out while raising your leg back up
- **TARGET:** 2 to 3 sets of 8 to 12 repetitions

Air Bike

- **EQUIPMENT:** Mat
- For this core exercise, lie on your back with your hands behind your head
- Bend at your knees and lift both of your feet so that your calves are held parallel to the floor
- Next bring one knee towards your chest while reaching to it with the elbow from the opposite side, you should look as though you are pedalling a bike
- Breathe normally
- **TARGET:** 2 to 3 sets of 30-second bursts resting for one minute between sets

Seated Twists

- **EQUIPMENT:** Mat, note this exercise is for a more advanced person
- For this core exercise, start by sitting on a mat
- Bend your body to an angle of about 45-degrees from the floor, with your arms across your chest, leaning back, then move forward and slowly twist your body to the left then lean back slowly twisting back to the starting position
- Breathe normally
- **TARGET:** 2 to 3 sets of 12 to 15 repetitions

Semi-sits

- **EQUIPMENT:** Chair
- For this core exercise, start your Semi-sits exercise by standing in front of a chair, gently pulling in your stomach muscles
- Next slowly lower your bum, and bend your knees as though you are about to sit back down on a chair making only light contact with the chair seat and then return back up to the starting standing position, this is one complete rep
- Breathe in as you slowly sit down, breathe out as you slowly stand back up
- **TARGET:** 2 to 3 sets of 8 to 12 repetitions

Lumbar Rotation

- **EQUIPMENT:** Mat
- For this core exercise, start by lying on the floor with your legs bent and with both knees together on the floor over on your left side
- Next, extend both your arms out, but keep your shoulders firmly on the ground, pull your stomach muscles in
- Keeping your body still slowly roll your knees from the left, over to the right until they touch the floor or get close to touching the floor, hold this position just for a few seconds and then roll back, repeat

- Breathe normally,
- **TARGET:** 2 to 3 sets of 5 to 8 repetitions each side

Kneeling Rear Leg Raise

- **EQUIPMENT:** Mat
- For this core exercise, start by getting down on your hands and knees and engage your core muscles
- Next, extend your right leg back holding it slightly off the floor, toes pointing
- Lift your leg straight up as high as you can and then lower your leg back to the starting position, be careful not to arch your back
- Repeat this exercise with your other leg
- **TARGET:** 2 to 3 sets of 8 to 12 repetitions each leg

Wood Chops

- **EQUIPMENT:** N/A
- For this core exercise, start the Wood Chop exercise with your feet wider than shoulder-width apart clasping together both hands in front
- Next, pull your arms up to be level with one side of your head
- Squat down while doing a chopping movement with your arms diagonally downwards to the opposite side of your body
- Repeat by performing the chopping action back up towards the top, this is one rep
- Breath normally
- **TARGET:** 2 to 3 sets of 8 to 12 repetitions each side

Crunches

- **EQUIPMENT:** Mat
- For this core exercise, start by lying down with your back flat on the floor
- Place both of your feet on the floor about hip-width apart
- Next, bend both your knees, place both your hands behind your head, elbows pointing forwards while breathing in
- Breathe out and lift your torso slightly keeping your head and neck neutral
- To finish breathe out and return your body to the starting position
- **TARGET:** 2 to 3 sets of 12 to 15 repetitions

Superman

- **EQUIPMENT:** Mat
- For this core exercise, start the Superman exercise by lying on your stomach with your arms stretched out fully
- Next, raise your head, neck, and your right arm, as well as your left leg 5 cm off of the floor, lower and repeat on your other side
- During the exercise pull your stomach muscles in
- Breathe normally
- **TARGET:** 2 to 3 sets of 8 to 12 repetitions each side

ACTIVITY TIME GUIDELINES: Older adults should aim to be active daily. Over a week, your activity should add up to at least 150 minutes of moderate-intensity activity in bouts of 10 minutes or more. One way to achieve this would be to do 30 minutes on at least 5 days of the week. Ideally, you should aim to build up a routine of 8 to 12 exercises that strength train the major muscle groups 2 to 3 times a week on non-consecutive days to allow for recovery.

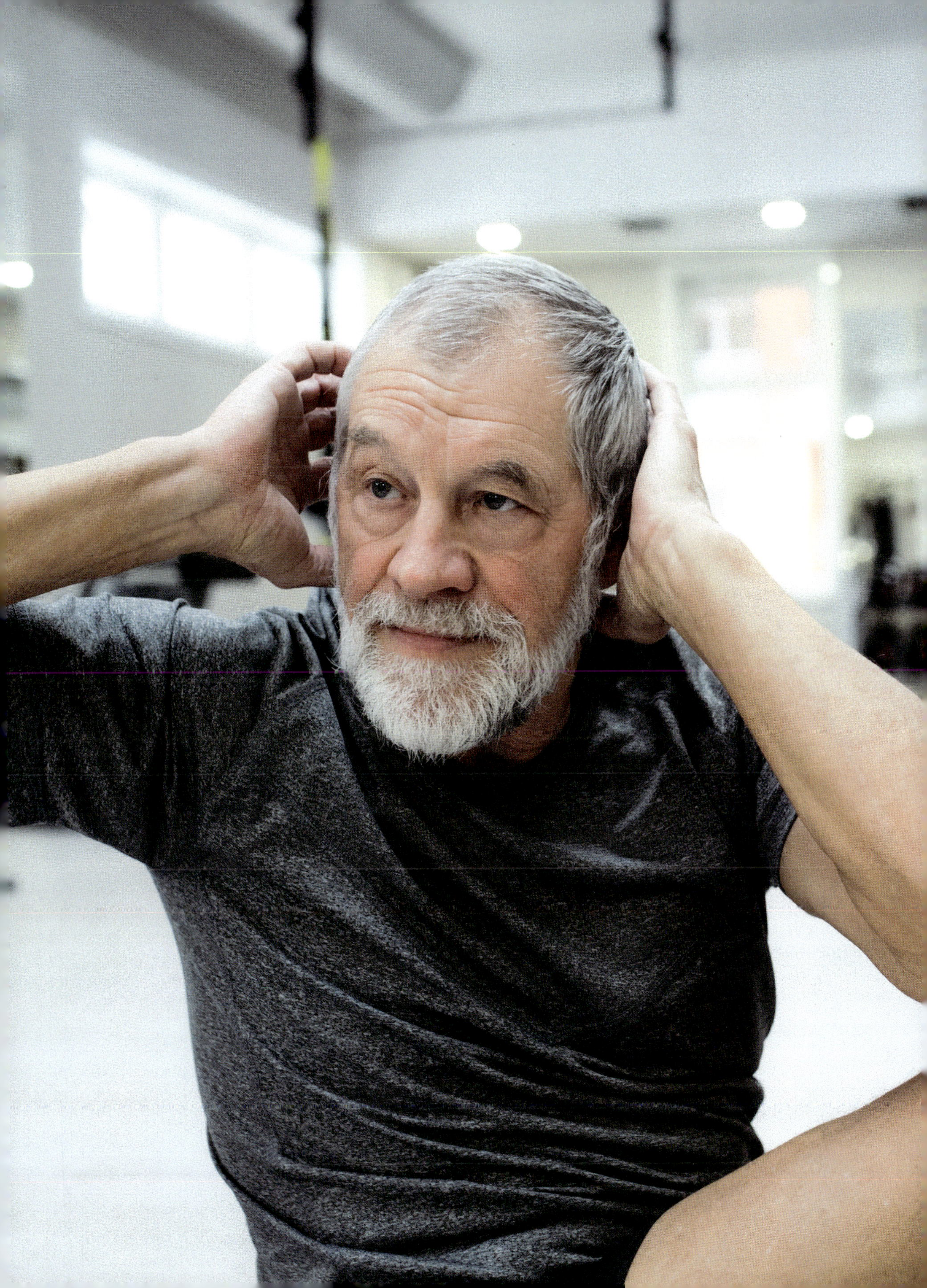

Step-By-Step Stretching Exercises

Hamstring Seated Stretch

- **EQUIPMENT:** Chair
- For this stretching exercise, sit on the chair
- Straighten out one leg and place both hands on this bent leg
- Lean gently forwards
- Hold the position for about 10 to 15 seconds and ease further forwards, after about another 10 to 15 seconds ease forward once again
- Repeat with the other leg
- Breathe normally

Hamstring Bent Knee Seated Stretch

- **EQUIPMENT:** Chair
- For this stretching exercise, sit on the chair
- Straighten one leg out but keep it slightly bent, place both your hands on the bent leg and lean gently forwards
- Hold the position for about 10 to 15 seconds and ease further forwards, after about another 10 to 15 seconds ease forward once again
- Repeat with the other leg
- Breathe normally

Back & Shoulder Stretch

- **EQUIPMENT:** Chair
- For this stretching exercise, begin seated clasp both hands together in front with your arms extended out, next drop your head and shoulders forward and then push hands away from your body as far as you can
- Hold for about 10 to 15 seconds
- Breathe normally

Obliques Reaching Up Standing Stretch

- **EQUIPMENT:** N/A
- For this stretching exercise, stand with your feet about hip-distance apart keeping your spine neutral
- Place one hand just below your hip and reach with your other arm up right up above your head
- Next, lean over to one side
- Hold for about 10 to 15 seconds
- Repeat on your other side
- Breathe normally

Arms Across Body Seated Stretch

- **EQUIPMENT:** Chair
- For this stretching exercise, sit on the chair, take one arm and fold it across the front of your body
- Place the palm of the other hand on the back of the upper arm and pull in and hold this position for about 10 to 15 seconds, release and then repeat on the other arm
- Breathe normally

Seated Chest Stretch

- **EQUIPMENT:** Chair
- For this stretching exercise, sit on the chair and place hands on small of your back
- Squeeze your shoulder blades so that they feel as though pinching together
- After about 10 to 15 seconds ease a little further into the stretch
- Breathe normally

Triceps Stretch

- **EQUIPMENT:** Chair
- For this stretching exercise, sit on the chair and place one hand above the head and bend at the elbow, hand touching the back of your shoulder, with your other hand on the back of upper arm apply pressure
- Hold for about 10 to 15 seconds
- Breathe normally

Quads Leg Stretch

- **EQUIPMENT:** Chair (optional)
- For this stretching exercise, stand with feet hip-distance apart, neutral spine
- Hold on to chair or counter if needed, stand on one leg
- Raise one heel towards your bum and hold in your hand, or hold your trouser hem if easier
- After 10 to 15 seconds pull in a little further and hold for another 10 seconds
- Breathe normally

ACTIVITY TIME GUIDELINES: Older people should aim to do flexibility (stretching) exercises at least twice a week, there is no set time given but a sensible target would be at least 15 minutes each time, using sustained stretches for each major muscle group.

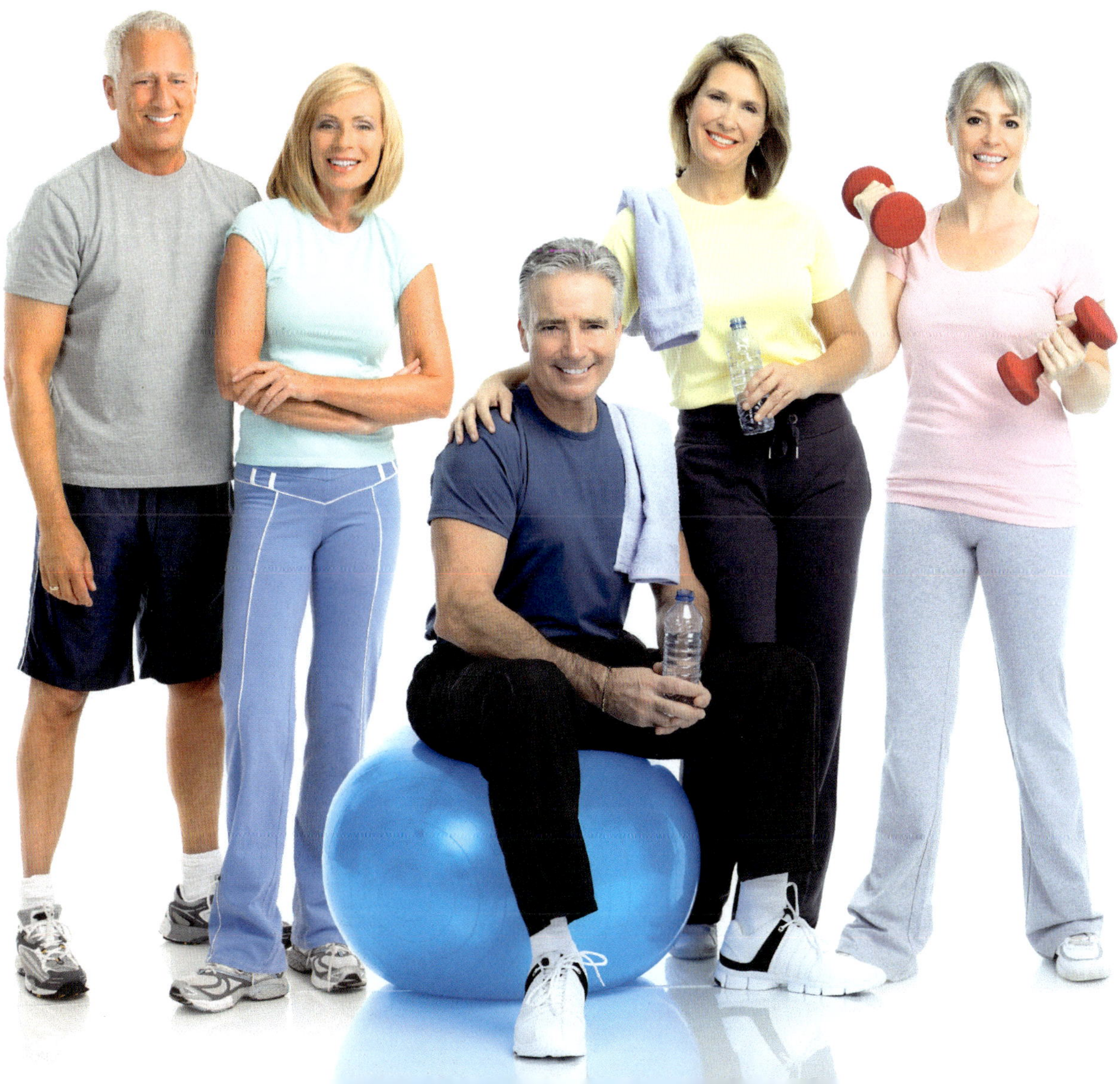

PUBLISHING
www.3fspt.co.uk

Printed in Great Britain
by Amazon

45557553R00159